MEDICAL GENETICS:

Principles and Practice

MEDICAL GENETICS:
Principles and Practice

James J. Nora, M.D.

Professor and Chairman, Department of Pediatrics
State University of New York
Chief of Pediatrics, State University Hospital
and Kings County Hospital
Downstate Medical Center
Brooklyn, New York

F. Clarke Fraser, Ph.D., M.D.C.M., F.R.S.C., D.Sc. (Acadia)

Professor of Medical Genetics, Department of Biology
Associate Professor, Department of Paediatrics
McGill University, Montreal;
Director, Department of Medical Genetics
The Montreal Children's Hospital
Montreal, Canada

Lea & Febiger

Philadelphia

1974

Library of Congress Cataloging in Publication Data

Nora, James J.
  Medical genetics.
1. Medical genetics. I Fraser, F. Clarke, 1920– joint author. II. Title. [DNLM: 1.
Genetics, Human. 2. Hereditary diseases. QZ50 N822m 1974]
RB155.N67   616′.042   73-16009
ISBN 0-8121-0373-4

Published in Great Britain by Henry Kimpton Publishers, London

Printed in the United States of America

To

Audrey Hart Nora, M.D. and Joseph J. Nora, M.D.,

and

Frank Fraser and Nan Fraser

PREFACE

The decision to write this book was reached in The Hague in September, 1969, at the Third International Conference on Congenital Malformations. The finished product will appear shortly after the Fourth International Conference in Vienna, in September, 1973.

The reason for undertaking this project was to provide within a single volume the basic genetic information and its application to the clinical problems that fall broadly within the sphere of medical genetics. Other texts vary widely in their emphasis on basic versus clinical material, depending on the authors' views of what is most suitable for the intended readers. Since pediatricians and obstetricians are more likely to become involved with genetic problems than other kinds of physicians, our examples are oriented in their direction. Nevertheless we hope that physicians from other disciplines and nonmedical genetic counselors will also find help in these pages. We are especially hopeful that this text is of appropriate breadth and depth to introduce medical students to the subject of medical genetics.

Our book does not attempt to be a catalogue of diseases with a more or less genetic basis—our choice of diseases has been limited by the dictates of practicality and by the bounds of our own knowledge and experience. We do not, moreover, presume it to be a general pediatric or medical text. Diagnostic criteria are discussed at a level that should warn physicians and counselors of diagnostic pitfalls, and methods of treat-

ment are dealt with only in sufficient detail to give the physician/counselor an idea of what may be involved for the family.

For more sophisticated discussion of genetic theory and more authoritative information on diagnosis and treatment, the reader is referred to more extensive texts of genetics, pediatrics or medicine, to be kept in office, home or library. We hope this volume will find a place in hospital wards, clinics, counseling centers and medical school classrooms.

James J. Nora
F. Clarke Fraser

ACKNOWLEDGMENTS

Many people have helped us in many ways, and should these paragraphs fail to acknowledge assistance we have received it is not because of lack of appreciation, but through oversight, trying to recall all of the support we have had during the four years from the conception of this book to its final form.

Dr. Audrey Hart Nora wrote Chapters 21, 23 and 28. Ms. Marilyn Preus was largely responsible for writing Chapter 19. Ms. Joy Weishuhn,, Ms. Peggy Baldwin, and Mr. Ralph Jackson produced many of the illustrations and line drawings. Ms. Weishuhn and Ms. Marilyn Peterson helped with library research. Ms. Mildred Meek, Ms. Nan O'Keeffe, Ms. M. Forster, and Ms. Peterson typed the manuscript.

Previously unpublished photographs of patients and cytologic material have been provided by a number of colleagues: Dr. Anil Sinha, Dr. Dan McNamara, Dr. Edward Singleton, Dr. Arthur Robinson, Dr. Herbert Lubs, Dr. Stephen Goodman, Dr. Arnold Greensher, Dr. David W. Smith, and Dr. Gerald Nellhaus. Drs. Robinson and Lubs kindly reviewed the chapters dealing with cytogenetics.

Agencies which have suggested studies that accounted for much of the material of the book and have provided support during preparation of this manuscript include:

The U.S. National Institutes of Health; the Medical Research Council, Canada; the Department of National Health and Welfare, Canada; The National Foundation; and the American Heart Association.

Finally we wish to acknowledge the many children and their parents who have cooperated in helping us to a better understanding of genetic diseases.

CONTENTS

SECTION II. SPECIAL TOPICS

SECTION III. SYNDROMES AND MALFORMATIONS

Section I.

Heredity and Disease

Chapter 1

HERITABILITY OF DISEASE

But this disease seems to me to be no more divine than others. . . .
Its origin is hereditary like that of other diseases. . . . what is to hinder
it from happening that where the father and mother were subject to
this disease, certain of their offspring should be affected also? Hippocrates: On the Sacred Disease.

From the very beginning of the history of Western medicine, the heritability of physical traits and diseases has been recognized. Hippocrates not only observed that blue eyes and baldness ran in families, but that diseases such as epilepsy followed a similar pattern. Before the early twentieth century, inheritance was considered to be a blending, a continuous variation—and this is probably what Hippocrates had in mind. However, the emphasis shifted away from blended inheritance following the rediscovery of Mendel and unit inheritance and the locating of the hereditary particles, the genes, in chromosomes. Indeed, among the earliest published examples of mendelian inheritance was the disease alkaptonuria, described by Sir Archibald Garrod in 1902.[1] A large number of diseases attributed to single mutant genes followed this remarkable observation, until the current catalog of disorders considered to have a firm

mendelian basis lists 866 conditions.[2] The terms "dominant" and "recessive" entered the medical vocabulary, and many diseases which have later been demonstrated to have no true basis in mendelian inheritance still carry such labels. If a disease was presumed to have a genetic basis, an effort at mendelian interpretation was made.

A further shift in emphasis began in 1959, when the first disorders were described that could be traced to abnormalities of chromosome number. During the next few years, several more syndromes associated with a chromosomal aberration were discovered. Then, in the minds of many students (and referring physicians), the erroneous idea took root that if a disease has a genetic basis, a chromosome karyotype must be ordered to establish the diagnosis. However, the consultant in genetics appreciates that a large percentage of the patients he is asked to see have disorders that can be attributed to neither a single mutant gene nor a chromosomal anomaly (see Table 1–1). If there is a genetic basis for these diseases, then we must return through the full circle to Hippocrates and discuss the hereditary aspect of disease in its earliest sense, that is, predisposition or *diathesis.*

A useful classification of diseases having a genetic background would thus be:
1. Single mutant gene (mendelian) syndromes
2. Chromosomal aberration syndromes
3. Diseases determined by multifactorial inheritance — genetic predisposition with environmental interaction.

TABLE 1-1. Diagnosis for 495 Families Referred to a Genetics Clinic for Counseling

Autosomal Dominant

Ullrich-Noonan syndrome	11
tuberous sclerosis	9
osteogenesis imperfecta	9
Huntington chorea	7
neurofibromatosis	6
Holt-Oram syndrome	5
Apert syndrome	4
retinoblastoma	4
ectodermal dystropy, hidrotic	3
Ehlers-Danlos syndrome	3
Crouzon disease	2
holoprosencephaly	2
Leber optic atrophy	2
lymphedema, hereditary	2
mandibulofacial dysostosis	2
Marfan syndrome	2
nerve deafness	2
Waardenburg syndrome	2
aniridia	3
polycystic kidneys	3
Other (1 each)	25
	108

X-Linked

Duchenne muscular dystrophy	11
hemophilia	5
agammaglobulinemia	2
Other (1 each)	4
	22

Autosomal Recessive

pancreatic cystic fibrosis	11
albinism	9
Friedreich ataxia	6
congenital deafness	5
Werdnig-Hoffman disease	4
cataracts	3
chondrodystrophia calcificans	3
cretinism	3
PKU	3
Tay-Sachs disease	3
thalassemia	3
ataxia telangiectasia	2
nerve deafness	2

Gaucher disease	2
Hurler syndrome	2
Larsen syndrome	2
Riley-Day syndrome	2
Other (1 each)	38
	103

Chromosomal

Down syndrome	43
D/D translocation	2
XO Turner syndrome	2
Other (1 each)	6
	53

Multifactorial or Unclear

congenital heart defects	44
neural tube defects	31
multiple congenital anomalies	21
mental retardation, nonspecific	19
convulsive disorders	16
limb malformations and mental retardation	5
microcephaly	5
de Lange syndrome	4
Goldenhar syndrome	4
leukemia, acute lymphoblastic	4
cerebral palsy	3
hemangioma	2
hydrocephalus	2
repeated abortion	3
omphalocoele	2
Robin syndrome	2
Rubinstein-Taybi syndrome	2
Other (1 each)	34
	203

Miscellaneous

consanguinity	17
racial ancestry	2
exposure to mutagens or teratogens	4
Other (1 each)	3
	26

To these may be added a fourth category: maternal-fetal incompatibility, an example of which is erythroblastosis fetalis. This category is not considered separately but is discussed in the context of blood groups (Chapter 21).

The clinical geneticist is asked to see patients for several different reasons. Often an infant or child is born with a common malformation and the parents are concerned about the risk of recurrence. Is the malformation inherited? Is there something that the parents did to cause this problem? What is the chance that this may recur and what can be done to prevent it?

Another category of patients referred to the clinical genetics consultant is a patient with a pattern of anomalies in search of a diagnostic label. The hope here is that naming a disease will explain it. In some cases this is true. Determining that a patient has the Marfan syndrome provides a reasonable basis for medical management, prognosis and counseling. Very often, however, suggesting a label for a group of anomalies implies a greater understanding of the disease than actually exists. The cause of the condition is uppermost in the minds of the anxious parents. Invoking a difficult-to-pronounce eponym makes the geneticist appear to be a scholar, but he is deceiving both himself and his patients unless he acknowledges the limits of his diagnostic label. Does naming this disease answer the question of etiology? Does it provide a reasonably firm basis for discussing prognosis in the patient and risk of recurrence in the family? And how precise is the diagnosis of the Balderdash syndrome, anyway? Could this be another condition entirely?

If the patient has a common malformation, the familial aspects of which have been well investigated (e.g., atrial septal defect), then meaningful genetic counseling may be offered. If the patient clearly has a specific syndrome about which there is usable etiologic and prognostic information (e.g., Hurler syndrome or 21 trisomy), it is possible for the geneticist to answer many urgent questions.

Knowledge in fundamental genetics has expanded explosively during the past decade to the point that it may be considered the central and unifying biologic science. The aim of this monograph is to explore the field of medical genetics following the map provided by investigation into the fundamental areas of genetics.

REFERENCES

1. Garrod, A. E.: The incidence of alkaptonuria: A study in chemical individuality. Lancet, 2: 1616, 1902.
2. McKusick, V. A.: Mendelian Inheritance in Man. Ed. 3. Baltimore, Johns Hopkins Press, 1971.

Chapter 2

CHROMOSOMAL BASIS OF HEREDITY

The general conceptions here advanced were evolved purely from cytological data, before the author had knowledge of the Mendelian principles. . . . As will appear hereafter they completely satisfy the conditions in typical Mendelian cases, and it seems that many of the known deviations from the Mendelian type may be explained by easily conceivable variations from the normal chromosomic processes. Walter S. Sutton: The chromosomes in heredity. Biological Bulletin, 4:231, 1903.

The word "chromosome" was introduced into the scientific vocabulary in 1888 by Waldeyer.[20] As is the case with so many important discoveries, the early recognition of the role of the chromosome as the carrier of the information of heredity must be credited to several investigators working in the late nineteenth and early twentieth centuries· Roux, Boveri, Wilson and Sutton, pursuing a course running parallel to that followed by genetic researchers, appreciated before the rediscovery of Mendel that the chromosomes could be the ultimate dividing units and carriers of heredity. However, it was the rediscovery of Mendel that provided the catalyst for the reaction that synthesized the discoveries of cytology and genetics into the discipline of cytogenetics. It became apparent to the cytologists that the behavior of the hereditary characters

of Mendel was reflected by the behavior of the chromosomes in meiosis. Sutton[18] and Boveri[1] independently proposed the chromosomal hypothesis of inheritance (the "Sutton-Boveri hypothesis").

The remarkable contributions to the chromosomal basis of heredity that were made over the next decades were, of necessity, derived from studies in lower animals, the drosophila proving to be a most useful subject. As early as 1910, T. H. Morgan[11] was able to locate a specific gene locus on a specific chromosome of *Drosophila melanogaster*. The human, however, is in many ways an unsatisfactory subject for genetics research. This has been especially true in the area of cytogenetics· It was not until 1956 that the diploid number of human chromosomes was demonstrated to be 46 by Tjio and Levan.[19] For the 33 years prior to this date, students of medicine and biology were taught that the human diploid complement was 48.[13] The reason for this discrepancy was not carelessness on the part of cytogeneticists. Rather, the determination of the correct diploid number had to await the development of techniques capable of accurately revealing the human chromosomes.

Recognizing that the hereditary material was carried by the chromosomes did not, of course, define the nature of the unit of inheritance, which Johannsen labeled the gene. The development of this line of investigation is undertaken in Chapter 5. It

is sufficient for this discussion to state that the chromosome consists of the hereditary material, desoxyribonucleic acid (DNA), embedded in a protein matrix (histone in the human). The units of inheritance, the genes, are segments of DNA. The number of genes distributed throughout the 46 chromosomes of the human cell has been estimated to be of the order of 100,000.

CHROMOSOMES

Chromosomes (*chromos* = color; *soma* = body) are not individually distinguishable except during cell division, at which time they may be seen under the light

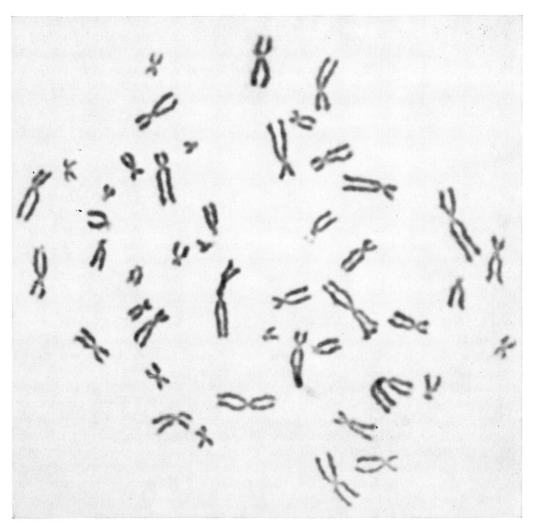

Figure 2-1. Human chromosomes in metaphase.

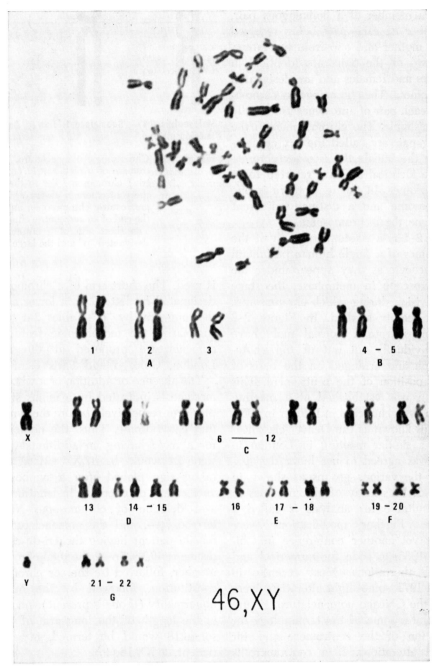

Figure 2-2. Chromosomes from a normal human male are shown as they appear in metaphase and as they are displayed in a karyotype for study. The chromosomes have been individually cut out of the photomicrograph and arranged on the basis of size and position of centromere.

clear identification of chromosomes 4, 5, 13, 14, 15, 17 and 18. It is the only method for identifying the late-replicating X chromosome. When tritiated thymidine is made available to the cell culture, the chromosome that replicates later than all others is the X chromosome (when more than one X chromosome is present). Chromosomes 19 and 20 are among the earliest to terminate DNA synthesis, but may not be distinguished from one another autoradiographically. Chromosome 18 appears to replicate later than the morphologically similar chromosome 17, as do chromosome 4 with respect to chromosome 5 and chromosome 13 as compared with the rest of group D. On the other hand, it is not possible to distinguish clearly chromosome 21 from 22 by morphologic or autoradiographic means (so that the attribution of Down syndrome to 21 trisomy was originally arbitrary). Also, with the exception of the late-

replicating X chromosome, it is not easy to differentiate between the individual chromosomes of group C.

Recognizing these deficiencies, it becomes obvious that more powerful tools are needed to derive the kind of information one would ideally require of chromosomal analysis. A recent innovation by Caspersson and colleagues[2] has provided one such tool: **quinacrine mustard (QM) fluorescence** ("Q-staining methods"). Quinacrine binds preferentially to certain regions of metaphase chromosomes to produce characteristic banding patterns ("Q-bands") (see Fig. 2–4). These banding patterns are sufficiently reproducible to enable the identification of each chromosome when these findings are added to the usual information such as centromere index and morphologic features.

By inspection alone, good fluorescent preparations reveal banding patterns ade-

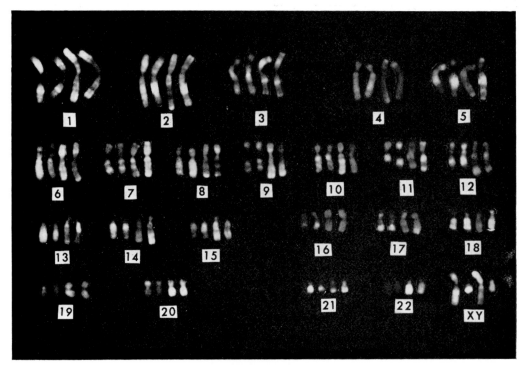

Figure 2-4. Human chromosomes by Q-staining methods revealing Q-bands and by a reverse-staining method (in this case, acridine orange) revealing R-bands. The Q-banded homologues are on the left. (From Lubs, H. A., *et al. In*: Prescott, D. M. (Ed.): Methods in Cell Physiology. New York, Academic Press. In Press.)

quate for distinguishing the chromosomes. A further refinement, the photometric recording of patterns, has been used by Caspersson in the development of the Q-staining methods. This refinement requires expensive equipment and is not used by most laboratories. Quinacrine fluorescence clearly differentiates between the G+Y group chromosomes, and taken with other cytogenetic findings, provides distinctions between the eight chromosomes of the C+X group not possible by earlier techniques.

Techniques that may be more easily employed by many laboratories are the **G-staining methods.** In one such method,[15] rather than staining with Giemsa at pH 6 (which has been a standard method for many years), the pH is altered to 9, and banding patterns ("G-bands") are revealed which with few exceptions are similar to those obtained with quinacrine fluorescence. Those laboratories that have used Giemsa at pH 6 (preferably with air-dried preparations) may now restudy their patients of the past decade by the new methods by

destaining their old slides and restaining with Giemsa 9 and quinacrine.

Figure 2–5 illustrates a computerized band analysis of chromosomes prepared by G-staining methods. The densitometric curves are similar to those obtained by the methods of Caspersson, except in this instance the entire operation is computerized and a metaphase cell is analyzed in about two minutes.

A variation on the G-staining methods is the **reverse-staining Giemsa method** ("R-staining methods"),[6] which gives patterns ("R-bands") opposite in staining intensity to the G-bands. Methods that demonstrate constitutive heterochromatin are the "C-staining methods"[3] and the chromatin stained, the "C-bands." At a number of laboratories throughout the world, research in banding techniques is being carried out, and many methods are being developed in addition to the ones described in this chapter. The selection of Q-, G-, R- and C-methods is based on the Paris Conference (1971).[14]

Appendix A gives details of the identi-

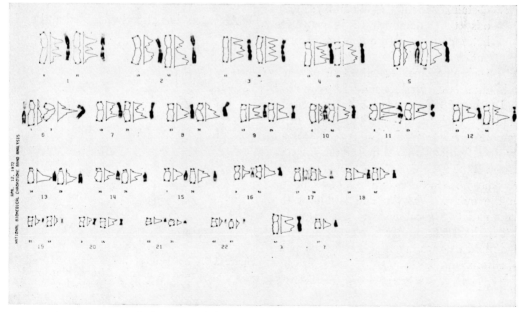

Figure 2-5.   Computerized chromosomal band analysis (Calcomp plot) of male karyotype. The chromosome is traced by the computer and the bands analyzed in about two minutes. (Courtesy R. S. Ledley and H. A. Lubs.)

fication system of chromosomes by the various banding techniques proposed at the Paris Conference. This descriptive material may be used with the illustrations in this text to appreciate the methods for identifying individual chromosomes. The summary of methods now being employed to identify chromosomes is:

1. Measurements and morphology by standard Giemsa 6 stain
    a. sum of the length of 22 autosomes and the X-chromosome expressed per thousand
    b. arm ratio, long arm:short arm
    c. centromere index
    d. morphologic features, satellites, secondary constrictions, etc.
2. Autoradiography
3. Q-staining methods (Q-bands): quinacrine mustard (or dihydrochloride) fluorescence.
4. G-staining methods (G-bands): Giemsa staining with altered pH (e.g., Giemsa at pH 9)
5. R-staining methods (R-bands): reverse-staining Giemsa methods (e.g., with temperature treatment)
6. C-staining methods (C-bands): methods that demonstrate constitutive heterochromatin (the constantly present fraction).

The chromosomal constitution of each individual is derived equally from mother and father, 23 chromosomes being contributed by each parent in the form of a **gamete** (ovum or sperm). The cell formed by the fertilization of the ovum by the sperm is the **zygote**. Each of the 23 paternal chromosomes in the sperm has a homologue in the ovum. Thus the end result of the fusion of two germ cells (gametes), each with a haploid number of chromosomes, is a diploid cell having 23 homologous pairs of chromosomes.

MITOSIS

Mitosis, or somatic cell division, is the means by which body cells reduplicate themselves for maintenance or growth of tissue. Cells that are not dividing are said to be in interphase. This is the normal condition in which cells are engaged in their designated functions. Also during interphase the genetic material duplicates itself, so that before cell division actually takes place, a double DNA content is present, which is then divided between the two daughter cells during mitosis. The chromosomes, which are metabolically active and greatly elongated during interphase, are not visible at this stage. They appear as formless granularity (Fig. 2-6).

In mitosis four stages are recognized: prophase, metaphase, anaphase and telophase. It is during this process that a precise sequence of events occurs that results in the production of two daughter cells, each having the exact chromosome complement and genetic material of the parent cell. The cytoplasmic material merely divides in half, but the nucleus undergoes the series of changes that characterize the stage of mitosis.

Prophase. This stage begins when the chromosomes, which have not been distinguishable in interphase, condense and become visible under light microscopy. The DNA content has already doubled and each

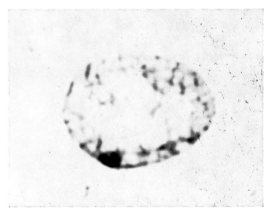

Figure 2-6. Nucleus of buccal mucosal cell in human female. Observe the formless granularity of chromosomes during interphase except for the darkly staining mass (Barr body) adjacent to the nuclear membrane at 7 o'clock. (See Chapter 4 for discussion of the significance of the Barr body.)

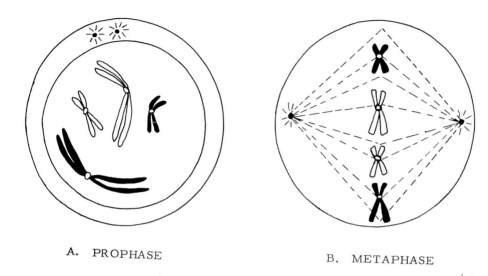

A. PROPHASE   B. METAPHASE

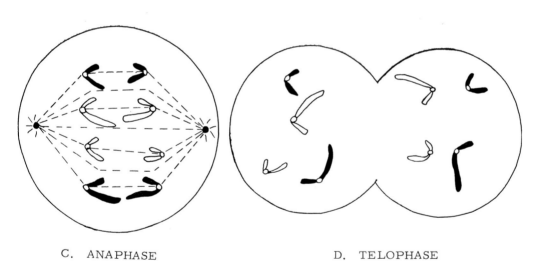

C. ANAPHASE   D. TELOPHASE

Figure 2-7. Mitosis. Two of 23 pairs of chromosomes are shown passing through the four stages. Observe that **single-stranded** chromosomes separate at cell division. See text.

chromosome is visualized as two parallel strands, **chromatids**, joined together in one place, the **centromere.** The nuclear membrane begins to disappear and two small bodies, the **centrioles**, start to migrate to opposite poles from a position immediately external to the nuclear membrane (Fig. 2-7A).

Metaphase. This is the stage during which the individual chromosomes are most clearly visualized. The karyotype, the display of human chromosomes for analysis, is taken from metaphase plates. As may be seen in Figure 2-7B, the nuclear membrane disappears and the chromosomes line up along an equator and are connected at their centromeres to the **spindle**, which consists of protein fibers radiating from the centriole.

Anaphase. The separation of the two

chromatids from each other signals the beginning of anaphase (Fig. 2-7C). The centromere divides longitudinally into two and the two daughter centromeres move toward opposite poles, dragging their chromatids with them. Thus, each pole of the dividing cell will receive a set of chromosomes identical with that of the original nucleus.

Telophase. The daughter chromosomes, which are now single-strand chromatids, arrive at the poles of the cells as the cytoplasm begins to divide in the area of the equatorial plane (Fig. 2-7D). The two daughter cells go on to separate as the chromosomes become less densely staining until they are indistinguishable. When the separation is complete, two new daughter cells are recognized in interphase.

MEIOSIS

Two critical events occur in **meiosis** (division of germ cells) that do not occur in mitosis (division of somatic cells): (1) pairing of the homologous chromosomes; (2) two successive divisions of nuclear material so that the resulting cells have only 23 chromosomes rather than 46. Bearing this in mind, the events of meiosis will now be considered.

First Meiotic Division

Prophase. This stage of division of germ cells may be seen as five clearly defined substages, the details of which can be found in cytology textbooks. The important events in meiotic prophase that do not occur in mitotic prophase are that the chromosomes pair (**synapse**) and that the strands of the paired chromosomes may break and recombine so that a piece of one homologous chromosome may be exchanged for a comparable piece of its homologue. This is known as **crossing-over.**

1. *Leptonema.* The chromosomes first become visible and appear to be single threads, although the DNA has already reduplicated (Fig. 2-8A).

2. *Zygonema.* Each chromosome now

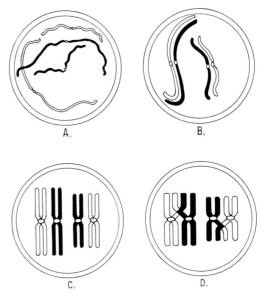

Figure 2-8. Prophase of the first meiotic division. Two of 23 pairs of chromosomes are shown in the stages of prophase: A. Leptonema; B. Zygonema; C. Pachynema; D. Diplonema. Diakinesis is not illustrated. Note that there is pairing of homologous chromosomes and crossing over. See text.

pairs with its counterpart in such a way that each part of one chromosome is associated with the identical part of its homologue. *These synapsed chromosomes, or* **bivalents,** *do not form in mitosis* (Fig. 2-8B).

3. *Pachynema.* Each chromosome is now visible as a double strand (Fig. 2-8C).

4. *Diplonema.* The two members of the bivalent now begin to move apart except where crossing-over has occurred, and the exchange of strands results in "X-like" formations, known as **chiasmata,** which hold the homologues together. Figure 2-8D illustrates one such chiasma in which the material from one chromatid (in black) has been exchanged with the homologous segment of material from a chromatid of its homologous chromosome (in white). Exchanges of genetic material by crossing-over adds almost infinite variety to the ultimate genetic makeup of a given individual.

5. *Diakinesis.* The final stage of prophase is characterized by the chromosomes becoming more condensed and darkly staining. It is not illustrated in the accompanying figures.

Metaphase. This stage is the same in meiosis as in mitosis except that the homologues are paired as bivalents. The nuclear membrane disappears and the chromosomes line up in an equatorial plane connected at their centromeres by protein fibers radiating from the centrioles (Fig. 2-9E).

Anaphase. The chromosomes, each still consisting of two chromatids joined at a centromere, now separate from their homologues and *23 double-stranded* chromosomes go into each of two daughter cells

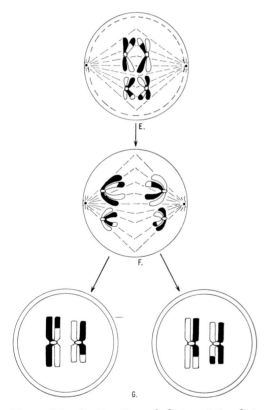

Figure 2-9. Continuation of first meiotic division: E. Metaphase; F. Anaphase; G. Telophase. Note that **double-stranded** chromosomes go into the daughter cells (23 randomly assorted double-stranded chromosomes instead of 46 single-stranded chromosomes as in mitosis). See text.

(Fig. 2-9F). Note the difference from mitotic anaphase, in which the two chromatids of each chromosome separate at the centromere and *46 single-stranded* chromosomes go into each cell. In first meiotic anaphase we find the chromosomal basis for two of Mendel's laws of inheritance: **segregation** and **independent assortment.** The separation of the homologous chromosomes, with either the maternal or paternal members of the pair going (after further divisions) to a given gamete, is the basis of segregation. The decision as to which pole gets the maternal and which the paternal homologue is independent for each pair. This is the physical basis of independent assortment.

Telophase in meiosis I is comparable to mitotic telophase except that there are 23 double-stranded daughter chromosomes that congregate at the poles of the cells rather than 46 single-stranded chromosomes (Fig. 2-9G).

Second Meiotic Division

An interphase in which the DNA is replicated does not occur between the first and second meiotic divisions. In fact, no interphase at all may separate the two meiotic divisions. As may be appreciated in Figure 2-10, the stages of metaphase, anaphase and telophase are essentially the same as those found in somatic cell mitosis except for the fact that *only 23 chromosomes are involved.* At metaphase, the 23 chromosomes, each consisting of two chromatids joined by a centromere, line up on the equator (Fig. 2-10H); at anaphase, the centromeres divide longitudinally and the single strands migrate to the poles (Fig. 2-10I); and at telophase, the chromatids arrive at the poles and the cytoplasm begins to divide. Four spermatids result from the successive meiotic divisions in spermatogenesis, and one ovum and three polar bodies are produced during oogenesis. The cytoplasm divides evenly in cells destined to become sperms, so that two equal spermatocytes are present after first meiotic

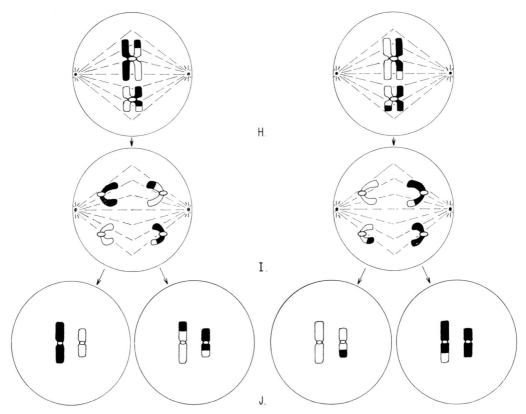

Figure 2-10. Second meiotic division: H. Metaphase; I. Anaphase; J. Telophase. The 23 double-stranded chromosomes now separate into 23 single-stranded chromosomes.

division (Fig. 2-9G) and four equal spermatids after second meiotic division (Fig. 2-10J). In the female, however, the cytoplasm is unevenly divided. After first meiotic division the major share of the cytoplasm goes to one cell, the secondary oocyte, and a polar body containing the full 23 chromosomes (but negligible cytoplasm) which divides before eventually being discarded. After second meiotic division the same unequal distribution of cytoplasm occurs, yielding an ovum and another polar body.

GAMETOGENESIS AND FERTILIZATION

The end-products of the events of meiosis are gametes and fusion of the maternal and paternal gametes during fertilization produces the first cell of the new individual, the **zygote.** Within this single cell resides all the genetic information required for growth and differentiation into a complex, multicellular human organism.

Spermatogenesis. This is the process through which the early male germ cells (**spermatagonia**) undergo a series of changes terminating in the previously described first and second meiotic divisions. Spermatogenesis occurs in the seminiferous tubules of the testes, and only takes place in the mature male. The entire process from spermatagonium through primary and secondary spermatocytes and spermatid to mature sperm requires 74 to 75 days.[9] The first and second meiotic divisions occupy approximately half of this time period. About 200 million sperms are normally present in an ejaculate, only one of which will participate in fertilization of the egg.

Oogenesis. This process by which the

early female germ cells (**oogonia**) differentiate into ova may consume from 12 to 45 years, depending on when during the reproductive life of the female the mature ovum is extruded. At about three months of intrauterine development the oogonia begin to differentiate into primary oocytes. At the time of birth of a female infant, it is thought that every oocyte she will ever possess is already present, although this concept has been challenged. These primary oocytes are already in first meiotic prophase and remain suspended in this stage until sexual maturity. In the sexually mature female a graafian follicle progresses to maturity each month and extrudes an oocyte which, having completed first meiotic division, continues through second meiotic division in transit through the fallopian tube.

Fertilization usually occurs in the lateral portion of the fallopian tube (Fig. 2-11), when one of the many sperm that surround the secondary oocyte penetrates it. The second meiotic division of the ovum usually is not completed until after fertilization. During fertilization the tail of the sperm rapidly disappears as the head is embedded in the ovum. Soon all that remains of the sperm is the pronucleus containing the 23 chromosomes. The sperm pronucleus makes its way into the pronucleus of the ovum, the nuclear membranes disappear and fusion occurs, producing a zygote that now has a single nucleus containing 46 chromosomes. The chromosomes now embark on a series of typical somatic cell mitotic divisions. At interphase there is replication of DNA; the usual mitotic sequence is followed through to the division into two cells, four cells, eight cells and so on through the blastula, gastrula and embryo stages, until finally a mature individual develops who is capable of reproduction and initiating a similar series of events.

CHROMOSOMAL ABERRATIONS

What are the possible errors in meiosis and early cell division of the zygote that can lead to abnormalities of chromosomes? First, some definition of terms is in order. The number of chromosomes in the gamete is 23 and this is the **haploid** (n) number. Forty-six is called the **diploid** (2n) number. Any exact multiple of the haploid number is called **euploid**. Therefore, haploid (n) and diploid (2n) numbers of chromosomes, which are multiples of 23, are euploid. However, if a patient has a chromosome number that is not an exact multiple of 23,

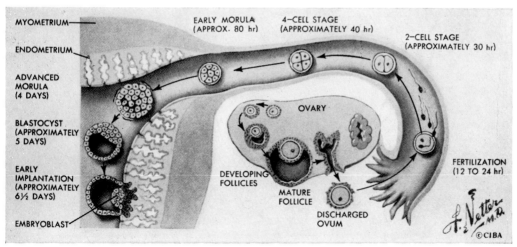

Figure 2-11. Fertilization and early mitotic cell divisions to implantation. (© Copyright 1969, CIBA Pharmaceutical Company, Division of CIBA-GEIGY Corporation. Reproduced, with permission, from THE CIBA COLLECTION OF MEDICAL ILLUSTRATIONS by Frank H. Netter, M.D. All rights reserved.)

as in Down syndrome with 47 chromosomes, the number is called **aneuploid.** A condition that is rarely encountered in humans except in abortuses, in certain differentiated cells and in tumors is **polyploidy.** This is a euploid condition (other than diploid) in which an exact multiple of the haploid state is present; 69 (3n) chromosomes is the triploid number; 92 (4n), the tetraploid, and so on through higher multiples.

An aneuploid state in which a third homologous chromosome is present in addition to the normal autosomal pair (as in Down syndrome) is called **trisomy.** Down syndrome is the eponym for 21 trisomy, the presence of chromosome 21 in triplicate rather than in duplicate. Absence of a chromosome is called **monosomy** for that chromosome. Although monosomy for the X chromosome in Turner syndrome is relatively common, monosomy for an autosome is almost nonexistent. As will be discussed in Chapter 4, whether there are 1, 2, 3 or more X chromosomes, only one X chromosome is fully active, so that monosomy for an X chromosome involves very little loss of vital genetic material. However, although the human can survive the amount of developmental confusion produced by the genetic information of an autosome being present in triplicate, he cannot withstand the absence of an entire autosome.

If only a piece of a chromosome is present in triplicate, as is found in **translocation,** this is termed partial trisomy. If a piece of a chromosome is missing, the terms partial monosomy or **deletion** may be used. In the following sections on numerical aberrations and structural alterations, further essential terms are defined.

Numerical Aberrations

Aneuploidy is a manifestation of a mistake in meiosis that may occur at first or second meiotic divisions or during a cell division of the zygote. The usual term for these mistakes is **nondisjunction** on the assumption that a homologous pair has failed to disjoin at first meiotic division or the double-stranded chromosome has failed to separate into single-stranded chromatids at second meiotic division or first somatic

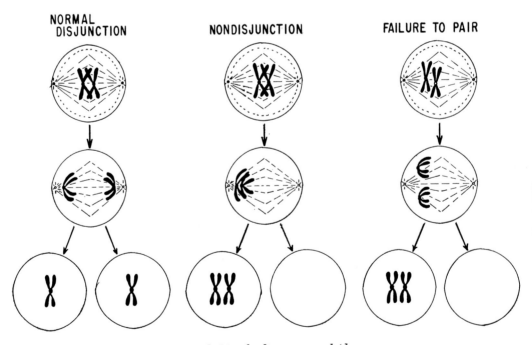

Figure 2-12. Mistakes in **first meiotic division** leading to aneuploidy.

cell division. It is generally recognized that nondisjunction may not be the actual mechanism underlying numerical aberrations in the majority of cases, and it has become accepted that when one uses the term nondisjunction one may also include failure to pair and anaphase lag.

Thus, in the strictest sense the term nondisjunction is probably incorrect for the most common mistake at first meiotic division. If the pair fails to disjoin, as may be visualized in Figure 2-12, both chromosomes of a homologous pair may end up in one daughter cell (24 chromosomes) and neither member of the pair in the other cell (22 chromosomes). But the same result occurs if the homologous chromosomes failed to pair and were randomly assorted between the two daughter cells. Experimental evidence favors the latter mechanism as being the more frequent error in first meiotic division.

In aneuploidy resulting from a mistake during second meiotic division (Fig. 2-13) there is a failure of the double-stranded chromosome to divide (disjoin) at the centromere into two chromatids migrating to separate poles and thus into separate daughter cells. There may also be a failure of a chromatid to move quickly enough during anaphase to become incorporated into a new daughter (**anaphase lag**). Such a chromatid is simply lost. Again the result is one cell having 24 chromosomes and the other, 22 chromosomes. Almost without exception the cell lacking an autosome is not viable. However, a cell lacking an X chromosome is frequently viable and capable of progressing through fertilization and differentiation, resulting in liveborn patients having the 45,X chromosomal constitution and the clinical features of Turner syndrome.

Thus, if a gamete gains or loses a chro-

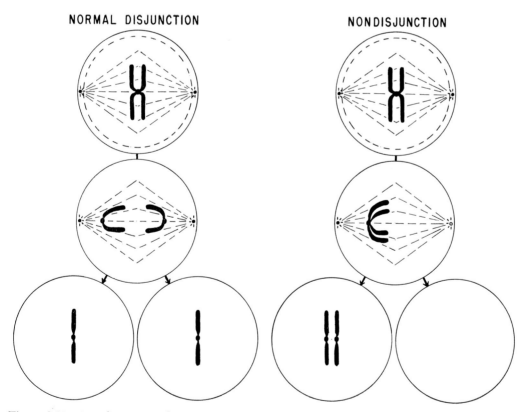

Figure 2-13. Mistake in **second meiotic division** leading to aneuploidy.

mosome at first or second meiotic division, when that gamete fuses with a gamete having the normal haploid number (23), aneuploidy results. If an autosome has been gained, as in Down syndrome, the aneuploid number is 47, and if an X chromosome has been lost, as in Turner syndrome, the aneuploid number is 45.

What happens at the second meiotic division may also occur during the first cell division of the zygote (Fig. 2-13), producing a viable cell line with an aneuploid number and a usually nonviable cell line. If nondisjunction occurs at the time of second or later cell division, then a different result is observed (Fig. 2-14). Two viable cell lines may be formed, one with a normal diploid number and one with an aneuploid number. This is called **mosaicism.** Mosaicism may result from nondisjunction at the third or fourth or subsequent cell divisions and the percentage of aneuploid cells compared with diploid cells depends on when the nondisjunction occurs. The capacity for establishing new cell lines leading to mosaicism is rapidly lost. The predominance of one cell line over another appears to affect the phenotypic features and severity of manifestation of the disorder. For example, a patient who has a cell line of 21 trisomic cells constituting 50% of his cell population is more severely affected than an individual having only 10% 21 trisomic cells.

Structural Aberrations

In the clinical setting, the commonly observed abnormalities of chromosome structure are **isochromosomes, deletions** (including **ring chromosomes**) and **transloca-**

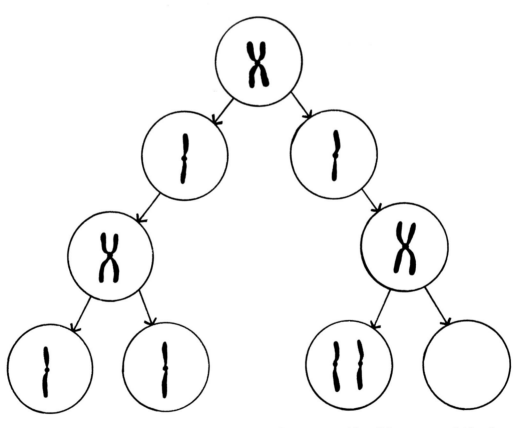

Figure 2-14. Nondisjunction at second cell division producing two viable cell lines, one euploid and one aneuploid (mosaicism).

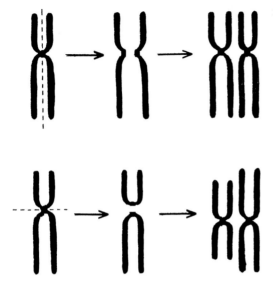

Figure 2-15. Isochromosome formation resulting from division of the chromosome in the plane of the short axis (below) rather than normal division in the long axis (above).

tions. **Inversions** and **duplications** may also be important in the human subject but will not be considered in this presentation.

Isochromosomes. These are the easiest of the structural aberrations to visualize. In Figure 2-15 the results of normal longitudinal division of the centromere are compared with what happens when division occurs at right angles to the long axis. The chromosomes produced by this abnormal division are one chromosome having the two long arms of the original chromosome, but no short arms, and the other chromosome consisting of the two short arms with no long arms. Each of these, called isochromosomes, constitutes a simultaneous duplication and deletion. If the isochromosome of the long arm of a chromosome is present in a diploid cell, the genes of the long arm are present in triplicate (trisomy of the long arm) and the genes of the short arm are only represented once (monosomy of the short arm). As an example, in the nomenclature of the Chicago and Paris Conferences, a female patient having an isochromosome of the long arm of the X chro-

mosome would be classified as 46,XX,i(Xq), with "q" being the abbreviation for long arm and "i" for isochromosome.

Deletion. A portion of a chromosome may break away and be lost. Only that portion retaining the centromere is able to orient on the spindle and be maintained through successive cell divisions. The break may be at an end (or both ends) or two breaks may occur within an arm so that a piece is removed from the middle. Where there is a break, the broken fragments are sticky and have a tendency to reunite. However, if there is no chromosomal material nearby to reunite with, the amputated end "heals" but sustains a loss of genetic material (Fig. 2-16A). If breaks occur at the ends of both arms, the two "sticky" ends may curl back and unite with each other, forming a ring chromosome (Fig. 2-16B),

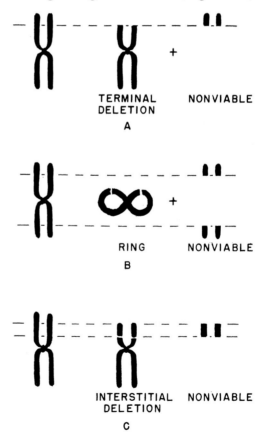

Figure 2-16. Deletions producing loss of chromosomal material.

which also results in a loss of genetic material. Finally, if two breaks take place within an arm and they are not properly reunited, the broken piece may fall out and the "sticky" proximal and distal ends reunite (Fig. 2-16C), causing a loss of gene loci. As illustrated earlier, the Chicago Conference nomenclature for a female having the deletion syndrome cri-du-chat would be 46,XX,5p— if the deletion of the short arm of chromosome 5 is "open." The same syndrome may occur if the deletion is in the form of a ring chromosome, and the nomenclature would be 46,XX,r(5).

Translocation. In this situation a broken piece of a chromosome is transferred to another chromosome. An example is the translocation of the long arm of a chromosome 21 to a chromosome 14 (Fig. 2-17). In a patient having 14/21 translocation mongolism, an unbalanced translocation, the affected individual has 46 chromosomes (a homologous pair of chromosome 21; a normal chromosome 14 and a structurally abnormal chromosome 14, which has an addition to the short arm consisting of the translocated long arm of chromosome 21). Such a patient is effectively trisomic for chromosome 21. A phenotypically normal patient could have a 14/21 balanced translocation, would be a translocation carrier and would have a chromosome count of 45 (one normal chromosome 14; one normal chromosome 21; and one abnormal chromosome made up of the long arms of chromosome 14 and 21). This patient would have almost all of the genetic material of a pair of chromosome 14 and a pair of

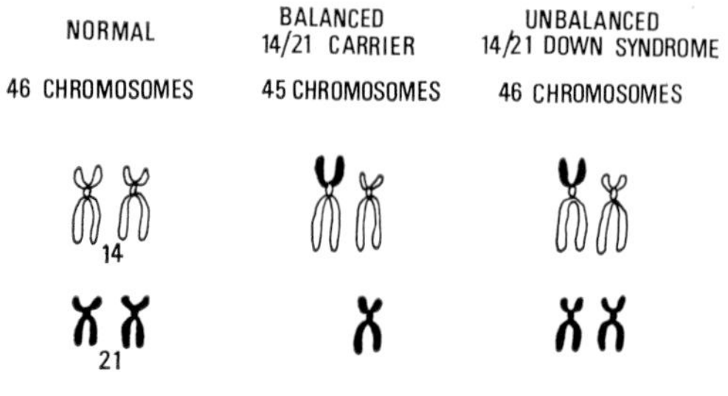

chromosome 21 and would thus be phenotypically normal.

The nomenclature for a male patient with 14/21 translocation Down syndrome would be 45,XY,—D,+t(14q21q). The patient has 46 chromosomes, 1 X and 1 Y chromosome, and is missing a normal D group chromosome (—D). This chromosome has been replaced by a chromosome made up of the long arm of a D group chromosome now known to be 14 and a G group chromosome identified as 21: +t(14q21q).

CLINICAL DISORDERS PRODUCED BY CHROMOSOMAL ABERRATIONS

Studies reveal that one infant in every 200 newborn has a recognizable chromosomal abnormality.[5,10,17,21] An investigation of therapeutic abortions between five and 20 weeks has shown that between 1.5% and 2.8% of specimens have gross chromosomal anomalies,[12] suggesting that the majority of conceptuses that have chromosomal aberrations do not survive to term. In support of this inference is evidence that 28% of first trimester spontaneous abortions have chromosomal anomalies.[16] A commonly used figure for the percentage of all pregnancies that end in recognizable spontaneous abortion is 15%.[22] (It has been suggested that perhaps 40% of fertilized ova are abnormal and probably result in early abortion, often unrecognized.)

The question that is uppermost in the minds of the parents of a patient with a chromosomal anomaly has still not been approached. What caused the chromosomal aberration? Tracing a patient's disease to a chromosomal aberration is not an insignificant accomplishment. It provides a firm diagnosis (which is the basis for subsequent clinical management), prognosis and recurrence risk data for genetic counseling. But why a specific chromosomal anomaly occurs in a specific patient can seldom be answered. The vast majority of aberrations are sporadic, although on rare occasions a chromosomal disorder is directly inherited (such as an unbalanced 14/21 transloca-

NORMAL	BALANCED 14/21 CARRIER	UNBALANCED 14/21 DOWN SYNDROME
46 CHROMOSOMES	45 CHROMOSOMES	46 CHROMOSOMES

Figure 2-17. 14/21 translocation, balanced and unbalanced.

tion transmitted from a balanced 14/21 translocation carrier).

There are some general underlying causes of these sporadic events. Late maternal age has certainly been implicated in mongolism. There also seems to be a slight familial predisposition to nondisjunction, with more than one "sporadic" aneuploidy occurring in first-degree relatives. Environmental agents such as radiation, chemicals and viruses have been demonstrated to cause chromosomal damage in experimental models. These environmental insults have been associated not so much with nondisjunction as with chromosomal "breakage." A particularly intriguing recent line of investigation has implicated an immunologic mechanism in nondisjunction through the discovery of antithyroid antibodies in mothers of infants with 21 trisomy.[7,8]

In Chapters 3 and 4 the commonly occurring autosomal and sex chromosomal anomalies are reviewed, emphasizing the clinical features leading the physician to arrive at the diagnosis as well as problems in management and ultimate prognosis.

REFERENCES

1. Boveri, T.: Ergebnisse uber die Konstitution der Chromatischen des Zellerns. Jena, Fischer, 1904.
2. Caspersson, T., Lamakka, G., and Zech, L.: The 24 fluorescence patterns of the human metaphase chromosomes—distinguishing characters and variability. Hereditas 67: 89, 1971.
3. Chen, T. R., and Ruddle, F. H.: Karyotype analysis utilizing differentially stained constitutive heterochromatin of human and murine chromosomes. Chromosoma, 34: 51, 1971.
4. Chicago Conference: Standardization in Human Cytogenetics. Birth Defects: Original Article Series, II: 2, 1966. New York, The National Foundation.
5. Court-Brown, W. M., and Smith, P. G.: Human population cytogenetics. Brit. Med. Bull. 25: 74, 1969.
6. Dutrillaux, B., and Lejeune, J.: Sur une nouvelle technique d'analyse du caryotype humain. C. R. Acad. Sci. (Paris), 272: 2638, 1971.
7. Fialkow, P. J.: Autoimmunity and chromosomal aberrations. Amer. J. Hum. Genet., 18: 93, 1966.
8. Fialkow, P. J., et al.: Familial predisposition to thyroid disease in Down's syndrome: controlled immuno-clinical studies. Amer. J. Hum. Genet., 23: 67, 1971.
9. Heller, C. G., and Clermont, Y.: Spermatogenesis in man: An estimate of its duration. Science, 140: 184, 1963.
10. Lubs, H. A., and Ruddle, F. H.: Chromosomal abnormalities in the human population: Estimation of rates based on New Haven newborn study. Science, 169: 495, 1970.
11. Morgan, T. H.: Sex limited inheritance in Drosophila. Science, 32: 120, 1910.
12. Nishimura, H.: Frequency of malformations in abortions. In Fraser, F. C., and McKusick, V. A. (eds.): Congenital Malformations. Proceedings of the Third International Conference, 1970. Amsterdam-New York, Excerpta Medica, p. 275.
13. Painter, T. S.: Studies in mammalian spermatogenesis. J. Zool., 37: 291, 1923.
14. Paris Conference (1971): Standardization in Human Cytogenetics. Birth Defects, Original Article Series, VIII: 7, 1972. The National Foundation, New York.
15. Patil, S. R., Merrick, S., and Lubs, H. A.: Identification of each human chromosome with a modified Giemsa stain. Science, 173: 821, 1971.
16. Polani, P. E.: Chromosome anomalies and abortions. Develop. Med. Child. Neurol., 8: 67, 1966.
17. Sergovich, F., et al.: Chromosome aberrations in 2159 consecutive newborn babies. New Eng. J. Med., 280: 851, 1969.
18. Sutton, W. S.: The chromosomes in heredity. Biol. Bull., 4: 231, 1903.
19. Tjio, J. H., and Levan, A.: The chromosome number of man. Hereditas, 42: 1, 1956.
20. Waldeyer, W.: Ueber Karyokinese und ihre Beziehungen zu den Befruchtungsvorgangen. Arch. mikr. Anat., 32: 1, 1888.
21. Walzer, S., Breau, G., and Gerald, P. S.: A chromosome survey of 2400 normal newborn infants. J. Pediat., 74: 438, 1969.
22. Warburton, D., and Fraser, F. C.: Spontaneous abortion risks in man: data from reproductive histories collected in a medical genetics unit. Amer. J. Hum. Genet., 16: 1, 1964.

Chapter 3

AUTOSOMAL CHROMOSOMAL ANOMALIES

Before abnormalities of human chromosomes could be recognized, satisfactory preparations and knowledge of normal human chromosomes were required. Tjio and Levan[27] provided the techniques for preparation and the definition of the normal number in 1956; and Lejeune and associates[16] followed, in 1959, with the first description of a chromosomal abnormality in the clinical disorder called Down syndrome or mongolism. Since then, a large number of chromosomal anomalies have appeared in the world literature. There are three well-established autosomal trisomy conditions and six other aberrations of autosomes that produce recognizable patterns of anomalies that appear to justify clinical description. The selection of these nine autosomal abnormalities for discussion is somewhat arbitrary and reflects the experience of the authors as well as the frequency with which these autosomal anomaly syndromes appear in the literature. There are, of course, reports of many numerical and structural aberrations of chromosomes that are not included in this chapter or are only briefly mentioned. Some general observations precede the description of specific syndromes.

GENERAL OBSERVATIONS

Partial Trisomy and Mosaicism. The complete or incomplete manifestation of an autosomal trisomy syndrome may be produced by partial trisomy or mosaicism. Many examples are available in Down syndrome when an unbalanced D/21 translocation results in the phenotypic pattern of 21 trisomy. Similarly, patients having mosaicism consisting of a 21 trisomy, aneuploid cell line and a euploid cell line may present with the full clinical expression of 21 trisomy or may have some features only mildly reminiscent of mongolism. Presumably this represents a quantitative reflection of the developmental confusion produced by greater or lesser amounts of genetic material in triplicate.

Trisomy Phenotypes Without Apparent Chromosomal Aberration. The diagnostic pattern of anomalies accepted for the clinical diagnosis of any one of the chromosomal syndromes may be found in patients having no demonstrable chromosomal abnormality. This is true not only for the less well-established deletion syndromes, but also for well-known trisomy syndromes. The classic manifestations of Down syndrome and 13 trisomy have been found in patients with normal karyotypes. One possible explanation for this phenomenon is that such patients have submicroscopic translocations or duplications of a segment of chromosome responsible for the phenotype of the syndrome. Undetected mosaicism may also be suggested, based on the possibility that the number of cells or the tissue studied in such patients may have been inadequate to reveal the aneuploid line responsible for the clinical abnormalities. Another suggestion is that such patients may represent phenocopies of an autosomal syndrome. The term phenocopy refers to the fact that patients with different genotypes (the total genetic makeup of an individual) may have similar phenotypes (the total physical makeup and appearance of an individual). A patient may have many of the stigmata of 21 or 13 trisomy because of a chromosomal anomaly, because of the interaction of another genotype with environmental factors, or even possibly because of a single mutant gene.

Double Aneuploidy and Familial Nondisjunction. One of the earliest reports of a chromosomal anomaly presented a patient with two separate trisomic aberrations, 21 trisomy and XXY.[3] Since this publication, a large number of other examples of double aneuploidy within a given individual have entered the literature. These may represent the effects of an error in distribution of one chromosome at cell division affecting the distribution of another chromosome, or may reflect some general predisposition to nondisjunction. In support of the latter concept are reports of families having an instance of one type of aneuploidy (e.g., Turner syndrome) in one offspring and a different aneuploidy (e.g., 13 trisomy) in another offspring. The genetic counselor appreciates that, although the chance of recurrence of a sporadic trisomic condition within a sibship is remote, a family already having a member with aneuploidy is at greater risk than a family in the general population. A commonly used estimate is that the risk of recurrence of sporadic aneuploidy in a sibship is about double the risk in the general

population. Recent data from amniocentesis material show that in Down syndrome the recurrence of "sporadic" trisomy may be as high as 2 to 3%.[18]

Isochromosomes. Although examples of isochromosome formation are not uncommon for the X chromosomes, these structural aberrations are rarely encountered in the autosomes. As will be remembered from Chapter 2 and Figure 2-15, an isochromosome is a misdivision at the centromere across the short axis rather than the long axis of the chromosome. Apparent isochro-

TABLE 3-1.   Features of 21 Trisomy

Area	Findings
General	Equal sex distribution, variable lengths of survival
Neurologic	Hypotonic, psychomotor retardation
Head	Characteristic facies—patients look more like other patients with 21 trisomy than like their sibs; flat occiput
Eyes	"Mongoloid slant," epicanthic folds, Brushfield spots
Ears	Small, frequently low-set
Nose	Low nasal bridge
Mouth and chin	Protruding fissured tongue secondary to maxillary hypoplasia and narrow palate
Neck	Broad; frequently webbed
Heart	Congenital heart lesions in 50%, ventricular septal defect and atrioventricular canal most common
Abdomen	Diastasis recti, umbilical hernia, duodenal atresia
Hands	Short hands and fingers, clinodactyly fifth finger
Feet	Gap between first and second toes with plantar furrow
Urogenital	Occasional cryptorchism
X-ray	Pelvic x-rays iliac index < 60°; hypoplasia midphalanx fifth finger
Dermatoglyphics	Simian line, distal axial triradius, ten ulnar loops or radial loops on fourth and fifth fingers
Incidence	1 in 660

mosomes of the long arm of a D group autosome (presumably 13) have been observed in patients having phenotypic stigmata of the 13 trisomy syndrome. Also, isochromosomes attributed to the G group have been found in patients with features of Down syndrome. All viable offspring of the balanced carrier should be expected to have a trisomic condition.

Ring Chromosomes. Ring chromosomes may be visualized as being formed when breaks occur in both arms of a chromosome and healing takes place by the "sticky" ends of both arms joining each other. The physician is interested in what happens to a patient possessing a ring autosome. The clinical features of such a patient usually reflect deletion, because there has been a net loss (partial monosomy) of genetic material. Thus, patients with a ring D chromosome [r(D)] have stigmata consistent with a D deletion syndrome (13q—), although curiously there have been reports of patients with ring D who have features more consistent with 13 trisomy.

21 TRISOMY (DOWN SYNDROME, MONGOLISM, G₁ TRISOMY)

This is the most common autosomal abnormality (see Table 3-1 and Fig. 3-1). An accepted frequency for the occurrence of mongolism in the general population is 1:660.[4] The clinical disorder was first recognized by Down in 1866,[10] and before techniques were available to demonstrate the cytogenetic abnormality, Waardenburg[29] suggested in 1932 that a chromosomal anomaly could be responsible for the features of the syndrome.

After Lejeune demonstrated that the underlying chromosomal anomaly was a trisomy of a small acrocentric chromosome, he designated that chromosome 21 was the autosome present in triplicate. By cytologic and autoradiographic evidence it was not possible to distinguish chromosome 21 from

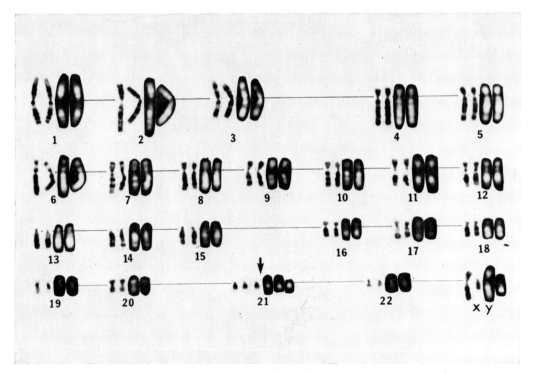

Figure 3-1. Karyotype of male infant with Down syndrome, 21 trisomy. Homologues on the left are by G-staining methods and on the right by Q-staining methods. (Courtesy G. Singh and H. A. Lubs.)

chromosome 22, so many preferred the term G or G_1 trisomy to 21 trisomy. Now, of course, with the newer banding techniques the G group chromosomes are readily distinguishable. The majority of patients who have Down syndrome have a complete 21 trisomy (Fig. 3-1). However, a significant number have translocation or mosaicism as the underlying aberration.

Complete 21 Trisomy. There does not seem to be a preponderance of patients of one sex over the other with this syndrome. The length of survival may be measured in weeks or decades, and a life expectancy approaching normal may be predicted for a well cared-for patient who does not have a congenital heart defect.

In infancy the patient is observed to have poor muscle tone and may appear to remain "floppy" for months or even years. Growth is poor. Those patients who have congenital heart lesions and frequent pneumonia do not thrive. However, patients without these complications also fail to achieve the height

of their sibs. Psychomotor development is the major area of concern, and there is a fairly broad spectrum of achievement. Although most patients are in the I.Q. range of 25 to 50, an occasional patient is educable and able to learn to read and write.

The facial appearance in Down syndrome is so typical that patients with 21 trisomy, whatever their racial origin, tend to have facial features more like other patients with 21 trisomy than their own sibs (Fig. 3-2). The palpebral fissures tend to slant upward at the lateral borders and there is an epicanthic fold which together contribute to the "mongolian" appearance. The iris is speckled with a ring of round, grayish Brushfield spots. The back of the head is somewhat flat and the nasal bridge is also flattened. The maxilla is small and the palate narrow, which makes the oral cavity inadequate to accommodate the tongue, which frequently protrudes and often has a fissured appearance. A third fontanelle is an important sign in the newborn.

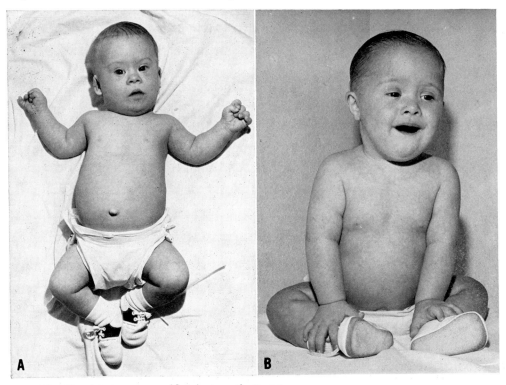

Figure 3-2.   Unrelated one-year-old infants with 21 trisomy.

Among the stigmata of many syndromes is webbing of the neck, which occurs in less than half of the patients with 21 trisomy. The abdominal wall may be inadequate; diastasis recti and umbilical hernias are common. Cryptorchism is frequent and the adult male mongol is sterile. Adult female patients have been reported to reproduce, and about 50% of their offspring have Down syndrome, as expected.

About half the patients with this aberration have congenital cardiac malformations. Ventricular septal defect is slightly more common than atrioventricular (AV) canal, but since the latter lesion is relatively uncommon in the general population, AV canal may be considered a characteristic cardiovascular anomaly of Down syndrome. A mongoloid child who has a pansystolic murmur and the electrocardiographic finding of left axis deviation should be suspected of having this particularly unfavorable heart lesion. Most of the other heart lesions occur, including atrial septal defect (ostium secundum) and patent ductus arteriosus, but transposition of the great vessels occurs less frequently than expected. The congenital heart malformation is responsible for much of the morbidity and early and late mortality in this syndrome.

The fingers are short and the fifth finger incurved. There is a gap between the first and second toes with a furrow extending down the plantar surface from this gap. Roentgenographic abnormalities include a decreased iliac index (Fig. 3-3). The normal mean value is 81° but in Down syndrome the mean value is 62°, and an iliac index of less than 60° strongly favors the diagnosis. Hypoplasia of the middle phalanx of the fifth finger is also observed on x-ray.

That certain dermatoglyphic patterns are characteristic of Down syndrome has been appreciated for over 30 years.[7] A bilateral simian line is found in about 30% of the palms of mongols and a bilateral distal axial triradius more frequently (82%). Ulnar loops on all ten fingers, which is rare in

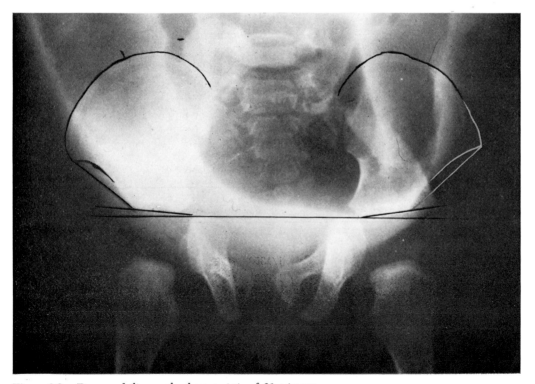

Figure 3-3. Decreased iliac angle characteristic of 21 trisomy.

the general population, is found in one-third of these patients. When present, a hallucal loop is the most useful discriminating feature, as it occurs in 72% of cases and less than 0.5% of controls. For further details, see Chapter 19.

For many decades physicians have recognized that there is a relationship between maternal age and the risk of having an offspring with Down syndrome. Although the overall frequency of Down syndrome in the general population is about 1:660, the risk increases precipitously from 1:1500 for mothers under 30 years of age to 1:50 for mothers over 45 years old[3] (see Table 3-2). Since cases resulting from translocations do not show the maternal age effect, they are relatively more frequent in younger mothers. Thus, in the absence of chromosome studies, the recurrence risk is greatly increased in the young mothers. A 50-fold increase in risk has been estimated for mothers under 25 years of age.

Previously undiagnosed normal/21 trisomy mosaicism in the mother has been implicated in some instances of 21 trisomic offspring being born to younger mothers. We have observed this situation in two teen-aged mothers of children with Down syndrome. Maternal thyroid disease and antithyroid antibodies in younger mothers of mongols has also been emphasized, and we have had examples of this situation in our clinic. This immunologic finding and the finding of the "Australia antigen" in 30% of patients with Down syndrome provide an area of continuing interest and speculation.

Translocation. At any maternal age the most frequent cause of Down syndrome is complete 21 trisomy. However, because there is such a clear relationship between increased age and increased frequency of offspring with Down syndrome, the affected infant of a young mother may be suspected of having an inherited translocation. For mothers under 30 years of age, translocation accounts for 9% of all patients with mongolism; one-fourth of these are inherited and three-fourths are sporadic translocations. So in the younger age groups there is only one chance in 11 that the mongoloid patient has a translocation Down syndrome, and even if he has a translocation, the chances are only one in four that it is inherited. *Thus, the overall chance that a baby with an unbalanced translocation Down syndrome born to a woman under 30 years of age inherited this aberration is only one in 50.*[34]

The translocations that occur most commonly involve D group chromosomes. Autoradiographic evidence suggests that the D chromosomes participating in the translocation do not belong to pair number 13, but evidence from QM fluorescence suggest

TABLE 3-2. Maternal Age and Risk of Down Syndrome

Age of Mother	Risk at Any Pregnancy	Risk after Birth of Down Syndrome*
15-19	1/1850	Increased 50×
20-24	1/1600	Increased 50×
25-29	1/1350	Increased 5×
30-34	1/800	Increased 5×
35-39	1/260	No apparent increase
40-44	1/100	No apparent increase
45+	1/50	No apparent increase
All ages	1/660	

* If chromosomal studies *not* performed on affected child. (Adapted from Carter, C. O., and Evans, K. A. Lancet, 2:785, 1961.)

that D/G translocations are usually 14/21, but may involve 13 (and not, as yet, 15). Translocation within the G group and isochromosome formation must also be considered. Patients having mongolism caused by an unbalanced translocation usually have the full features of 21 trisomy. However, an occasional patient will have a less complete expression of the syndrome, which may be related to the quantity of extra genetic material.

The Chicago and Paris Conference abbreviation for a male infant who has a D/G unbalanced translocation is 46,XY,—D,+t (DqGq). The patient has 46 chromosomes, but one of the D chromosomes is missing (—D) and is replaced by a chromosome made up of the long arm of a D chromosome and the long arm of a G chromosome [+t(DqGq)]. Although the chances are only one in four of this being inherited translocation, let us assume that the mother is a balanced carrier. The nomenclature for her chromosome complement would be 45, XX,—D,—G,+t(DqGq). She would have 45 chromosomes, a missing D chromosome (—D) and a missing G chromosome (—G); the long arms of these are united in a single chromosome that contains essentially all of the genetic information of the D and the G chromosomes.

The next observations would not have been predicted. It had been expected, on the basis of random segregation, that one in three viable offspring of either parent who was a balanced D/G translocation carrier would have translocation Down syndrome (one in three would be a carrier and one in three would be normal). The empiric data from different series reveal that between 6% and 20% of offspring of a mother who is a balanced translocation carrier have Down syndrome, and only 2% of offspring of a father with a balanced translocation are mongoloid. Comparable recurrence risk figures have been suggested for the G/G translocation also.

Therefore if a patient has an inherited translocation, subsequent sibs have a rela-tively high recurrence risk, but a lower risk than had been previously thought. With amniocentesis and antenatal diagnosis of chromosomal aberrations being more common, this risk may be further reduced. Therapeutic abortion can be recommended if an unbalanced translocation is demonstrated following amniocentesis. One caution: the rarely encountered isochromosome 21 or 21/21 translocation, if transmitted by a balanced carrier, will produce mongolism in all viable offspring. Isochromosome 21 is now distinguishable from 21/22 translocation by banding techniques, but cannot, even by this method, be differentiated from 21/21 translocation.

Mosaicism. Patients having a normal cell line and a 21 trisomy cell line have the widest range of ultimate intellectual and physical attainment. Estimates that mosaicism is found in only 1.5% of patients with Down syndrome appear to be too low. There may be a sizeable number of patients with minimal findings to suggest Down syndrome who are 21 trisomy mosaics. It has not been uncommon in our experience for a pediatrician to ask for a chromosomal evaluation of a baby or child who may have few stigmata (or perhaps no clear stigmata) of mongolism and to find that the patient is a G trisomy mosaic (presumably 21 trisomy mosaic). These are frequently patients we would have predicted not to be particularly good bets for chromosomal anomalies.

Patients with 21 trisomy mosaicism may have the classic appearance of Down syndrome or may look essentially normal, presumably depending on the preponderance of the abnormal cell line. The realization of this is important to the genetic counselor, who should maintain a fairly high index of suspicion regarding the intellectually dull normal young mother of a patient with 21 trisomy. If a parent has a mosaicism, the risk of 21 trisomy in future offspring is significantly increased. In fact, one may speculate that unrecognized mosaicism may account partially, if not completely, for the occasional high-risk family attributed to a "predisposition to nondisjunction."

One further point of interest, which has profound cytogenetic implications, is the disappearance of or "selection against" the abnormal (or normal) cell line in a mosaic patient as reported by Taylor[26] and others. In our clinic we have observed one such patient[19] who had a mosaicism consisting of 50% G trisomic cells out of eight cells karyotyped from the peripheral blood at six months of age. At this initial visit, at which she was referred to as being mongoloid, her development was judged to be at the three-month level, and she had a few stigmata that were suggestive of Down syndrome (Fig. 3-4). During the next few months her development appeared to accelerate to such an extent that the cytogenetic diagnosis was questioned. Three more chromosomal evaluations were performed between 16 and 26 months of age. Of the 137 cells from the peripheral blood that were karyotyped, all were normal. The patient's developmental age at 24 months was estimated to be between 24 and 30 months. It would seem that the G trisomic cell line has dis-

appeared in this patient and that there has been a normalizing of development. The latter statement is offered with extreme caution because of the difficulty in making reliable developmental evaluations at these early ages. Continued observation and verbal I.Q. testing will be required to further assess these unusal findings.

Counseling. The counseling of a family with a child having Down syndrome proceeds from the establishment of the cytogenetic diagnosis. It is difficult to argue convincingly for the need to karyotype for counseling purposes the infant with classic stigmata of Down syndrome whose mother is over 40 years of age, is multiparous and does not intend to have more children. Protocols differ. Many geneticists may be reluctant to karyotype infants with Down syndrome born to mothers over 30 years old, knowing that an inherited translocation probably does not occur more frequently than one in 300 cases in this age group. Some have expressed the minority opinion that even infants with Down syndrome of mothers under 30 years of age need not be karyotyped, because only one in 50 has an

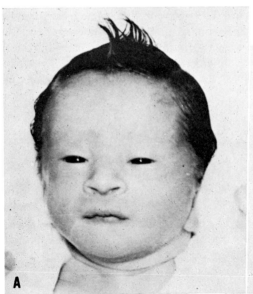 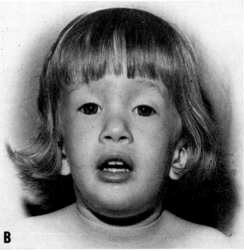

A   **B**

Figure 3-4. Patient (at birth and at 26 months) who had G trisomy mosaicism at six months of age. The abnormal cell line could not be detected in three different chromosomal evaluations between 16 and 26 months.

inherited translocation. Acknowledging that there are differences of opinion in this area, we personally prefer to karyotype all infants with Down syndrome for clinical, humanitarian and investigative purposes. It simply seems to be more humane to tie up laboratory facilities doing karyotypes on 49 or 299 patients who are negative with respect to the question of inherited translocation than to permit parents to experience the grief of having another child with Down syndrome or to live with the anxiety of not knowing the risk of recurrence. From the research point of view, there still is not enough information to be confident of the recurrence risks to parents when one has a balanced D/G or G/G translocation. The data are reasonably acceptable that if the father is the carrier the risk is only 2%, but there is a great difference between the suggested risks of 6% and 20% if the mother is a D/G balanced translocation carrier. More data are still needed.

The first step is to obtain a diagnosis in which confidence can be placed. The next step is to ascertain the risks as closely as possible. The risks for translocation have been reviewed. A mother with a balanced translocation who has living normal children may not wish to have more pregnancies. However, a young mother who has a mongol as her only child is likely to desire more pregnancies. Such future pregnancies should only be considered if facilities are available to obtain reliable karyotypes from amniotic fluid. The opportunity to abort an affected fetus must be present.

What of the risk to the young mother of a patient with a complete 21 trisomy? In general, with two reservations, the risk is small, perhaps 2 to 3% (which is actually higher than previously thought). The first reservation is that the not-too-bright young mother of a mongol may, herself, be a mosaic and need karyotyping. This event is rare, but it occurs. The second reservation is related to the thyroid status of these young mothers. At the time of this writing, a second child with Down syndrome has

not been reported to have been delivered to a mother who has been discovered to have antithyroid antibodies. However, if this factor has etiologic relevance, increased risk should eventually be demonstrated.

Having discussed the diagnosis, the cause (as is best understood) and the chances of recurrence, there is still a child to treat and a family crisis to be weathered. Half of the children with 21 trisomy have congenital heart lesions and may spend more time in the hospital than out during the first year of their lives. Yet many of the heart lesions, such as patent ductus arteriosus and ventricular septal defect, are subject to complete or palliative repair at any age. Other lesions, such as atrioventricular canal, are not so easily managed. The point is that the choice between having a constantly hospitalized child and a reasonably healthy child who stays at home depends on appropriate medical and surgical management.

Which introduces the next consideration: Do you keep a child with mongolism at home or try to place him in an institution? How does a family live with this problem? First of all, in most places it is not possible to place such a child immediately in a tax-supported institution, and many families lack the financial resources to pay for a good private institution (which may have a waiting list). So even the family that does not seem to be able to accept what has happened must, at least for a while, take the affected baby home and live with him. Some parents verbalize their rejection of the baby, some reject while making a great display of their concern and acceptance (sometimes by constantly calling the pediatrician, cardiologist and geneticist for every sneeze, snort and stool), and some appear to accept the baby honestly and openly and make him a part of the family from the very beginning. Most parents and siblings eventually accept the baby and develop a genuine love and concern. For the family or individual parent whose stability is borderline, having a mongoloid baby may be the

last straw. Time and again divorce has resulted and not infrequently psychiatric
assistance, including hospitalization, has
been required. Support from the involved
physicians, social workers, other family
members and clergymen is unquestionably
necessary. The crisis is survived in the
great majority of cases, and the patient with
Down syndrome spends his childhood at
home as an equal, loved and accepted
member of the family. Many parents emphasize how unusually affectionate and
agreeable these children can be.

Medical center and community resources
need to be mobilized to handle the special
problems of patients with this disorder.
Developmental evaluation and special training should be afforded as indicated. Many
children with complete 21 trisomy are train-
able and an occasional patient is educable.
This is some of the information that is required to answer the early questions regarding prognosis.

One aspect that must be continually emphasized to the parents is that they set
realistic goals for the level of achievement
of their child. This is all part of acceptance.
The infant and young child with Down
syndrome may reach occasional developmental milestones at a normal age. Indeed,
by many objective criteria, the developmental age of these patients appears to be
more advanced in the early years than their
ultimate level of attainment will be. The
parents must recognize this. It is good for
them to work with their child and with professional guidance to develop the child's
potential to maximum—as long as the goals
are realistic. Frequent trips to distant cities
for special treatments that have not been
generally incorporated into the standard
therapeutic armamentarium may place an
unwarranted or even disastrous burden on
a family and deprive the normal siblings
of their rightful share of the family's financial and emotional resources.

There are certain ingredients in every case
of genetic counseling: diagnosis, recurrence
risks, prognosis, etiology, treatment of the
patient and support of the family. Many of
the steps described in the approach to the
patient with Down syndrome could apply
to a patient with another chromosomal
aberration, a single mutant gene syndrome,
a malformation determined by multifactorial inheritance or a syndrome of undetermined etiology. However, each patient
like each disease is a special and unique
case.

TABLE 3-3. Features of 18 Trisomy

Area	Findings
General	Female sex preponderance (M, 1:F,3); low birth weight for gestational age; failure to thrive, early death
Neurologic	Mental and growth retardation, hypertonic
Head	Prominent occiput
Eyes	Epicanthic folds, small palpebral fissures
Ears	Low-set, malformed
Mouth and chin	Micrognathia, narrow palatal arch, microstomia; infrequently, cleft lip and/or palate
Thorax	Short sternum, eventration of diaphragm
Heart	Congenital heart anomalies in 99%, most often ventricular septal defect or patent ductus arteriosus
Abdomen	Meckel's diverticulum, inguinal hernia
Hands	Third and fourth fingers clenched against palm with second and fifth fingers overlapping them
Feet	Rocker-bottom shape, great toe dorsiflexed
Pelvis	Small pelvis, limited hip abduction
Urogenital	Renal anomalies, cryptorchism
X-ray	Hypoplastic sternum, thin tapered ribs, hypoplastic mandible, "antimongoloid" pelvis
Dermatoglyphics	Characteristic digital pattern of six to ten low arches, high axial triradius, single flexion crease on digits
Incidence	1 in 3500

18 TRISOMY (E TRISOMY, 17 TRISOMY, 16-18 TRISOMY, EDWARDS SYNDROME)

In the same issue of *The Lancet* in 1960, two teams of investigators described the phenotypic abnormalities produced by a trisomy for a chromosome in the E group. Edwards and his colleagues[11] described in detail the findings in a female child and designated that the extra chromosome was a number 17. Patau, Smith and co-workers[20] presented a preliminary description of this trisomic condition in two patients in a report that also included the first recognition of a patient with trisomy in the D group. In their full presentation of the clinical findings of the E group trisomy, Smith and associates considered the extra chromosome to be homologous with pair 18,[24] and it has since been accepted that this is the appropriate assignment of the extra chromosome on the basis of centromere indexes, autoradiography, and, more recently, fluorescence patterns (Fig. 3-5).

This appears to be the second most common of the autosomal trisomy syndromes, with a frequency of 1:3500 live births in a North American population A preponderance of patients have been reported as being female (78% in the review by Smith),[16] although this may reflect the longer-term survivors. Growth and developmental retardation and early death, usually before six months, are typical of the course, but some patients may survive for years. The

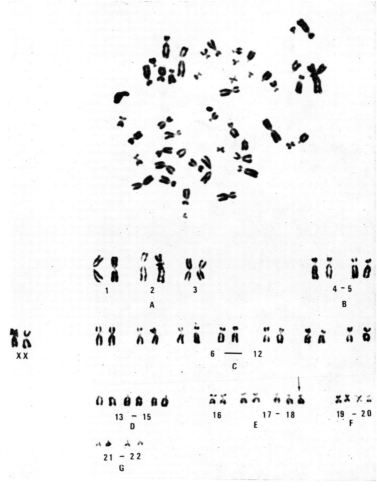

Figure 3-5. Conventional karyotype of 18 trisomy by Giemsa 6 method.

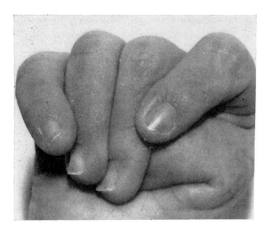

Figure 3-6. Typical conformation of hand in 18 trisomy.

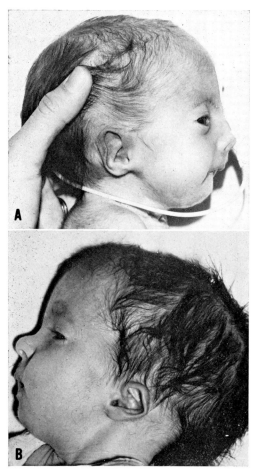

Figure 3-7. Two infants illustrating craniofacial characteristics of 18 trisomy (prominent occiput, low-set malformed ears and small chin).

affected individual is usually hypertonic and holds her hands in the peculiar manner illustrated in Figure 3-6; the third and fourth fingers are clenched tightly against the palm and the second and fifth fingers overlap them. There is a prominent occiput, low-set malformed ears and a small chin (Fig. 3-7). A short sternum, small pelvis with limited hip abduction and rocker-bottom feet are common (Figs. 3-8, 3-9). All patients in the literature with the exception of one have had congenital heart lesions, most often ventricular septal defect and patent ductus arteriosus. The dermatoglyphics in 18 trisomy provide useful diagnostic evidence (see Chapter 19). In addition to the bilateral distal axial triradius (t″) in 25% and single flexion crease on digit 5 (40%) and simian crease (25%) encountered in many syndromes, there is a characteristic preponderance of low arches on the fingers; 80% of cases have seven or more (see Table 3-3) whereas this occurs in less than 1% of normal individuals.

As with Down syndrome, a patient having the stigmata of 18 trisomy most often has a complete trisomy, but may have a partial trisomy or mosaicism consisting of a normal cell line and a +18 trisomic line. The phenotypic expression may be complete or incomplete in these patients, presumably related to the quantity of genetic information appearing in triplicate. Double aneuploidy has also been reported in patients

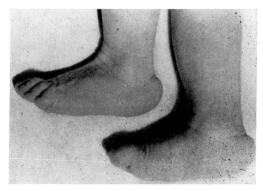

Figure 3-8. Rocker-bottom foot of infant with 18 trisomy.

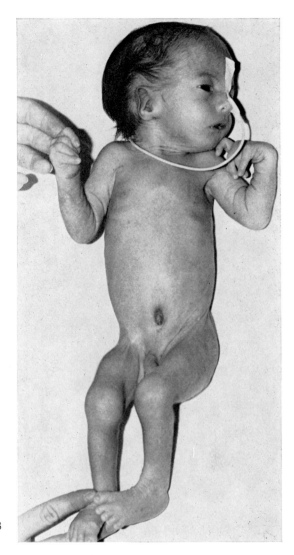

Figure 3-9. Full body view of infant with 18 trisomy.

with 18 trisomy who have had an additional trisomy of the X chromosome, chromosome 21 or chromosome 13. It should also be noted that in this syndrome, as in other chromosomal disorders, classic stigmata of 18 trisomy may be found in patients who do not have a *demonstrable* chromosomal anomaly.

Unbalanced translocation is rare in this syndrome. The parents of a patient with 18 trisomy should be reassured that this has been a sporadic event that occurs in one infant in 3,500, and that the likelihood of a recurrence in their family is negligible.

13 TRISOMY (D₁ TRISOMY, D TRISOMY, 13-15 TRISOMY, PATAU SYNDROME)

Although the pattern of anomalies found in 13 trisomy has been traced back through 300 years of the world literature, the first report that these abnormalities were associated with a chromosomal aberration was presented by Patau, Smith and colleagues in 1960.[20] A detailed clinical description by Smith *et al.* followed.[25] To indicate that this was the first clinically recognizable disorder involving trisomy of a D group chromosome, the term D_1 trisomy was used. Subsequent autoradiographic and fluores-

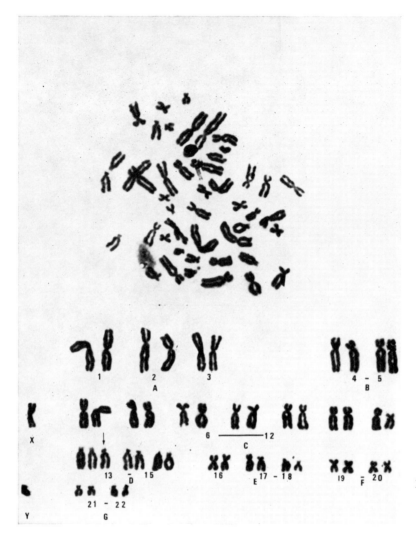

Figure 3-10. Conventional karyotype of patient with 13 trisomy.

cence studies have provided evidence that the trisomic chromosome in this syndrome is homologous with pair 13 (Fig. 3-10). Of the three major autosomal trisomy syndromes, this is the least common, occurring in approximately 1:7000 live births.

A patient with this syndrome has the appearance of being more severely malformed than patients having the other two trisomic syndromes (Table 3-4 and Fig. 3-11). Most 13 trisomic patients have cleft lip and palate and eye abnormalities, which range from colobomata of the iris through microphthalmia to complete absence of the eye. Seventy-five percent of the patients

have defects of the midface and forebrain, including arhinencephaly and holoprosencephaly (Fig. 3-12). The head is small and the forehead sloping. Those patients not having cleft lip and palate have a characteristic midfacial appearance (Fig. 3-13). The ears are low-set and malformed and the chin small. Polydactyly is common and the hands are often held clenched as in 18 trisomy with the second and fifth fingers overlapping the third and fourth.

Although the cardiovascular lesions most frequently encountered are ventricular septal defect and patent ductus arteriosus, rotational cardiovascular malformations are

TABLE 3-4. Features of 13 Trisomy

Area	Findings
General	Equal sex distribution, failure to thrive, apneic spells, early death
Neurologic	Mental and motor retardation; hypertonic or hypotonic; defects of the forebrain (holoprosencephaly, arhinencephaly)
Head	Sloping forehead, scalp defects, microcephaly
Eyes	Colobomata, microphthalmia, anophthalmia
Ears	Low-set, malformed
Mouth and chin	Usually cleft lip and/or palate; micrognathia
Heart	Congenital heart lesions in 88%, most often ventricular septal defect, patent ductus arteriosus and rotational anomalies
Abdomen	Rotational anomalies, hernias, absent spleen, accessory spleens
Hands	Polydactyly; frequently third and fourth fingers clenched against palm with second and fifth fingers overlapping; hyperconvex nails
Feet	Polydactyly, frequently rocker-bottom shape
Urogenital	Polycystic kidneys, hydronephrosis, cryptorchism, bicornuate uterus
Dermatoglyphics	Ridge hypoplasia, radial loops and arches, high triradius, single palmar flexion crease; hallucal arch fibular or fibular-S pattern
Incidence	1 in 7000

highly characteristic of this lesion (e.g., dextroposition of the heart without abdominal situs inversus). These rotational anomalies usually include complex intracardiac lesions, such as the combination of single ventricle with L-loop transposition, single atrium and anomalous pulmonary venous return. In these situations the spleen may be absent or there may be accessory spleens. Urogenital anomalies are common.

The dermatoglyphics are diagnostically useful. Although the finger patterns may be difficult to see because of ridge hypoplasia, there is an excess of arches (25% have more than three) and radial loops on digits other than no. 2 (50%). A high triradius (81%) and simian crease (58%) are frequently found. On the foot there may be a hallucal fibular loop or arch (43%) or a tibial loop (34%). An S-shaped fibular arch pattern is quite specific for D_1 trisomy. (See Chapter 19 for further details.)

The majority of patients having the stigmata of 13 trisomy have a complete trisomy. However, it is not an uncommon experience to obtain a karyotype on a patient who has the phenotypic features of 13 trisomy but no detectable chromosomal anomaly. Balanced and unbalanced familial translocations involving a D group chromosome (presumably 13) are among the most common chromosomal aberrations. The frequency in the North American population of balanced D group translocations may be as high as 1:1000. Clinical features of patients with unbalanced D group translocations usually reflect the full expression of the 13 trisomy syndrome. Mosaicism (normal/13 trisomy) also occurs.

Parents of a patient with complete 13 trisomy may be counseled that the incidence of 13 trisomy is about 1:7000 in the general population. The risk of recurrence of nondisjunction in their family, although higher than the general population, should be very small (of the order of 1:3500). If the patient has an unbalanced translocation, chromosomal evaluation of the parents is required. Often the unbalanced translocation proves to be a sporadic event, but if a balanced translocation is found in a parent, the frequency of affected offspring of such balanced carriers is high enough to justify antenatal chromosomal studies of subsequent pregnancies by amniocentesis.

In Chapter 16 a clinical example of a D/D translocation family is reviewed. As in 21/D translocation-Down syndrome, the occurrence of affected offspring is less than anticipated. Likely explanations are that

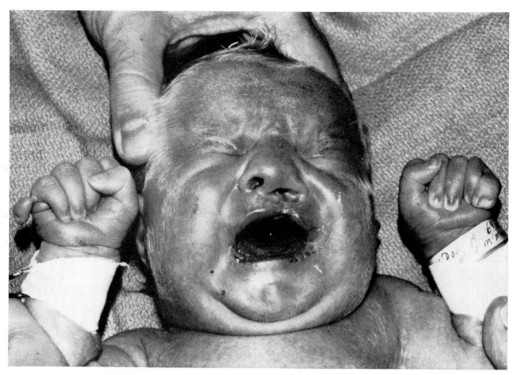

Figure 3-11. Note cleft lip and palate, polydactyly and microphthalmia typical of 13 trisomy.

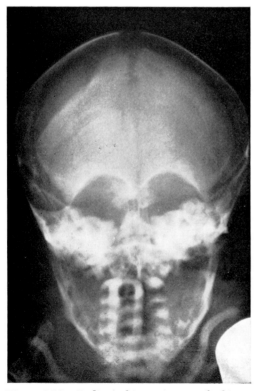

Figure 3-12. Radiographic appearance of arhinen-chephaly in 13 trisomy.

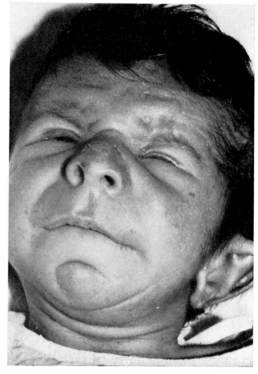

Figure 3-13. Midfacial appearance of infant with 13 trisomy but without cleft lip and palate.

the majority of pregnancies with embryos and fetuses having unbalanced translocations terminate in spontaneous abortion or that there is some form of prezygotic selection. It has been suggested that the risk to a balanced D/D translocation carrier of having a liveborn offspring with an unbalanced translocation is only of the order of 1%. Personal experience with a very limited series leads us to place the risk somewhat higher.

22 TRISOMY

Prior to banding techniques with quinacrine fluorescence and other methods, it was not possible to distinguish with confidence between chromosomes 21 and 22. Certainly the overwhelming majority of patients with G trisomy have classic stigmata of mongolism. However, there are a few reports of patients with G trisomy who do not have the features of Down syndrome. At the time of this writing, there were no reports discovered of banding techniques employed in patients with G trisomy who did not have the features of 21 trisomy

and who did have the features of 22 trisomy. Despite this, there are enough similarities between cases published as presumed 22 trisomy to lead one to conclude that there is a distinct syndrome.[14] (See Table 3-5 and Fig. 3-14.) Further, there is some evi-

TABLE 3-5. Features of 22 Trisomy

Area	Findings
General	Preponderance of females; failure to thrive
Neurologic	Mental and growth retardation
Head	Microcephaly
Ears	Low-set, angled, malformed; preauricular tags
Nose	Anteverted nares
Mouth and chin	Cleft palate, micrognathia
Neck	Redundant skin folds
Heart	Anomalies in 50%
Extremities	Abnormal thumbs (fingerized or broad), cubitus valgus, dislocation of the hip
Dermatoglyphics	Excess of whorls, distal axial triradius
Incidence	Unknown

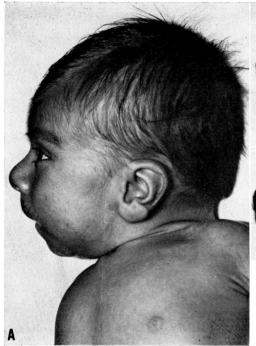

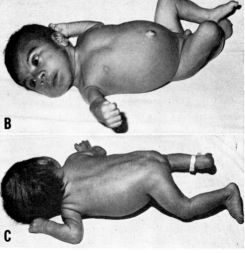

Figure 3-14. Three views of patient with additional small acrocentric chromosome—presumed to be 22 trisomy. Note redundant skin folds of neck, low-set ears and micrognathia.

dence (which is not reviewed here) that this small acrocentric chromosome is not a fragment of another chromosome, such as a D chromosome. Obviously a study of presumed 22 trisomy patients by banding techniques would resolve doubts about the identity of this extra chromosome.

There appears to be a distinct similarity of facial features in patients with presumed 22 trisomy: anteverted nares, frequent epicanthic folds, low-set angled and malformed ears, preauricular tags, micrognathia, microcephaly and occasional cleft palate. Redundant skin folds of the neck, abnormal malopposed thumbs and congenital dislocation of the hip are prominent features. Cardiac anomalies have been detected in over half of the patients reported. In a number of patients whose dermatoglyphics were studied, there was an excess of whorls.

These patients, who have been female in the majority of cases, have growth and mental retardation and significant failure to thrive. Sufficient long-term follow-up data are not available to discuss the natural history of the disease. It is known that some patients do not survive infancy.

OTHER STRUCTURAL AND NUMERICAL ABERRATIONS OF AUTOSOMES

Group B

Cri-Du-Chat (5p—) Syndrome. This clinical condition was first attributed to a chromosomal aberration in 1963 by Lejeune and co-workers.[17] On morphologic grounds the chromosomal anomaly was interpreted as being a deletion of the short arm of chromosome 5. Autoradiographic evidence has since added support that the deletion involving the earlier-replicating B group chromosome (5) was associated with the clinical features of this syndrome.[31] The fluorescence patterns are very different and provide the clearest distinction between the B group chromosomes.[6] The incidence of this lesion in the general population has been estimated as being about 1:50,000.

The striking clinical manifestation of this syndrome, which apparently affects girls more commonly than boys, is the cry—a mewing, plaintive cry that sounds like that of a kitten in distress. The physical features are not as diagnostic in this disorder as in the major autosomal trisomies (Fig. 3-14).

TABLE 3-6. Features of Cri-du-chat (5p—) Syndrome

Area	Findings
General	Female preponderance (M,1:F, 2); mewing cry in infancy and early childhood; variable lengths of survival
Neurologic	Mental, motor and growth retardation
Head	Microcephaly, moon-faced, paradoxic alert expression
Eyes	Epicanthus, antimongoloid slant, hypertelorism
Mouth and chin	Retrognathia
Heart	Congenital cardiovascular anomalies in 50%, most often ventricular septal defect or patent ductus arteriosus
Dermatoglyphics	Distal axial triradius (t′), increased whorls, high ridge count
Incidence	1 in 50,000

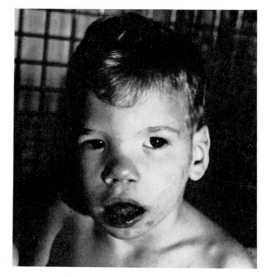

Figure 3-15. Patient with the cri-du-chat syndrome. The eyes are widely spaced with an inner canthic fold, but there is nothing pathognomonic about the facial features of this syndrome.

However, the appearance of the face is often round; the expression may be paradoxically alert; and the head is small. The eyes are widely spaced and chin is frequently receding. A congenital heart defect is present in about half of the patients, ventricular septal defect and patent ductus arteriosus being the most common lesions. These patients are, of course, severely retarded. The dermatoglyphic analysis usually discloses a distal axial triradius (t′, 80%) and a preponderance of digital whorls, which are responsible for a high ridge count (see Table 3-6). Parents should be reas-

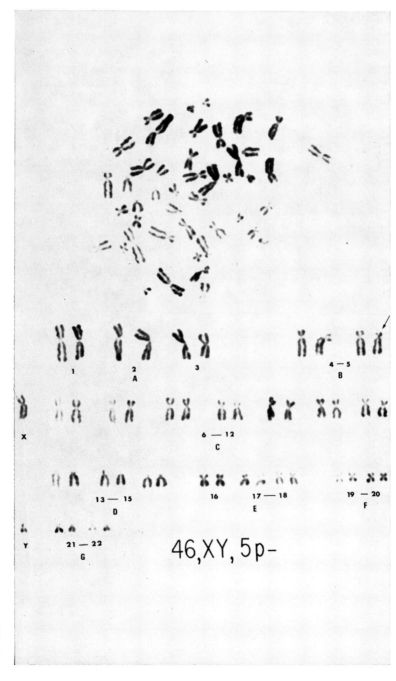

Figure 3-16. Conventional karyotype of patient with the cri-du-chat syndrome.

sured that this is a rare sporadic event that is not likely to recur. However, familial translocation[8] and ring chromosome cases have been recognized.

4p— Syndrome (Wolf Syndrome). A number of patients have been observed who have a deletion of a B group chromosome but who do not have the features of the cri-du-chat syndrome. This deletion appears to be in the short arm of the later-replicating B chromosome, and thus has been called a 4p— anomaly.[13,33] This designation has been occasionally assigned to the cri-du-chat syndrome in the literature, but this probably represents a difficulty in distinguishing between the two group B chromosomes by morphologic criteria. If the 5p— syndrome is seen in one patient in 50,000, then this syndrome, which has been said to account for no more than one-sixth of the B group short arm deletions, is very uncommon.

Males and females appear to be affected equally in this condition, which is characterized by severe mental retardation and a midline facial defect consisting of marked hypertelorism, a broad nose, root and bridge and a prominent glabella. Colobomata, ptosis, low-set ears with preauricular dimples or tags, carp-mouth, cleft lip and/or palate, and midline scalp defects complete the abnormalities of the head and face. There are also anomalies involving nails and ossification of carpal bones. A cat-cry is probably not present in patients with this constellation of anomalies. The dermatoglyphics of a patient with the 4p— syndrome do not show any unusual features other than dysplastic dermal ridges (in contrast with the high ridge count and frequent whorls in the 5p— syndrome). This chromosomal anomaly has not been reported to recur in families (Table 3-7 and Fig. 3-17).

TABLE 3-7. Features of 4p— Syndrome (Wolf Syndrome)

Area	Findings
General	Equal sex distribution, variable length of survival
Neurologic	Mental, motor and growth retardation; seizures, hypotonic
Head	Microcephaly, prominent glabella, broad nasal root, moon-face, midline scalp defects
Eyes	Colobomata, stasis, nystagmus, strabismus, epicanthus
Ears	Large, floppy, low-set; pre-auricular tags
Nose	Misshapen
Mouth and chin	High-arched palate, micrognathia, occasional cleft lip and/or palate
Heart	Congenital anomalies in 33%
Extremities	Clubbed feet, deformities of fingers and nails
Dermatoglyphics	Distal axial triradius, low ridge count, frequent arches, hypoplastic dermal ridges
Incidence	Undertermined

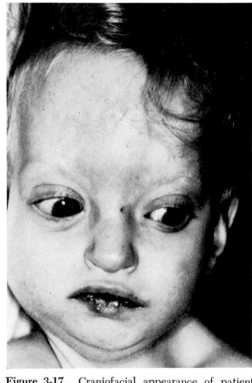

Figure 3-17. Craniofacial appearance of patient with 4p— syndrome. Note prominent glabella and widely spaced eyes with inner canthic folds.

Trisomy C Mosaicism (and Partial C Trisomy)

Since the first report in 1962 of a retarded male patient with multiple congenital anomalies,[21] subsequent reports have attempted to specify diagnostic phenotypic features of patients with trisomy C mosaicism.[28] This mosaicism consists of a normal cell line and a cell line having an extra group C chromosome. The Chicago-Paris classification for such a male patient would be 46,XY/47,XY,+C. The frequency of this chromosomal aberration has not been determined. Although it is rare it has been reported from several clinics.

A consistent pattern of anomalies has not emerged to the satisfaction of some observers. Two very good reasons for this apparent lack of pattern may be suggested. First, different group C chromosomes may be involved in the different patients reported; second, the predominance of one cell line over another may be expected to

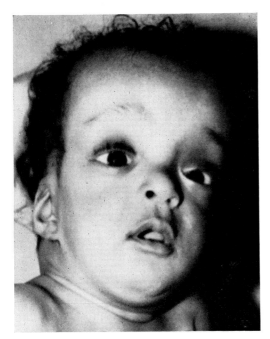

Figure 3-18. Patient with facial features shared by some patients reported as having C-trisomy mosaicism. (From Sinha, A. K., Nora, J. J., and Pathak, S.: Isochromosomes arising from a human 'C'-autosome. Hum. Hered., 21: 231, 1971.)

alter phenotypic expression. However, certain features have been shared by patients with trisomy C mosaicism (and partial C trisomy) that may be suggestive of the aberration, if not diagnostic (Fig. 3-18). There is no apparent sex preponderance. The patients are retarded. Phenotypic features include a large head with frontal prominence associated with nonprogressive hydrocephalus. The eye abnormalities include widely spaced eyes, lower inner canthic fold with antimongoloid slant, proptosis, strabismus, elliptic and eccentric pupils and corneal opacities. The ears are low-set and malformed, and the tapering fingers have dysplastic nails and joint limitations. Congenital heart defects are frequently found. Recurrence risk predictions for future sibs of an affected individual should take into consideration parental karyotypes in the partial C trisomy. Offspring of a C trisomy mosaic are, theoretically, at risk for the transmission of complete C trisomy. These considerations have little clinical importance since the fertility and survival to reproductive age in this syndrome remains to be demonstrated. There is one reported instance of the familial occurrence of the phenotypic abnormalities of this syndrome, and that involved a Cq+ partial trisomy.

The problem of trying to decide whether a single syndrome is produced by mosaicism of one specific C group chromosome or whether several syndromes are produced by mosaicism of different C group chromosomes should be resolved by banding techniques. (Most recent evidence from banding techniques, as of March 1973, suggests that the C group chromosome involved in patients with trisomy C mosaicism and partial C trisomy is chromosome number 8.)

Group D

Deletions of the long arm of a D group chromosome, presumably number 13 (13q−),[2] have been repeatedly described. Short arm deletions (13p−) and ring chromosomes [r(D)] have also been reported. A recognizable pattern of anomalies cannot be confidently attributed to the 13p— aberrations, but similar diagnostic features may be suggested for the 13p— syndrome and some patients with r(D).

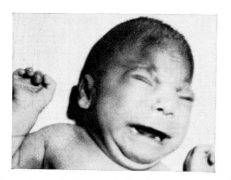

Figure 3-19. Trigonocephaly in patient with 13q— syndrome.

13q— Syndrome. A sufficient number of reports have been introduced into the literature to establish phenotypic similarities in patients having a loss of chromosomal material from the long arm of a group D chromosome, either as 13q— deletion or a ring chromosome 13. There are equal numbers of males and females and the length of survival is variable. Patients with the syndrome are severely retarded and have poor muscle tone. The head is small and a midline facial abnormality, trigonocephaly, is appreciated (Fig. 3-19). The root and bridge of the nose are broad. Hypertelorism and epicanthic folds are noted. Two eye anomalies observed in 13 trisomy are also found in the 13q— deletion: colobomata and microphthalmia. Retinoblastoma has occurred in a number of patients

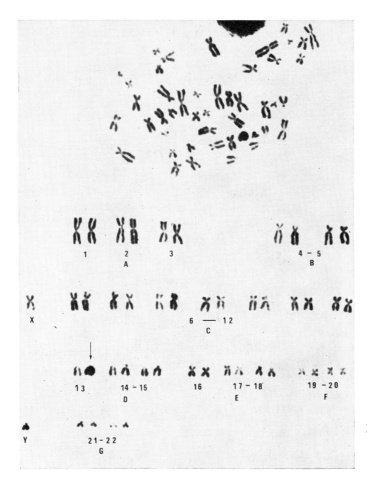

Figure 3-20. Karyotype showing ring chromosome in D group from patient with stigmata of 13q— syndrome.

with 13q— and r(13), but this chromosomal anomaly in patients having only retinoblastoma has not been detected. Other features (see Table 3-8) include large, low-set ears, frequent webbing of the neck, congenital heart lesions, imperforate anus and hypoplastic or absent thumbs.

The midline facial prominence, colobomata and some of the other anomalies seen in 13q— patients are also found in 4p— patients, just as the clenched fist and rocker-bottom feet are found in both 18 trisomy and 13 trisomy. Clinical experience and discrimination are required to distinguish these malformation syndromes. The dermatoglyphic patterns are useful, although not entirely reliable, in this syndrome. A distal axial triradius (t') and a high ridge count with a preponderance of whorls in 13q— contrasts with the low ridge count and frequent arches found in 4p— patients.

Group E

Structural abnormalities including deletions of the long arm (18q—),[9,32] short arm (18p—), and rings [r(18)] have been reported for group E chromosomes. The pattern of anomalies is more uniform in patients with deletions of the long arm than in those with deletions of the short arm, so only the 18q— syndrome is discussed in detail. Some 18p— patients have features that are difficult to distinguish from Turner stigmata, while others have varying patterns of abnormalities that are not consistent.

18q— Syndrome. Patients with a long-arm deletion of chromosome 18 are retarded and may survive periods ranging from months to many years. In infancy they are hypotonic and have a low-pitched voice. Soon it becomes apparent that the middle of the face is retracted and that the mouth is broad and down-turning (carpmouth). With further growth the jaw becomes jutting, which accentuates the re-

TABLE 3-8. Features of 13q— Syndrome

Area	Findings
General	No apparent sex preponderance (M,1:F,1); variable lengths of survival
Neurologic	Psychomotor retardation, hypotonic
Head	Microcephaly, facial asymmetry, midline facial prominence of glabella with broad nasal root and bridge (trigonocephaly)
Neck	Frequently webbed
Eyes	Hypertelorism, microphthalmus, epicanthus, ptosis, colobomata, retinoblastoma
Ears	Low-set, large, malformed
Mouth and chin	Micrognathia
Heart	Congenital heart defects in 50%
Hands	Hypoplastic or absent thumbs, short fifth fingers
Urogenital	Hypospadias, cryptorchism
Anus	Occasionally imperforate
Dermatoglyphics	Distal axial triradius (t'), high ridge count with preponderance of whorls, simian lines
Incidence	Undetermined

TABLE 3-9. Features of 18q— Syndrome

Area	Findings
General	Equal sex distribution; variable length of survival; low-pitched voice
Neurologic	Mental, motor and growth retardation; hypotonic
Head	Microcephaly, midface hypoplasia
Eyes	Hypertelorism, epicanthus, nystagmus, fundoscopic abnormalities
Ears	Prominence of helix, antihelix and/or antitragus; atretic canals with impaired hearing
Mouth and chin	Downward-turned "carpmouth"; jutting jaw
Heart	Congenital malformations in 40%
Extremities	Long tapering fusiform fingers; dimpled knuckles, elbows, knees, club feet
Urogenital	Cryptorchism
Dermatoglyphics	High ridge count, preponderance of whorls (> 5)
Incidence	Undetermined

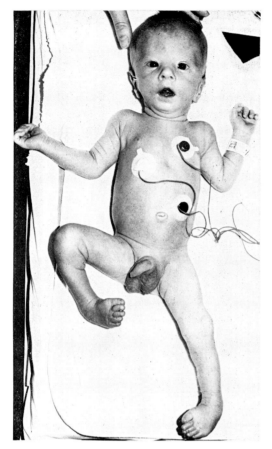

Figure 3-21. Infant with 18q— syndrome. Note midface hypoplasia, epicanthus, strabismus, carp-mouth and club feet.

traction of the middle of the face. The head is small and the eyes widely spaced. Epicanthic folds and nystagmus are common. The ears are frequently large and, in contrast, the ear canal may be small or sometimes not patent. Long tapering fingers and dimples of the knuckles, elbows and knees are occasionally found. The dermatoglyphic pattern most often reveals a high ridge count with a preponderance of whorls. A number of cases of 18q— have been reported with absent IgA. Patients with this syndrome usually represent sporadic events, although there is at least one report of occurrence of this syndrome in sibs (Table 3-9 and Fig. 3-21).

Group G

Several structural and numerical aberrations of group G chromosomes have been described other than the anomalies producing Down syndrome and its variants and 22 trisomy. Abnormalities reflecting loss of chromosomal material include long arm deletions (21q—), ring chromosomes [r(21)], and in at least three reports, a complete absence of a G group chromosome (45,—G).

It was stated in Chapter 2 that the human cannot easily survive the loss of an entire autosome. Small additions of chromosomal material and even smaller deletions of chromosomes are compatible with survival, although responsible for maldevelopment. (As will be discussed in Chapter 4, numerical and structural alterations of the X chromosome represent a different situation, because only one X chromosome is normally "completely active" in an individual no matter how many X chromosomes may be present.) Therefore, if one were to try to predict which autosome an individual could survive the loss of, the prediction would be an autosome with the least amount of genetic information (i.e., the smallest). And this has proved to be the case. Monosomy for a G group chromosome has been reported in three patients; mosaicism involving a normal cell line and a 21 monosomy cell line (46,XX/45,XX,—21) has also been reported.

On the assumption that the monosomy involved the chromosome which, in triplicate, produces Down syndrome, Lejeune proposed that monosomy leads to the "contre-type" of polysomy.[15] Although *some* features of a patient with a monosomy may be the opposite of a patient with a polysomy, there is no justification based on present knowledge of differentiation and development for the concept of contre-type or "antimongolism," except as clinical descriptions of physical findings. Thus, certain findings in complete[1] or partial monosomy[22] of chromosome 21 may be the opposite of findings in complete or partial trisomy. The patient with 21 monosomy (complete, partial or mosaic) is generally hypertonic rather than hypotonic, has an antimongoloid slant to the eyes, an elevated nasal bridge and an elongated skull. Micrognathia, hypospadias and pyloric stenosis are also found. The dermatoglyphic patterns have not been consistent; however, a proximal (normal) axial triradius has been repeatedly observed. These disorders are rare sporadic events.

One final association with partial deletion of a G group chromosome is leukemia with the Philadelphia chromosome. The leucocytes of a large percentage of patients who have chronic granulocytic leukemia have a deletion of the long arm of a G group chromosome (Gq−), the Philadelphia chromosome. When these patients are in remission the G chromosomes appear to be normal, but the deletion reappears when the patient is in relapse. Recently, it has been established by quinacrine fluorescence that the Philadelphia chromosome is number 22.[5]

REFERENCES

1. Al-Aish, M., et al.: Autosomal monosomy in man. Complete monosomy G (21-22) in a four-and-one-half-year-old mentally retarded girl. New Eng. J. Med., 277:777, 1967.
2. Allderdice, P. W., et al.: The 13q− deletion syndrome. Amer. J. Hum. Genet., 21:499, 1969.
3. Carter, C. O., and Evans, K. A.: Risk of parents who have had one child with Down's syndrome (mongolism) having another child similarly affected. Lancet, 2:785, 1961.
4. Carter, C. O., and MacCarthy, D.: Incidence of mongolism and its diagnosis in the newborn. Brit. J. Soc. Med., 5:83, 1951.
5. Caspersson, T., et al.: Identification of the Philadelphia chromosome as a number 22 by quinacrine mustard fluorescence analysis. Exp. Cell Res., 63:238, 1970.
6. Caspersson, T., Lindsten, J., and Zech, L.: Identification of the abnormal B group chromosome in the "cri du chat" syndrome by QM fluorescence. Exp. Cell Res., 61:475, 1970.
7. Cummins, H.: Dermatoglyphic stigmata in mongoloid imbeciles. Anat. Rec., 73:407, 1939.
8. DeCapoa, A., et al.: Translocation heterozygosis: A cause of five cases of the cri-du-chat syndrome and two cases with a duplication of chromosome number five in three families. Amer. J. Hum. Genet., 19:586, 1967.
9. De Grouchy, J., et al.: Deletion partielle du bras long du chromosome 18. Path. Biol., 12:579, 1964.
10. Down, J. L.: Observations on the ethnic classification of idiots. Lon. Hosp. Clin. Lec. Rep., 3:259, 1866.
11. Edwards, J. H., et al.: A new trisomic syndrome. Lancet, 1:787, 1960.
12. Ford, C. E., et al.: The chromosomes in a patient showing both mongolism and the Klinefelter syndrome. Lancet, 1:709, 1959.
13. Guthrie, R. D., et al.: The 4p− syndrome. Amer. J. Dis. Child., 122:421, 1971.
14. Hsu, L. Y. F., Shapiro, L. R., and Gertner, M.: Trisomy 22: A clinical entity. J. Pediat., 79:12, 1971.
15. Lejeune, J.: Types et contre-types. J. Genet. Hum., 15(Suppl.):20, 1966.
16. Lejeune, J., Gautier, M., and Turpin, R.: Étude des chromosomes somatique de neuf enfants mongoliens. C. R. Acad. Sci. (Paris), 248:1721, 1959.
17. Lejeune, J., et al.: Trois cas de deletion partielle du bras court d'un chromosome 5. C. R. Acad. Sci. (Paris), 257:3098, 1963.
18. Nadler, H. L.: Indications for amniocentesis in the early prenatal detection of genetic disorders. Birth Defects: Original Article Series 7, No. 5: 5, 1971.
19. Nora, J. J., and Sinha, A. K.: Unpublished data.
20. Patau, K., et al.: Multiple congenital anomalies caused by an extra autosome. Lancet, 1:790, 1960.
21. Pfeiffer, R. A., Schellong, G., and Kosenow, W.: Chromosome anomalies in the blood cells of a child with multiple anomalies. Klin. Wschr., 40:1058, 1962.
22. Reisman, L. E.: Anti-mongolism. Studies in an infant with a partial monosomy of the 21 chromosome. Lancet, 1:394, 1966.
23. Smith, D. W.: Autosomal abnormalities. Amer. J. Obstet. Gynec., 90:1055, 1964.
24. Smith, D. W., et al.: A new autosomal trisomy syndrome: multiple congenital anomalies caused by an extra chromosome. J. Pediat., 57:338, 1960.
25. ———: The D₁ trisomy syndrome. J. Pediat., 62:326, 1963.
26. Taylor, A. I.: Cell selection in vivo in normal/G trisomic mosaics. Nature, 219:1028, 1968.
27. Tjio, J. H., and Levan, A.: The chromosome number of man. Hereditas, 42:1, 1956.
28. Van Eys, J., Nance, W. E., and Engel, E.: C autosomal trisomy with mosaicism: A new syndrome? Pediatrics, 45:665, 1970.
29. Waardenburg, P. J.: Das menchliche Auge und seine Erbanlagen. The Hague, Nijoff, 1932.
30. Walker, N. F.: The use of dermal configurations in the diagnosis of mongolism. Pediat. Clin. N. Amer., 5:531, 1958.
31. Warburton, D., et al.: Distinction between

chromosome 4 and chromosome 5 by replication pattern and length of long and short arms. Amer. J. Hum. Genet., 19:399, 1967.

32. Wertelecki, W., and Gerald, P. S.: Clinical and chromosomal studies in the 18q— syndrome. J. Pediat., 78:44, 1971.

33. Wolf, U., *et al.*: Defizienz an den kurzen Armen eines Chromosoms Nr. 4. Humangenetik, 1:397, 1965.

34. Wright, S. W., *et al.*: The frequency of trisomy and translocation in Down's syndrome. J. Pediat., 70:420, 1967.

Chapter 4

SEX CHROMOSOMAL ANOMALIES

In 1959, the year the first autosomal anomaly was described, two sex chromosomal anomalies were reported. Jacobs and Strong[13] recorded a patient who had the clinical features of Klinefelter syndrome and had an XXY (47,XXY) sex chromosomal constitution, and Ford and co-workers[9] demonstrated monosomy for a C group chromosome in a patient having the stigmata of Turner syndrome and inferred that the missing chomosome was an X.

Two earlier events are important in the history of human sex chromosomes. The first is the investigations of Painter[21,22] regarding the presence of a Y chromosome in the human male. Strangely enough, it was not Painter's conclusion that the human chromosome complement was 48 that provoked a challenge, but rather the question of the role of the Y chromosome. Early investigators believed that it was the number of X chromosomes that determined the sex of the individual. The sex-determining function of the Y chromosome was established by the previously mentioned studies of Jacobs and Ford and their associates. The second historical event was the recognition of nuclear sex and development of the technique for the study of sex chromatin.

NUCLEAR SEX

Barr and Bertram[2] observed, in 1949, that there was a distinguishing difference in the interphase cells of males and females. The observation, first made in the nerve cells of cats, was that the female possessed a dense mass of chromatin in the nuclei of a significant percentage of cells that was not present in the male. An extension of this investigation, through several species of mammals to the human, provided a simple yet powerful clinical tool. In the human, a light scraping of cells from inside the mouth (buccal mucosa) is spread on a slide, fixed and stained to reveal the presence or absence of sex chromatin (Barr body), which distinguishes the female from the male—or, more precisely, determines whether an individual has more than one X chromosome.

Depending on the staining technique and other factors, a normal female possessing an XX chromosomal constitution will have a mass of densely staining chromatin pressed against the inner surface of the nuclear membrane in 20 to 60% of her buccal mucosal cells (Fig. 4-1). A normal XY male, having only one X chromosome, will not have sex chromatin, but 1 to 2% of his cells may contain darkly staining masses that could be mistaken for Barr bodies.

3

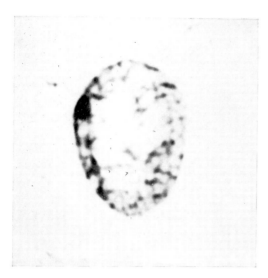

Figure 4-1. Barr body. Note that this densely staining mass lies against the nuclear membrane.

TABLE 4-1. Number of Barr and Fluorescent Y Bodies in Selected Conditions

Conditions	Barr Bodies	Fluorescent Y
Normal Male (XY)	0	1
Normal Female (XX)	1	0
Turner Syndrome (XO)	0	0
Ullrich-Noonan Syndrome (XX)	1	0
Ullrich-Noonan Syndrome (XY)	0	1
Klinefelter (XXY)	1	1
XYY	0	2
XXYY	1	2
XXX	2	0
XXXXY	3	1
XXXXX	4	0

Of less clinical importance is the finding of a "drumstick" in the nuclei of polymorphonuclear leucocytes. The drumstick is a projection from the nucleus that occurs in only about 5% of mature polymorphonuclear cells in the female, and does not occur in the male. It is often difficult to distinguish from other nuclear structures, and therefore has limited diagnostic value.

The buccal smear for Barr bodies is a useful screening procedure in patients in whom an X chromosomal anomaly is suspected. The rule is that the number of Barr bodies is one less than the number of X chromosomes; thus, a normal male has no Barr bodies, a normal female or an XXY male has one, an XXX female has two, and so on. There is no relationship of Barr bodies to the number of Y chromosomes. Table 4-1 lists the normal male and female chromosome constitutions and several common sex chromosomal anomalies together with the number of Barr bodies that one would expect to find in a proportion of buccal mucosal cells. Some cells of a chromatin-positive individual will have no Barr bodies and other cells may have fewer than the expected number of chromatin masses.

The phenotypic sex of the individual is determined (with few exceptions) by the presence or absence of a Y chromosome. Although a patient who has the XO Turner syndrome (45,X) has only one X chromosome, as does the normal male, she does not possess a Y chromosome, and is thus phenotypically female. A patient with Klinefelter syndrome (47,XXY) has two X's, like the normal female, but also has a Y chromosome, and is therefore a phenotypic male. The absence of Barr bodies (normal for male) in the buccal smear of the female patient with the XO Turner syndrome and the presence of Barr bodies (normal for female) in the male patient with Klinefelter syndrome merely reflects the number of X chromosomes possessed by the patient. It does not imply that the individual with XO Turner syndrome is not a female or the Klinefelter patient is not a male.

In addition to numerical aberrations of X chromosomes producing numerical aberrations of Barr bodies, structural anomalies of X chromosomes may produce structural differences in Barr bodies. An example of this is the patient who has an X isochromosome involving the long arm of an X chromosome, 46,X,i(Xq). The patient has 46 chromosomes, including a normal X chromosome and an abnormal X chromosome. The abnormal X chromosome is an isochromosome consisting of two long arms (q) of an X chromosome and no short arms (p). The abnormal X chromosome, the isochromosome, is consistently "inactivated." The patient has a loss of chromosomal material from the short arms of the X chromosomes and therefore has many phenotypic features of the XO Turner syndrome. (This concept will be developed later.) However, because the patient has two X chromosomes there will be a positive buccal smear; i.e., a Barr body will be present but it will be larger than normal, presumably because it consists of more chromosomal material (two long arms). Conversely, a patient with a deletion of part of an X chromosome may have a Barr body smaller than normal.

What precisely is the Barr body or sex chromatin mass? Ohno and Hauschka[20] observed in female cells at prophase a darkly staining (heteropyknotic) chromosome about the size of a Barr body which they assumed to be an X chromosome. In the normal male no such heteropyknotic chromosome is seen. Autoradiographic studies using tritiated thymidine, which is incorporated into the DNA of replicating chromosomes, demonstrate that one chromosome replicates later than all the others. This chromosome is located at the periphery of the nucleus where the Barr body is found. Individuals such as the normal XY male and the patient with the XO Turner syndrome do not have late-replicating X chromosomes and do not have Barr bodies. As will be discussed in the section on the single-active-X hypothesis, this late-replicating X chromosome is considered to be essentially inactive.

The work of Caspersson and colleagues[5] has shown that fluorescent alkylating agents such as quinacrine mustard bind most avidly to the Y chromosome in metaphase preparations. Pearson and co-workers[23] found that, in interphase cells obtained by buccal smear, a brightly fluorescing body may be found in normal males and two fluorescent bodies in patients with the XYY constitu-

tion. The number of fluorescent Y bodies has already become a standard technique for identifying the number of Y chromosomes possessed by an individual. This provides a useful adjunct to the Barr body analysis in determining nuclear sex from cells obtained at amniocentesis, from Wharton jelly[11] or from buccal smears. The two procedures should be used together to confirm each other and to provide information about the number of X chromosomes (Barr bodies minus one) and the number of Y chromosomes (number of fluorescent Y bodies). Findings in selected X and Y chromosomal constitutions are summarized in Table 4-1.

Two cautions should be advanced. First, in addition to the brightly fluorescing Y chromosome, chromosomes 3 and 13 are

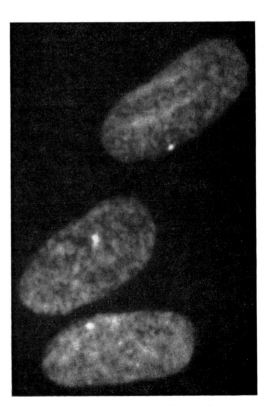

Figure 4-2. Fluorescent Y bodies in three interphase nuclei. Observe that the Y bodies are smaller than the Barr body in Figure 4-1 and that more often they are not against the nuclear membrane.

also bright when treated with quinacrine mustard. However, as a rule there is little difficulty in identifying the fluorescent Y body in cells treated with quinacrine hydrochloride (Fig. 4-2). Second, quinacrine hydrochloride fluorescence of white blood cells is disappointing in its reliability, at least in some hands. The percentage of cells with fluorescent Y bodies decreases from 80 to 90% in fibroblasts and Wharton jelly cells to 70% in buccal mucosal cells to less than 50% in white blood cells. In the white cells, the fluorescent Y is often difficult to distinguish.

SINGLE-ACTIVE-X HYPOTHESIS (LYON HYPOTHESIS)

In 1961, a concept was advanced by Mary Lyon and independently by several other workers. The hypothesis, as stated by Lyon[16] in 1962, is as follows:

1. The hyperpyknotic X chromosome is genetically inactivated.
2. It may be either paternal or maternal in origin in different cells in the same animal.
3. Inactivation occurs early in embryonic life (and persists in all descendants of the cell in which it occurs).

This hypothesis was based on genetic and cytologic observations in the mouse. In female mice heterozygous for sex-linked coat color genes, the coat appeared to be made up of patches of two different colors, each similar to the color of the respective homozygous parent. The same effect on coat pattern is found in the female tortoise shell cat, but not in the male cat or the male mouse carrying sex-linked mutant coat color genes.

The single-active-X hypothesis could explain how a female having two X chromosomes does not make twice as much product of X-linked genes as the female who has only one X: there is only one active X chromosome in any given cell. This could be a reasonable mechanism of "dosage compensation." Every female is, in effect, a mosaic for any X-linked gene for which she is heterozygous. Which X chromosome, paternal or maternal, becomes inactivated is apparently determined by about the sixteenth day of gestation, at which time the sex chromatin (Barr body) may be found.

Many studies support the single-active-X hypothesis. One interesting line of cytologic evidence was obtained from the mule (a cross between a horse and a donkey).[17] The horse X chromosome and donkey X chromosome are readily distinguishable on morphologic grounds. Examination of female mule karyotypes demonstrated that the late-replicating (inactive) X chromosome was of either horse or donkey origin in different cells. Among the human studies confirming the Lyon hypothesis are those derived from investigations of G6PD deficiency[3] and X/X chromosome translocation.[19]

If only one X chromosome is completely active, then why should patients with the XO Turner syndrome or XXY Klinefelter syndrome have any abnormalities? Why should increasing numbers of X chromosomes, as found in patients with XXX, XXXX, XXXY and XXXXY, be accompanied by progressively greater abnormality? The individual with XXY Klinefelter syndrome may graduate from high school or even go to college, but the patient with the XXXXY syndrome has an I.Q. in the 20 to 50 range and is not educable. Russell[26] has suggested, from studies on the mouse, that portions of the "inactivated" X chromosome may not be inactivated. The inactive X chromosome may contain loci that are required to be present in duplicate if normal development and function is to take place. Ferguson-Smith[7] has proposed that there are loci on the Y chromosome homologous with certain loci on the X chromosome, and thus the normal XX female and normal XY male have these loci in duplicate. The XO Turner syndrome would be deficient in these loci and the patient with XXY Klinefelter syndrome would have these loci in triplicate. Some such modification of the single-active-X hypothesis seems to be required to comply with the clinical observations.

SEX CHROMOSOMES

The X Chromosome. The X chromosome ranks between numbers 7 and 8 in total length and short arm length, making it one of the larger chromosomes. The banding pattern by fluorescence is distinctive, with a band in the short arm separated by a broad paracentric dark area from an intense band in the long arm. It would be expected that a large chromosome should contain a large number of genes, and this appears to be the case. Almost 100 genes have already been assigned to the X chromosome. To reiterate, the normal human female possesses two X chromosomes, one of which is "inactive" in each cell. The normal male has only one X chromosome and this chromosome is active in every cell. The X chromosome in the human assumes a passive role in the determination of sex. In the absence of a Y chromosome, the sex of an individual is female no matter what the number of X chromosomes may be.

The Y Chromosome. The Y chromosome, by contrast, is one of the smaller chromosomes, and is most similar to the G group chromosomes in length and morphology. However, it is readily distinguished from chromosomes 21 and 22 because it has the most intense fluorescence found in any chromosome (located at the distal long arm). The Y chromosome takes the active role in sex determination and its presence produces the male phenotype regardless of the number of X chromosomes an individual may possess. (Rare exceptions such as testicular feminization will be discussed later.) Other than determining "maleness" no significant role for the Y chromosome has been determined. A few decades ago several so-called Y-linked genes were described, but this number has been reduced to one inconsequential gene—the gene for hairy ears.

THE XO TURNER SYNDROME (TURNER SYNDROME, STATUS BONNEVIE-ULLRICH, GONADAL DYSGENESIS)

Most of the phenotypic features of what is now called the Turner syndrome were described in 1930 by Ullrich,[31] who reported a combination of anomalies in an eight-year-old girl which included webbing of the neck, cubitus valgus, congenital lymphangiectatic edema, prominent ears, ptosis, small mandible, dystrophy of the nails and hypoplastic nipples. In 1938, Turner[30] observed webbing of the neck and cubitus valgus together with sexual infantilism in young women. These three findings have become the cardinal signs of Turner syndrome. Ullrich did not describe sexual infantilism in his first or subsequent reports because his patients were children, whereas Turner's patients were young adults. An additional observation of Ullrich's,[32] not appreciated by Turner, was that the same stigmata (webbing of the neck, etc.) occurred in both girls and boys. When these multiple stigmata are found in the female, the designation that has eventually received the widest acceptance in the literature is Turner syndrome. In Chapter 7 some further distinction will be made in discussing the XX and XY Turner phenotype (Ullrich-Noonan syndrome).

In 1959, Ford and colleagues[9] performed a cytogenetic evaluation of a 14-year-old girl with clinical evidence of Turner syndrome, found that she had only 45 chromosomes, and suggested that the missing chromosome appeared to be an X. From this point on, patients with gonadal dysgenesis and Turner stigmata who have a 45,X chromosomal constitution have been said to have Turner syndrome (Fig. 4-3). To distinguish these patients from individuals who have similar stigmata and a normal 46,XX chromosome constitution, we elected to specify the chromosomal makeup of the individual as well as the phenotypic appearance. So, a female patient having Turner stigmata and a 45,X(O) chromo-

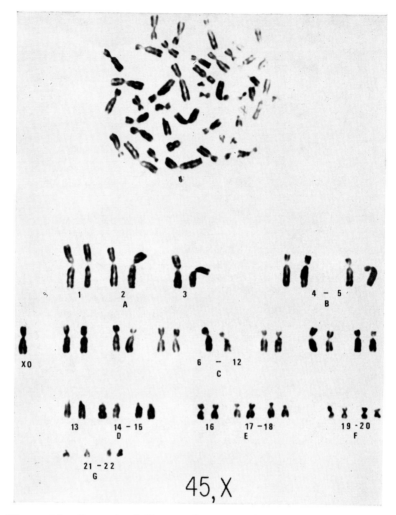

Figure 4-3. Conventional Giemsa 6 karyotype of patient with XO Turner syndrome.

some complement was said to have the XO Turner syndrome, and a patient with a 46,XX constitution and Turner stigmata was termed "XX Turner phenotype." This seemed to provide a clear distinction, but in an effort to reduce the number of alternative eponyms for a most common dominantly inherited syndrome, we have since abandoned the designations "XX and XY Turner phenotype" in favor of "Ullrich-Noonan syndrome."

The incidence of XO Turner syndrome in the newborn population is approximately one in 5,000 or about one in 2,500 females as estimated by chromatin-negative buccal smears.[29] However, the frequency with which the XO Turner syndrome is encountered in spontaneous abortions (as high as 7.5%) suggests that perhaps as few as one in 50 conceptions with the XO Turner syndrome is live-born.[25] A distinct maternal age factor has not been demonstrated in this syndrome.

Normal life expectancy is the rule, but this may be affected by associated lesions, such as coarctation of the aorta and renal disease. The most constant feature of the XO Turner syndrome is shortness of stature.

TABLE 4-2. Features of the XO Turner Syndrome*

Area	Findings
General	**Female**. Normal life expectancy may be altered by cardiovascular or renal disease. **Invariably small stature** for age with eventual height attainment rarely exceeding 60 inches; chromatin-negative
Neurologic	Intellectual development is generally good but is usually below the attainment of siblings; perceptive hearing loss is common
Skin	Frequent pigmented nevi
Head	Characteristic facies, narrow maxilla, small mandible
Eyes	Frequent epicanthic folds; occasional ptosis; infrequent hypertelorism
Ears	Usually prominent and low-set
Mouth	Shark-like—curved upper lip, straight lower lip.
Neck	Low posterior hairline; webbed in about 50% of patients
Chest	Shield shaped; widely-spaced hypoplastic nipples; underdevelopment of the breasts
Cardiovascular	Anomalies in approximately 35%; **coarctation of the aorta** is most common; pulmonic stenosis rarely if ever occurs; occasional idiopathic hypertension
Extremities	Cubitus valgus; lymphedema of dorsum of hands and feet in infancy; dystrophic nails; short fourth and fifth metacarpals; short fifth finger with clinodactyly; medial tibial exostosis
Urogenital	**Ovarian dysgenesis with infertility** (only two reported instances of fertility)
X-ray	Hypoplasia of lateral ends of clavicles and sacral wings; platyspondylia; metaphyseal dysplasia of long bones; "positive metacarpal sign" (short fourth and fifth metacarpals)
Dermatoglyphics	Distal axial triradius in 20 to 30%; higher than average ridge count
Incidence	1:5,000 (1:2,500 females)

*Many findings are similar to or identical with those observed in the Ullrich-Noonan syndrome. (See Table 7-2.) Features that help to distinguish between the syndromes are in **bold face**.

Eventual height attainment rarely exceeds 60 inches and appears to be related to "midparent" height. A patient with the XO Turner syndrome whose parents are tall is likely to reach 59 or 60 inches in height, whereas a patient whose parents are short may only grow to 53 or 54 inches. Intellectual development also appears to be related to midparent intelligence. In general, the patient with the XO Turner syndrome will be somewhat less gifted intellectually than her sibs, as well as significantly shorter. However, it is not unusual for these patients to finish college and to earn graduate degrees.

The appearance of the face is distinctive. A narrow maxilla, small chin, "shark" mouth, low-set malformed or prominent ears, epicanthic folds and ptosis comprise the typical facies. Only about 50% of patients have webbing of the neck, which is considered to be the characteristic anomaly of the syndrome (Fig. 4-4). Excessive looseness of the skin of the neck may be observed in infancy (Fig. 4-5), which may not necessarily produce obvious webbing in childhood. A low posterior hairline and pigmented nevi are frequently found.

A shield-shaped chest and widely-spaced hypoplastic nipples are common features. Approximately 35% of these patients have cardiovascular disease. Although many different cardiac lesions may be found, a diagnostically useful dichotomy in cardiovascular pathology exists between the XO Turner syndrome and Ullrich-Noonan syndrome.[19] In the XO Turner syndrome, coarctation of the aorta is the most common lesion, accounting for 70% of malformations. No patient with the XO Turner syndrome confirmed by chromosomal analysis has been reported to have cardiac catheterization data supporting a diagnosis of pulmonic stenosis. The opposite is essentially true of the Ullrich-Noonan syndrome, in which the characteristic cardiac lesion is pulmonary valve stenosis and for which there are only a few reports of patients with coarctation of the aorta. The differential diagnosis between the XO Turner syndrome and the Ullrich-Noonan syndrome may thus be made with a high degree of confidence if either coarctation of the aorta or pulmonic stenosis is present.

Cubitus valgus or increased carrying angle of the arms was emphasized by both Ullrich and Turner. However, the puffiness (lymphedema) of the hands and feet was recognized only by Ullrich (Fig. 4-6), because it diminishes and disappears during

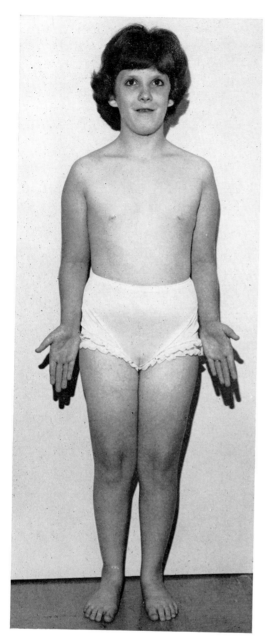

Figure 4-4. Fourteen-year-old girl with XO Turner syndrome. Note that she has the facies and somatic features of the disorder, but like 50% of patients with Turner syndrome she does not have webbing of the neck. Her height at this age was 55 inches.

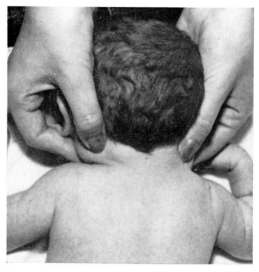

Figure 4-5. Prominent webbing of the neck and low posterior hairline in newborn with XO Turner syndrome.

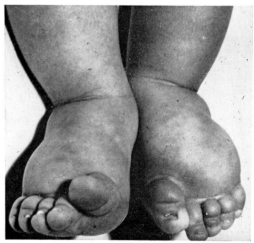

Figure 4-6. Pedal lymphedema and nail dysplasia of XO Turner syndrome.

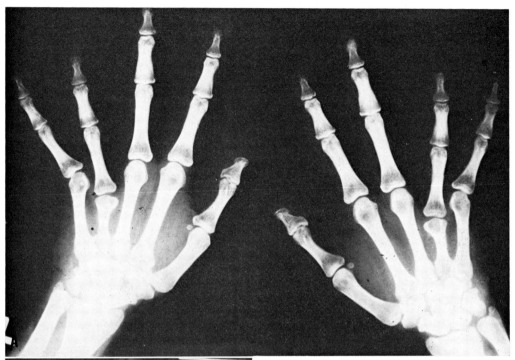

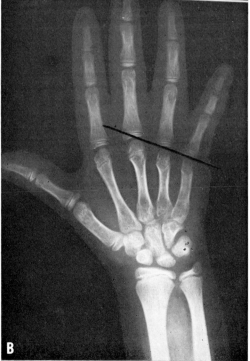

Figure 4-7. Unusually short fourth metacarpal and less strikingly short fourth and fifth metacarpals. Both types of skeletal anomalies are common in Turner syndrome.

infancy and childhood (and Ullrich's patients were infants and children). Ullrich's attempts to synthesize the finding of lymphedema in the human subject with similar observations by Bonnevie in the mouse led to the eponym "Bonnevie-Ullrich syndrome," which is still commonly applied to these patients. Short fourth and fifth metacarpals (Fig. 4-7), short fifth fingers with clinodactyly and medial tibial exostosis are other abnormalities of the extremities.

Wilkins and Fleischmann[33] found in 1944 that patients with Turner syndrome had, in place of normal ovaries, streaks of ovarian stroma without follicles. This they considered to be the important pathologic defect in Turner syndrome, at a time when the XO Turner syndrome could not be distinguished cytogenetically from the Ullrich-Noonan syndrome. Only two reports in the literature[1,18] provide evidence that a patient with the XO Turner syndrome had sufficient ovarian function to reproduce and give birth to a normal infant.

The dermatoglyphic patterns differ, on the average, between patients with the XO Turner syndrome and those with Ullrich-Noonan syndrome, but not sharply enough to be diagnostic in the individual case. For instance the ridge count is usually higher than average in XO Turner syndrome patients and lower than average in those with Ullrich syndrome. About 28% of patients with XO Turner syndrome have a ridge count of 200 or more as compared to about 6% of controls and one of 12 patients with Ullrich-Noonan syndrome. A quick estimate of the ridge count may be made by merely looking at the fingertips through a magnifier or with the unaided eye and seeing how many arches there are. The precise count will require a careful dermatoglyphic print.

The next step in the differential diagnosis is to obtain a buccal smear. The absence of Barr bodies (chromatin-negative) confirms the diagnosis of the XO Turner syndrome. If Barr bodies are present, the Ullrich-Noonan syndrome is the most likely diagnosis. However, patients with structural

anomalies of the X chromosome or mosaicism will also have Barr bodies. The final diagnosis awaits karyotypic analysis of a sufficient number of cells to define with confidence the chromosomal constitution of the patient.

X CHROMOSOME MOSAICS

A patient bearing Turner stigmata may have more than one cell line, one of which

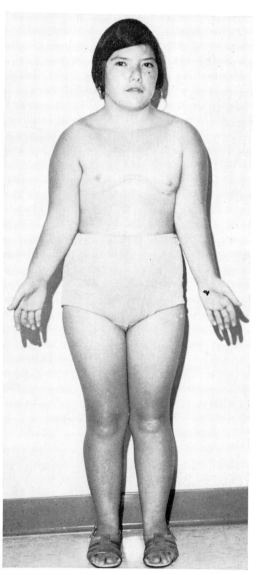

Figure 4-8.   Patient with XO/XX mosaicism and multiple stigmata of Turner syndrome.

is XO. A variety of mosaics have been reported including XO/XX; XO/XXX; XO/XX/XXX; and XO/X,i(Xq). These patients may have the same stigmata as the XO Turner syndrome although, in general, the expression of the phenotype is modified by the presence of cell lines other than XO. An XO/XX mosaic *may* thus have fewer and less striking Turner stigmata and a more normal female appearance (Fig. 4-8). Shortness of stature is still found in the vast majority of these patients, but is not invariable. The heart lesion has been pulmonic stenosis in the patients we have studied,[19] and coarctation of the aorta in the series of Emerit and colleagues.[6] XO/XY mosaicism is also found; these patients all have abnormal gonadal development and may have been reared as males or females depending on the degree of masculinization. There is a risk of gonadoblastoma in such patients.

STRUCTURAL ANOMALIES OF THE X CHROMOSOME

This group includes isochromosomes of the long arm [X,i(Xq)] and short arm deletions (XXp—); isochromosomes of the short arm [X,i(Xp)]; long arm deletions (XXq—); and ring chromosomes [X,r(X)].

Patients with an isochromosome of the long arm, 46,X,i(Xq), have the normal number of chromosomes, but have a structurally abnormal X chromosome and have sufficient Turner stigmata to suggest a diagnosis of the XO Turner syndrome or the Ullrich-Noonan syndrome. Barr bodies are found in the buccal smear, but to the experienced observer they are larger than usual. The karyotype reveals 46 chromosomes, one of which is an unusually large metacentric (mediocentric) chromosome that appears to be made up of two long arms of an X chromosome. This chromosome is always inactivated, so on buccal smear this larger amount of chromosomal material is appreciated as a larger Barr body

What is absent in this large "inactivated" isochromosome are the loci of the short arm. There is, in effect, monosomy for the short

arm of the X chromosome. Ferguson-Smith observed that patients with the isochromosome [46,X,i(Xq)] and the short arm deletion (46,XXp—) were most like the XO Turner syndrome in their overall clinical picture of multiple stigmata and shortness of stature. He hypothesized that Turner syndrome is due to monosomy of the short arm of the X chromosome, and further, that these loci in the short arm of the X chromosome are homologous with loci in the Y chromosome. This concept has been alluded to in earlier sections and will be developed further in the sections on the Ullrich-Noonan syndrome.

Isochromosomes of the short arm, 46,X,i(Xp), have rarely been encountered. Individuals with this anomaly apparently are not short and have few Turner stigmata. However they have primary amenorrhea. These patients are most like the more commonly found patients with long arm deletions (46,XXq—) in whom shortness of stature and multiple Turner stigmata are notably absent, but who have streak gonads and infertility. Ferguson-Smith proposes that infertility and gonadal dysgenesis are more a function of monosomy for the long arm, and shortness of stature and the multiple Turner stigmata are more related to monosomy of the short arm of the X chromosome.

Ring-X chromosomes have been found in mosaics, 45,X/46,X,r,(X), and in general their features are comparable to those of typical mosaics, 45X/46XX.

XXY KLINEFELTER SYNDROME

Klinefelter and co-workers[15] recognized, in 1942, a pattern of abnormalities that do not become evident until adolescence. These include small testes, absent spermatogenesis, high urinary excretion of gonadotrophins, and frequently eunuchoid habitus and gynecomastia (Fig. 4-9). Jacobs and Strong[13] observed an XXY chromosome complement (Fig. 4-10) in a patient with Klinefelter syndrome in 1959. The same year, Ford and coworkers[8] reported the

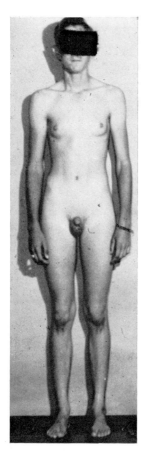

Figure 4-9. "Classic" phenotypic features of XXY Klinefelter syndrome (although gynecomastia is found in only 25% of patients with the XXY anomaly).

simultaneous chromosomal anomalies of Klinefelter and Down syndrome in the same patient.

Although this syndrome is apparently the most common of the X chromosomal anomalies (with a population incidence of perhaps 1:1,000), it is not diagnosed in infancy or childhood unless the patients are detected through a survey study of buccal smears or karyotypes. The buccal smear is chromatin-positive—a single Barr body is found. Children with Klinefelter syndrome do not look abnormal. It is not until adolescence and young adult life that the syndrome discloses itself, at which time gynecomastia or inadequate sexual development may prompt medical consultation.

The gynecomastia, although occurring in perhaps no more than 25% of XXY patients, may be particularly disturbing. Surgical ex-

TABLE 4-3. Features of XXY Klinefelter Syndrome

Area	Findings
General	Phenotypic males with chromatin-positive buccal smear; no detectable somatic abnormality in childhood; diagnosis usually made in adolescence or adult life; tall eunuchoid habitus is common
Neurologic	Intellectual development is fair to good but usually less than that of sibs
Chest	Frequent gynecomastia
Urogenital	Small testes in adolescence and adult (< 2 cm. in length); infertile
Dermatoglyphics	Average ridge count is low
Incidence	Approximately 1:1,000 (1:500 males)

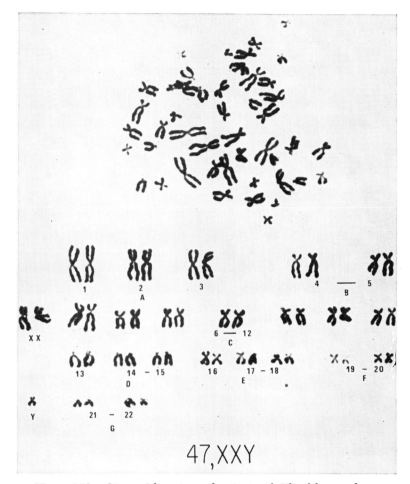

47,XXY

Figure 4-10. Giemsa 6 karyotype of patient with Klinefelter syndrome.

cision of excess breast tissue is required not infrequently. Body hair is often sparse and the patient may seldom have to shave. A long-legged, eunuchoid physical habitus is also common. However, none of these somatic features are invariable in a patient with an XXY sex chromosome constitution (see Table 4-3).

What is invariable is the small size of the testes, which usually do not exceed 2 cm. in length. Spermatogenesis is rare. Biopsy reveals hyalinized seminiferous tubules or small, immature tubules lined with Sertoli cells and Leydig-cell hyperplasia. Dermatoglyphic patterns reveal an excess of arches with a low ridge count. Thus, 15% have three or more arches, compared to 4% of

controls, but this is not a useful method of discrimination in the individual case. Intellectual attainment is generally below that of siblings. Some of these patients may go to college and some may be found in institutions for the retarded. Patients with Klinefelter syndrome have been ascertained in prison populations. The disturbing physical features of their disorder may contribute to sociopathic behavior.

As in most chromosomal anomalies, there are patients who have all of the stigmata of Klinefelter syndrome but who have apparently normal chromosomal constitutions. There are also patients with an XXXY chromosome complement who have the clinical features of Klinefelter syndrome ex-

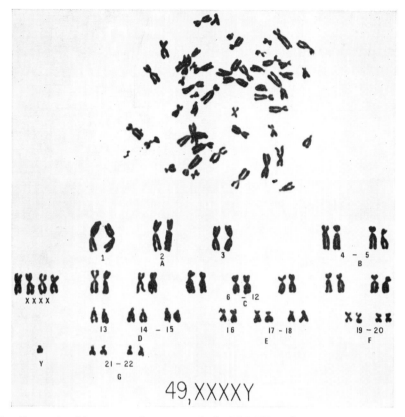

49,XXXXY

Figure 4-11. Conventional karyotype of patient with the XXXXY syndrome.

cept for a greater degree of retardation and a lesser degree of sexual development. XXXY patients are more severely affected and have some manifestations of the XXXXY syndrome, such as radioulnar synostosis, which illustrates the increasing disability that is found with increasing numbers of X chromosomes. These patients have a chromatin positive buccal smear that contains two Barr bodies. In the presence of three X chromosomes, all but one is "inactivated," yielding two Barr bodies.

THE XXXXY SYNDROME

This syndrome was first reported by Fraccaro and colleagues in 1960.[10] These male patients with the XXXXY chromosomal anomaly (Fig. 4-11), although on a continuum of increasing severity of disease with Klinefelter syndrome, present with a distinctive pattern. This relatively uncommon

disorder is diagnosed in infancy and childhood. The incidence has not been determined.

Retardation is significant and in the same I.Q. range (25 to 50) as patients who have 21 trisomy. These patients are also sometimes confused with patients having Down syndrome because of certain facial similarities: low nasal bridge, inner epicanthic folds, mongoloid slant and occasional Brushfield spots (Fig. 4-12 and Table 4-4). However, they can be clearly distinguished by the lack of dermatoglyphic features seen in Down syndrome. They often have strabismus, prominent chin and short neck with occasional webbing. Congenital heart lesions have been observed, including patent ductus arteriosus.

Limited pronation at the elbow is common and x-rays often reveal radioulnar synostosis. Knock-knees and incurved fifth fingers are frequently found. The genitalia are underdeveloped. Small penis, small testes, cryptorchism and occasionally a bifid scrotum may sometimes make the genitalia appear superficially ambiguous. Fertility has not been described. Dermatoglyphic evaluation reveals a low ridge count, on the

TABLE 4-4. Features of the XXXXY Syndrome

Area	Findings
General	Phenotypic males may have some genital ambiguity; small stature
Neurologic	Retarded: I.Q. between 25 and 50; moderate hypotonia and joint laxity
Head	Characteristic facies (often confused with mongoloid); low nasal bridge; protruding mandible; occasional flat occiput
Eyes	Epicanthic folds, mongoloid slant; occasional Brushfield spots; strabismus
Ears	Malformed; low-set
Neck	Short; occasionally webbed
Cardiovascular	Occasional congenital heart lesions (e.g., patent ductus arteriosus)
Extremities	Limited elbow pronation; genu valgum; clinodactyly of fifth finger
Urogenital	Small penis and testes; frequent cryptorchism
X-ray	Radioulnar synostosis
Dermatoglyphics	Average ridge count is low (< 60); frequent low arches; occasional simian line
Incidence	Undetermined; relatively uncommon

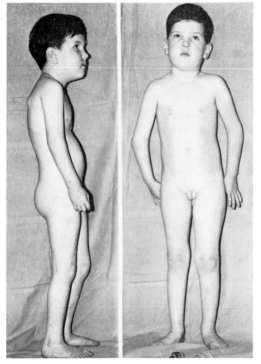

Figure 4-12. Five-year-old boy with the XXXXY syndrome. His I.Q. was 50. Note the arm deformity of severe radioulnar synostosis.

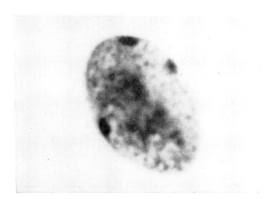

Figure 4-13. Three Barr bodies in patient with the XXXXY syndrome.

average, with an excess of low arches and an occasional simian line. The buccal smear is chromatin-positive and, because there are four X chromosomes, there are three Barr bodies (Fig. 4-13).

THE XYY SYNDROME

The first report of a male with the 47,XYY chromosomal constitution was published by Sandberg and co-workers in 1961,[27] but it was not until 1965, when Jacobs et al.[12] discovered that men in maximum security hospitals had the XYY complement (Fig. 4-14) in numbers that could not be attributed to chance, that attention was attracted to these patients. These XYY males appear to be taller and more aggressive than normal XY males, though it is not

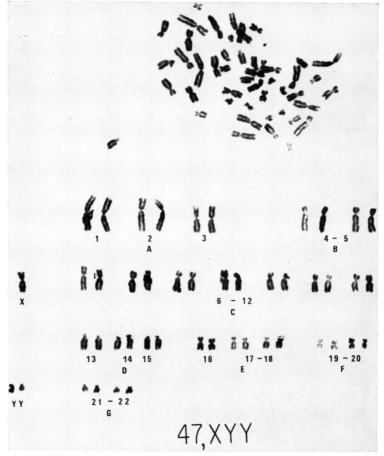

Figure 4-14. Conventional karyotype of XYY male.

clear how consistent this feature is. The aggressiveness and antisocial behavior of XYY males leading to imprisonment may be one of the more important discoveries in human behavioral genetics. Certainly this aspect of the syndrome has been popularized in the lay press and is even explored in the contemporary novel.

Recent population cytogenetics surveys place the incidence between 1:500 and 1:3,000. The only reliable ways to diagnose the syndrome in infancy are through a cytogenetic survey or by looking at Wharton jelly or buccal smear specimens for two fluorescent Y bodies (Fig. 4-15). Certain features (such as radioulnar synostosis and early and severe acne) have been recorded in XYY patients ascertained by these meth-

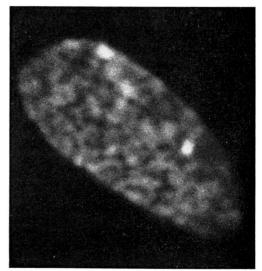

Figure 4-15. Two brightly fluorescing Y bodies from buccal smear of XYY male.

ods, but a precise diagnostic pattern is not yet evident. The diagnosis in childhood might be suspected in the large aggressive, prepubertal child in conflict with authority, as some reports have documented. However, there are also reports of XYY children who are normal in size, intelligence and behavior. Aggressiveness, violence and lawbreaking may increase with age, resulting eventually in imprisonment. Fertility may be impaired, and hypogonadism is not infrequent. As yet there are no reports of XYY offspring of XYY fathers.

A young man, 6'8" tall, referred himself to our clinic, having made a self-diagnosis after reading a report of the syndrome in *Time* magazine. He said that he was frankly worried that he might kill someone in a fit of uncontrolled rage. He frequently engaged in barroom brawls, some of which he claimed he did not instigate but, because of his great size, he was a natural target for "small drunks who wanted to feel big." This individual fulfilled the popular conception of the XYY male and we frankly lacked the courage to request a picture for publication.

The intellectual achievement appears to be fair to good. Although some XYY males have been discovered in institutions for the retarded, others have gone to college. EEG abnormalities have been reported, as have seizures, cardiovascular and skeletal disorders (Table 4-5). The adjustment to society is not invariably unfavorable. If the syndrome is as common as recent surveys suggest, there are probably a large number of undiagnosed XYY males who are neither in prisons nor in frequent barroom brawls. A particularly acceptable social adjustment that occurs to the authors would be as a pro-football linebacker, but it is also quite possible that the majority of individuals with XYY chromosomes are not sufficiently large or aggressive for this vocation.

OTHER ABERRATIONS OF SEX CHROMOSOMAL NUMBER

Many combinations of X and Y chromosomal numerical aberrations have been

TABLE 4-5. Features of the XYY Syndrome

Area	Findings
General	Many reported cases are taller and more aggressive and antisocial than average XY males and have been ascertained in prison populations with a frequency that exceeds expectation
Neurologic	Intellectual development is moderately impaired or normal; seizures and EEG abnormalities have been reported
Skin	Acne is common and found even in the infant and young child
Cardiovascular	Occasional congenital heart lesions; occasional prolongation of PR interval
Extremities	Arthropathies; radioulnar synostosis
Urogenital	Frequent hypogonadism; undescended testes, hypospadias and subfertility
X-ray	Radioulnar synostosis
Dermatoglyphics	Normal to slightly reduced ridge count
Incidence	Approximately 1:1,500 (1:750 males)

reported: XO; XXX; XXXX; XXXXX; XXY; XXXY; XXXXY; XYY; XXYY; XXXYY and so on. In each of these anomalies, the more X chromosomes the greater the degree of disability. A somewhat complementary proposal with regard to the Y chromosome might also be advanced. At least in terms of adjustment to our contemporary society, an extra Y chromosome may be accompanied by behavioral disability.

Two further syndromes deserve a brief acknowledgement. The first is the XXX syndrome, or **superfemale**. The term "superfemale" is derived from drosophila genetics. However, in the human species, the female with three X chromosomes is hardly "super." Retardation and infertility are common, but far from invariable. Many of these patients may appear to be perfectly normal intellectually, have no somatic malformations and may be fertile. Two Barr bodies are observed in the buccal mucosal cells.

No XXX daughter of an XXX mother has been reported. The incidence of this disorder is not known.

The patient with four X chromosomes is more retarded than the XXX individual and the patient with five X chromosomes, the **penta-X syndrome,** is severely retarded. Down syndrome was the initial diagnosis attached to patients with penta-X syndrome described in the literature,[4,14] because of the somewhat mongoloid appearance of the face (upward-slanting palpebral fissures). Both patients had patent ductus arteriosus and failure to thrive. One patient had epicanthic folds, hypertelorism, colobomata and simian lines. The presence of four Barr bodies rules against the slightly suggestive somatic features of Down syndrome in these patients; the diagnosis is further confirmed by a chromosomal analysis showing five X chromosomes.

INTERSEX

Hermaphrodites. A true hermaphrodite (Hermaphroditos, the son of Hermes and Aphrodite) is an individual who has both male and female gonadal tissue. The diagnosis is made when testicular and ovarian tissue are recovered either from separate organs or from a single ovotestis. The sex chromatin may be positive or negative and the chromosomal analysis may reveal mosaicism. The appearance of the external genitalia is variable.

Pseudohermaphrodites. These are individuals who have normal chromosomes and buccal smear for one sex, but have ambiguous sex characteristics that make them appear to be of the opposite sex.

Male Pseudohermaphrodites. A 46,XY male with a chromatin-negative buccal smear who is female in external appearance is a male pseudohermaphrodite. An example of this category is the **testicular feminization syndrome.** These patients usually have genitalia and secondary sex characteristics of the female and are an exception to the earlier statement that a Y chromosome produces the male phenotype. Medical attention is sought by these individuals because of infertility, amenorrhea, or sometimes inguinal hernia. The inguinal hernia may contain a testis or the testis may remain in the abdomen. (See discussion in Chapter 9.)

Female Pseudohermaphrodites. A 46, XX female with a chromatin-positive buccal smear who has an external appearance suggestive of a male is a female pseudohermaphrodite. Excess circulating sex hormone of maternal origin and the administration of progestational agents to pregnant women to prevent miscarriage may alter the appearance of the external genitalia of the female, producing clitoral hypertrophy and even fusion of the labia major.

The **adrenogenital syndrome** (virilizing adrenal hyperplasia) causes female pseudohermaphroditism. This disease and its different enzymatic forms is discussed in Chapter 8.

REFERENCES

1. Bahner, F., Schwarz, G., Heinz, H.A. and Walter, K.: Turner-syndrom mit voll ausgebildeten sekundaren Geschlechts-merkmalen und Fertilitat. Acta Endocr. (Kbh.), 35:397, 1960.
2. Barr, M. L., and Bertram, E. G.: A morphological distinction between neurones of the male and female, and the behavior of the nucleolar satellite during accelerated nucleoprotein synthesis. Nature, 163:676, 1949.
3. Beutler, E., Yeh, M., and Fairbanks, V. F.: The normal human female as a mosaic of X-chromosome activity: studies using the gene for G-6-PD deficiency as a marker. Proc. Nat. Acad. Sci., 48:9, 1962.
4. Brody, J., Fitzgerald, M. G., and Spiers, A. S.: A female child with five X chromosomes. J. Pediat., 70:105, 1967.
5. Caspersson, T., Zech, L., and Johansson, C.: Differential binding of alkylating fluorochromes in human chromosomes. Exp. Cell Res., 60: 315, 1970.
6. Emerit, I. J., de Grouchy, J., Vernant, P., and Crone, P.: Chromosomal abnormalities and congenital heart disease. Circulation, 36:886, 1967.
7. Ferguson-Smith, M. A.: Karyotype-phenotype correlations in gonadal dysgenesis and their bearing on the pathogenesis of malformations. J. Med. Genet., 2:142, 1965.
8. Ford, C. E., et al.: The chromosomes in a patient showing both mongolism and the Klinefelter syndrome. Lancet, 1:709, 1959.

9. ———: A sex-chromosome anomaly in a case of gonadal dysgenesis (Turner's syndrome). Lancet, 1:711, 1959.

10. Fraccaro, M., Kayser, K., and Lindsten, J.: A child with 49 chromosomes. Lancet, 2:899, 1960.

11. Greensher, A., Gersh, R., and Peakman, D.: Screening of newborn infants for abnormalities of the Y chromosome. J. Pediat., 79:305, 1971.

12. Jacobs, P. A., *et al.*: Aggressive behavior, mental subnormality and the XYY male. Nature, 208:1351, 1965.

13. Jacobs, P. A., and Strong, J. A.: A case of human intersexuality having a possible XXY sex-determining mechanism. Nature, 183:302, 1959.

14. Kesaree, N., and Wooley, P. V.: A phenotypic female with 49 chromosomes, presumably XXXXX. A case report. J. Pediat., 63: 1099, 1963.

15. Klinefelter, H. F., Reifenstein, E. C., and Albright, F.: Syndrome characterized by gynecomastia, aspermatogenesis without A-Leydigism and increased excretion of follicle stimulation hormone. J. Clin. Endocr., 2:615, 1942.

16. Lyon, M. F.: Sex chromatin and gene action in the mammalian X-chromosome. Amer. J. Hum. Genet., 14:135, 1962.

17. Mukherjee, B. B., and Sinha, A. K.: Single-active-X hypothesis: cytological evidence for random inactivation of X-chromosomes in a female mule complement. Proc. Nat. Acad. Sci., 51:252, 1964.

18. Nakashima, I., and Robinson, A.: Fertility in a 45,X female. Pediatrics, 47:770, 1971.

19. Nora, J. J., Torres, F. G., Sinha, A. K., and McNamara, D. G.: Characteristic cardiovascular anomalies of XO Turner syndrome, XX and XY Turner phenotype and XO/XX Turner mosaic. Amer. J. Cardiol., 25:639, 1970.

20. Ohno, S., and Hauschka, T. S.: Allocycly of the X-chromosome in tumors and normal tissues. Cancer Res., 20:541, 1960.

21. Painter, T. S.: The Y chromosome in mammals. Science, 53:503, 1921.

22. ———: Studies in mammalian spermatogenesis. J. Exp. Zool., 37:291, 1923.

23. Pearson, P. L., Bobrow, M., and Vosa, C. G.: Technique for identifying Y chromosomes in human interphase nuclei. Nature, 226:78, 1970.

24. Penrose, L. S.: Fingerprint pattern and the sex chromosomes. Lancet, 1:298, 1967.

25. Polani, P. E.: Chromosome anomalies and abortions. Develop. Med. Child. Neurol., 8: 67, 1966.

26. Russell, L. B.: Another look at the single-active-X hypothesis. Trans. N.Y. Acad. Sci., 26:726, 1964.

27. Sandberg, A. A., Koepf, G. F., Ishihara, T., and Hauschka T. A.: An XYY human male. Lancet, 2:488, 1961.

28. Sinha, A. K., and Nora, J. J.: Evidence for X/X chromosome translocation in humans. Ann. Hum. Genet., 33:117, 1969.

29. Smith, D. W.: Recognizable Patterns of Human Malformation. Philadelphia, W. B. Saunders, 1970.

30. Turner, H. H.: A syndrome of infantilism, congenital webbed neck and cubitus valgus. Endocrinology, 23:566, 1938.

31. Ullrich, O.: Uber typische Kombinationsbilder multipler Abartungen. Z. Kinderheilk., 49: 271, 1930.

32. ———: Turner's syndrome and status Bonnevie-Ullrich: A synthesis of animal phenogenetics and clinical observations on a typical complex of developmental anomalies. Amer. J. Hum. Genet., 1:179, 1949.

33. Wilkins, L., and Fleischmann, W.: Ovarian agenesis; pathology associated clinical symptoms and the bearing on theories of sex differentiation. J. Clin. Endocr., 4:357, 1944.

.

Chapter 5

GENETIC BASIS OF HEREDITY

Elementary, my dear Watson. Arthur Conan Doyle

THE STRUCTURE AND FUNCTION OF THE GENE

One of the most exciting discoveries in biology, and indeed, science of the last two decades has been the biochemical nature of the gene and how it works in precise biochemical terms. The details can be found in textbooks on molecular genetics[7]; only a summary of the current view of the gene's biochemical structure and functions will be presented here.

In bacteria, the genetic material is a strand of deoxyribonucleic acid or DNA. The brilliant work of Watson and Crick[7] showed that this material consists of a double-stranded helix, as in a rope ladder in which the ropes are made up of alternating deoxyribose and phosphate molecules and the rungs consist of pairs of nucleotide bases; the ropes are twisted into a double helix. The nucleotides are guanine (G), cytosine (C), adenine (A), and thymidine (T), and the physicochemical restrictions are such that G on one strand can pair only with C on the other, and A with T. Thus the base sequence on one strand bears a complementary relationship

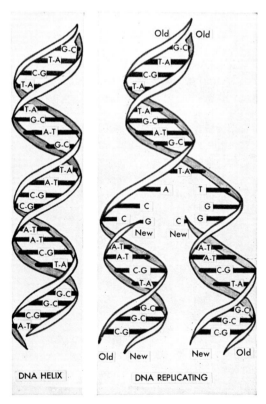

Figure 5-1. Diagram of the DNA double helix and DNA replicating.

73

to that on the other. When the DNA replicates the two strands separate, and each lays down a new complementary strand, so that two new double helices are formed, identical in base sequence with the original (Fig. 5-1).

In higher organisms the DNA is associated with proteins, particularly histones, to form the microscopically visible chromosomes depicted in Chapter 2. The ultrastructural organization of mammalian chromosomes is still not clear—though they look multistranded by the usual methods of inspection, they may contain a single strand of DNA, as in bacteria, but intensively folded.

It is now well established that genes act by controlling the amino acid sequences of polypeptides and, thereby, the structures and properties of proteins. For each polypeptide being synthesized there is a corresponding region of a chromosome in which the sequence of base pairs in the DNA determines the amino acid sequence of the polypeptide, and that particular area of the DNA is said to be the gene for the polypeptide. A mutant gene results in an altered amino acid sequence, which may alter the structure of the polypeptide and hence its properties, thus leading to a genetically determined defect in the corresponding protein, be it an enzyme as in the inborn errors of metabolism, or other protein as in the abnormal hemoglobins.

This concept was first suggested by the observation that in sickle cell anemia the mutant gene causing the disease resulted in an abnormal hemoglobin. Sickle-cell hemoglobin differs from normal hemoglobin only in that the sixth amino acid from the C-terminal end is a valine instead of a glutamic acid. Thus a single gene difference was associated with a single amino acid substitution in a particular polypeptide. Evidence from microbial genetics has confirmed that **a gene is that portion of the DNA responsible for the primary structure of a particular polypeptide.**

The means by which a gene determines the amino acid sequence of its polypeptide is briefly described in the following (see Fig. 5-2). The sequence of bases in the DNA constitutes a code for the amino acid sequence of the polypeptide, a triplet of three bases (or **codon**) corresponding to one amino acid. For instance, the triplet CTT at a particular place on the DNA codes for glutamic acid at the corresponding place on the polypeptide.

The translation of the DNA code into protein is done by means of a special type of ribonucleic acid, or RNA, called **messenger RNA or mRNA**. RNA differs from DNA in being single-stranded, with ribose instead of deoxyribose, and the nucleic acid uridine (U) instead of thymidine. The mRNA is synthesized on the DNA strand (by the action of the enzyme RNA synthetase) with the same kind of complementary pairing as the two DNA strands; for instance a CTT triplet in the DNA would correspond to a GAA triplet in the RNA. Thus the mRNA has a sequence of bases determined by that of the corresponding DNA strand. The mRNA migrates from the nucleus to the cytoplasm, and becomes associated with a ribosome (which contains another kind of RNA, the **ribosomal RNA**), where it acts as a mold or template on which the amino acids are assembled into polypeptides.

A third type of RNA, the **transfer RNA, or tRNA,** exists in the cytoplasm in 20 varieties, one for each amino acid. These serve to bring the amino acids to the messenger for incorporation into the polypeptide. To do this the transfer RNA must be able to recognize a specific amino acid, on the one hand, and a specific place on the mRNA, on the other. Thus each species of tRNA has one site—the recognition site—which combines specifically with a particular amino acid, and another site with a particular triplet—an "anticodon"—which can attach to the appropriate codon on the messenger.

As the messenger RNA strand moves along the ribosome, each codon in turn

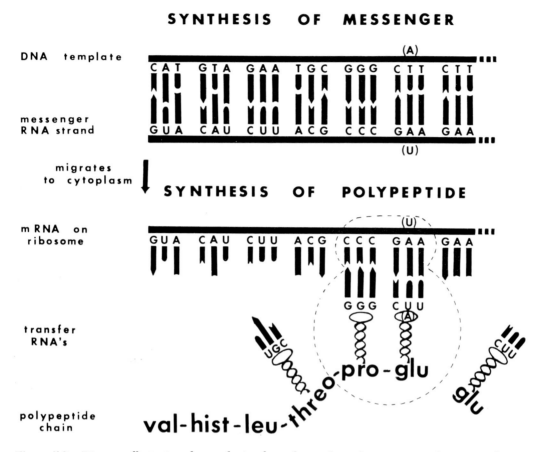

Figure 5-2. Diagram illustrating the synthesis of a polypeptide with a sequence of amino acids corresponding to a sequence of nucleotide triplets in the DNA.

is brought into a position where it can (with the aid of appropriate enzymes) combine with the anticodon on a molecule of the corresponding tRNA so that the amino acid is brought into position to be attached to the growing polypeptide chain. Thus if the codon is a GAA triplet on the messenger RNA, it will combine with a tRNA having the anticodon CUU, which brings a glutamic acid into position to be attached to the growing polypeptide chain. If the next codon triplet is a GUA, it will combine with a tRNA that has a CAU anticodon, and a valine will be brought into position and attached to the chain. In this way the amino acids are lined up on the template in an order specified by the sequence of triplets in the mRNA, which in

turn was specified by the sequence of triplets in the DNA. The mutation from the gene for normal hemoglobin beta chains to sickle beta chains presumably involved a change in the sixth triplet of the gene from CTT to CAT, so that the mRNA would carry GUA instead of GAA, and would therefore place valine in the sixth amino acid position instead of glutamic acid.

To recapitulate, the information coded in the DNA sequence of the gene is *transcribed* to the messenger RNA, which carries the information to the ribosome site where it is *translated* into a specified amino acid sequence in the corresponding polypeptide (Fig. 5-2).

The foregoing description is somewhat

oversimplified but conveys the basic concept. In fact, there may be more than one tRNA triplet specific for a particular amino acid; that is, the code is redundant. There are specific triplets that initiate transcription at the beginning of the gene, and presumably some that terminate it. Certain regions of the DNA transcribe ribosomal RNA and others the transfer RNA. In higher organisms there is more DNA than appears to be necessary for the known functions. The reason for the "redundant" DNA is not clear; perhaps it has something to do with the regulation of gene activity.

Regulation of Gene Activity. Since not all genes are active in all cells, there must be a way of suppressing the activity of certain genes and initiating that of others; the changes may be permanent, as in embryonic differentiation, or intermittent, as in the cyclic production of a specific protein by a certain cell type. The first understanding of how this may occur came from bacterial genetics, with the formulation of the "operon" concept by Jacob and Monod. The **operon** is a group of genes arranged in linear order that produces a series of enzymes all concerned with the same biosynthetic pathway. The first gene in the series contains the **operator,** which initiates the activity of the whole group. The operator can be activated or suppressed by another gene, the **regulator,** elsewhere on the genome. The product of the regulator gene can be modified by specific molecules in the cytoplasm, so that it will activate or suppress, as the case may be, its own operon. This provides a control mechanism whereby the group of genes responsible for a group of enzymes that metabolize a sugar, for instance, will produce the enzymes only when the sugar is present in the environment, thus making the cell more efficient. Further details are found in Chapter 12.

This is a matter of great importance, because some genetic diseases and defects may result from faulty gene regulation rather than the production of abnormal proteins, and this suggests an approach to treatment. A disease resulting from inactivity of a gene, rather than structural abnormality, could be cured by any treatment that led to reactivation of the gene. There may also be important implications of gene regulation in neoplastic change. Furthermore, the induction of enzymes by hormones, drugs and other agents may involve differential gene activation, and it is possible in tissue culture to stimulate the activity of specific genes (e.g., in orotic aciduria).

SINGLE MUTANT GENES

Dominant and Recessive Genes. We have said that a gene may be altered by mutation, which changes one of its nucleotide bases, resulting in a corresponding change in its mRNA and the polypeptide for which it codes. Thus a given gene locus can exist in one of several different states. Alternative forms of the same gene are called **alleles.** Each individual carries two sets of genes, one from the mother and one from the father. If the two members of a pair of genes are alike the individual is said to be **homozygous** for this locus; if they are different the individual is **heterozygous.** A heterozygous individual will make two kinds of mRNA for that gene, and therefore two kinds of the corresponding polypeptide.

Consider what happens in the case of a gene that codes for an enzymatic protein and a mutation that renders the protein enzymatically inactive. If an individual inherits the inactive allele from both parents, he will not make any active enzyme, the corresponding reaction will not occur, and thus the homozygous mutant individual will be abnormal. On the other hand, an individual who is heterozygous will make about half as much enzyme as one who is homozygous for the normal allele. Reducing the amount of enzyme by half is usually not enough to reduce the rate of the corresponding reaction, and so the heterozygote will function normally. In this case, the mutant allele is said to be **recessive** to the normal allele, since it does not produce any outward effect in the presence of the normal allele. Conversely, the normal allele is said to be **dominant** to the mutant allele. A recessively inherited disease, then, is one that is caused only by a homozygous mutant gene.

If the mutant gene can produce a disease or defect in the heterozygote, the corresponding disease or defect is said to show dominant inheritance. This may occur because the mutant gene results in the production of an abnormal protein, such as keratin, which results in an abnormal structure even in the presence of the normal protein produced by the normal allele. In such cases an individual homozygous for the mutant gene would probably be much more severely affected than the heterozygote, since there would be none of the normal protein. When the heterozygote is intermediate between the two homozygotes with respect to the trait in question, dominance is said to be **intermediate,** and if the heterozygote resembles the mutant homozygote, the mutant is said to show **complete** dominance.

Most deleterious dominant genes in man are so rare that homozygous mutants are never observed, since matings between heterozygotes almost never occur, so there is no opportunity to decide whether the given gene shows intermediate or complete dominance. In medical genetics, therefore, the term "dominant" is used for **any mutant gene that is outwardly expressed in the heterozygote,** regardless of whether dominance is intermediate or complete.

Finally the heterozygote may express the phenotype of both genes. For instance, a person of the AB blood group is heterozygous for an allele that produces antigen A and an allele that produces antigen B. When each gene is expressed, irrespective of the other, they are said to be **codominant.**

Models other than a mixture of normal and abnormal structural proteins will also account for the dominance of some mutant genes. For instance, a mutation may render an enzyme insensitive to feedback inhibition, or an operator gene that is normally suppressed by some cytoplasmic regulator may be rendered insensitive to the regulator. In either case there will be excessive activity of the corresponding enzyme(s). Acute intermittent porphyria and certain forms of gout may be examples of this kind of disorder. Another possibility would be that the mutant gene alters the specificity of the enzyme, allowing it to attack a different substrate or to assemble macromolecular material in the wrong way. Much remains to be discovered about the biochemical basis of dominance.

It must be made clear that the concept of dominance is an operational one and does not reflect any intrinsic property of the gene. Take, for example, the mutant gene for sickle cell hemoglobin. At the *clinical level,* the homozygote has a severe anemia but the heterozygous individual is not anemic under normal circumstances, so the mutant gene would be considered recessive. However, when the red blood cells from a heterozygote are put under reduced oxygen tension, they become sickle-shaped. Thus, at the *cellular level* the mutant gene can express itself when heterozygous, though not as strongly as when homozygous. This would be considered intermediate dominance. Finally, at the *molecular level,* the red cell from a heterozygote contains both normal and sickle hemoglobin, and the alleles are codominant. Whether a gene is dominant or recessive may, therefore, depend on the level at which one looks for its effect.

The fact that a mutant gene can be recessive and not produce any outward effect means that two outwardly similar persons may be genetically different. If we consider a gene a^D and mutant form, a^R, which is recessive, both homozygous $a^D a^D$ and heterozygous $a^D a^R$ individuals will be outwardly normal but genetically different. The outward appearance is referred to as the **phenotype** and the underlying genetic constitution as the **genotype**. Because of recessive genes and other irregularities to be mentioned later, one cannot always deduce the genotype from the phenotype.

MENDELIAN PEDIGREE PATTERNS

Autosomal Dominant Inheritance. As we have seen, a dominant gene is considered to be one that produces an effect in every individual who inherits it, irrespective of the state of the other allele. Thus the transmission of a dominantly inherited disease in a family is a direct reflection of the transmission of the gene. Each individual who inherits the gene will have the disease. Since (except in the case of fresh mutation) each affected individual inherits the gene from an affected parent, the first characteristic of autosomal dominant inheritance is that **every affected individual has an affected parent**; sporadic cases are presumed to have arisen by fresh mutation.

As deleterious mutant genes are rare, the affected individual will almost always inherit the mutant gene from one parent only, and a normal allele from the other parent— that is, he or she (let us assume it is he) will be heterozygous. He will probably marry an unaffected mate. His children will therefore inherit a normal allele from his spouse and either the normal or the mutant allele from him. This then, is the second rule of mendelian dominant inheritance: If the spouse is normal, **the affected individual's children will each have a 1:1 chance of inheriting the mutant gene and having the disease.**

Figure 5-3 is a pedigree of hereditary "cold urticaria" illustrating the autosomal dominant pedigree pattern. (See Appendix B for description of pedigree symbols.) Note that from any affected individual the disease can be traced to an affected parent, grandparent and so on as far back as information is reliable up to the point of first appearance in the family. The ratio of affected to unaffected offspring of affected individuals is 19:20, which is compatible with a 1:1 expectation for each individual. For instance, the proband inherited the mutant gene, which we will call a^D, from her mother and a normal allele, a^R, from her father. Figure 5-4 (left) shows the expectation for her children: each son and each daughter have a 1:1 chance of being affected.

If two heterozygotes mate, the offspring can draw either the normal or the mutant allele from each parent and will be either homozygous normal (one chance in four), heterozygous (two chances in four) or homozygous mutant (one chance in four), since the heterozygotes and homozygous

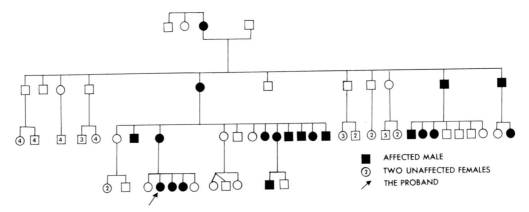

AFFECTED MALE
TWO UNAFFECTED FEMALES
THE PROBAND

Figure 5-3. A pedigree of hereditary "cold urticaria" illustrating autosomal dominant inheritance. There are approximately equal numbers of males and females (8:12) and among the offspring of affected individuals there are 18 affected to 20 unaffected (excluding the proband), which is close to the expected 1:1 ratio.

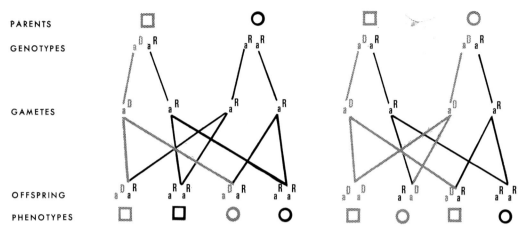

Figure 5-4. Segregation of an autosomal dominant gene in a mating of heterozygous and homozygous normal individuals (left) and between two heterozygotes (right). The shaded symbols represent the mutant genes and phenotypes.

mutants will both be affected (Fig. 5-4, right).

Finally, in the rare case in which an affected person was homozygous for the mutant gene and had a normal mate, all the offspring would inherit the mutant gene and be affected.

In summary, the pedigree pattern of autosomal dominant inheritance is characterized by the following features:

1. Each affected individual has an affected parent, to the point in the ancestry where the mutant gene arose by fresh mutation.

2. Each offspring of an affected person (with one affected and one unaffected parent) and a normal mate will have a 50:50 chance of being affected.

3. Unaffected relatives of affected persons will not have affected offspring.

Autosomal Recessive Inheritance. A recessive deleterious gene only produces its disease in the homozygote, so affected individuals must receive one mutant gene from each parent. Since deleterious genes are relatively rare in the population, almost all homozygous affected individuals arise from a mating of two heterozygous unaffected parents. Figure 5-5 (left) illustrates the types of offspring to be expected from a mating of two heterozygotes. The off-

spring may get the normal allele from both parents and be unaffected, or a normal allele from the father and a mutant allele from the mother and be unaffected but heterozygous, or a mutant allele from the father and a normal allele from the mother—also an unaffected heterozygote, or the mutant allele from both parents and be affected with the disease. Thus **each child of parents who are both heterozygous for a mutant gene has one chance in four of being homozygous and having the mutant phenotype.** Since the average family size in most populations is less than four, and the recurrent risk for siblings is one in four, most cases of recessively inherited disease will be sporadic. That is, the majority of cases will not have affected siblings even though the disease is inherited.

Occasionally an affected individual may marry a heterozygote, in which case the offspring will have an equal chance of being heterozygous unaffected or homozygous affected, thus simulating dominant inheritance (Fig. 5-5, right).

Since affected individuals usually arise from matings between heterozygotes, a recessive mutant gene may be transmitted through many generations without ever becoming homozygous. Thus it is characteristic of recessive inheritance that **the disease**

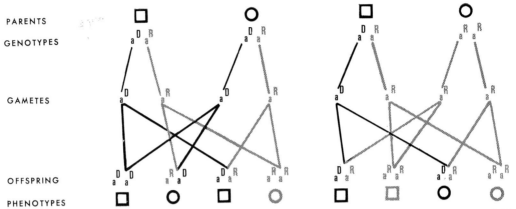

Figure 5-5. Segregation of autosomal recessive genes in a mating between two heterozygotes (left) and between a heterozygote and a homozygous affected individual (right). The shaded symbols represent the mutant genes and phenotypes.

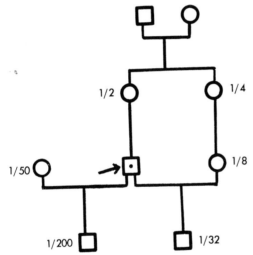

Figure 5-6. The significance of parental consanguinity. If the proband is heterozygous for a recessive gene carried by one in every 50 people, the chance that his first child by an unrelated spouse will be affected is 1/4 × 1/50 = 1/200. The chance of being heterozygous for the mutant gene is 1/2 for his mother (since he got the gene either from her or his father), 1/4 for her sister, and 1/8 for his first cousin, so the risk for the first child by his first cousin would be one in 32.

parents being heterozygous for a mutant allele are increased if they are related and have a common ancestry from which they may inherit the same recessive mutant gene. If such a gene was carried by, say, one of every 50 individuals in the population, the chance that a heterozygote would marry an unrelated heterozygote would be one in 50, but if a heterozygote married his first cousin, the chance that she would also carry the mutant gene would be one in eight, a considerably higher risk (Fig. 5-6). It follows that **children with a recessively inherited disease are more likely than average to have related parents.** The rarer the disease the more likely it is that the diseased individual will have consanguineous parents.

Figure 5-7 illustrates the effect of ancestral consanguinity on cystic fibrosis in a French-Canadian kindred. The gene must have been carried by one of the parents of the three sibs in generation I. Its descendants were transmitted to the four individuals in generation IV (IV-4 × IV-5 and IV-8 × IV9) who married their third cousins, and the disease appeared in the two first-cousin sibships in generation V.

In summary, the autosomal recessive pedigree pattern is characterized by the following features:

1. Almost always the disease is not pres-

usually does not appear in the ancestors or collateral relatives of affected individuals.

Exceptions may occur in families where there is inbreeding. The chances of two

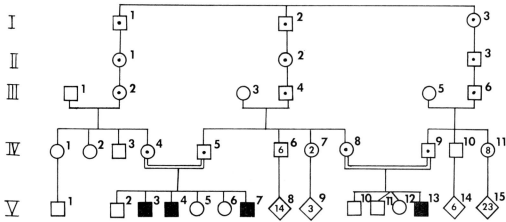

Figure 5-7. A pedigree of cystic fibrosis illustrating the effect of parental consanguinity in bringing recessive mutant genes together.

ent in the parents, ancestry or collateral relatives.

2. The sibs of an affected child have one chance in four of being affected, irrespective of sex.

3. The parents of affected children are more likely to be related to each other than are parents of normal children; the rarer the disease the greater the frequency of parental consanguinity.

4. In small families there will be more sporadic than familial cases.

Sex-linkage. *X-linked Recessive Inheritance.* Genes on the X chromosome can be dominant or recessive just as those on the autosomes, but the fact that females have two X chromosomes and males only one X and a Y leads to characteristic differences in the pedigree patterns of diseases caused by X-linked genes. In females the dominance relations of mutant and normal alleles are just as they are on the autosomes (with certain exceptions related to Lyonization, as discussed in Chapter 4). However, the Y chromosome, for the most part, is not homologous to the X—that is, most genes on the X chromosome do not have a corresponding locus on the Y. (Such genes on the X chromosome are said to be **hemizygous,** rather than hetero- or homozygous.) A mutant gene on the X chromo-

some will therefore always be expressed, even though it may behave as a recessive in the female. This accounts for the characteristic "criss-cross" pedigree pattern of diseases showing X-linked inheritance, the gene usually being transmitted by unaffected females and producing the disease in males.

The most characteristic mating is that of a female heterozygous for a recessive mutant gene on the X chromosome (X^R) and its normal allele (X^D) mated to a normal male (X^DY). She will give either X^D or X^R to each of her daughters, who will receive a normal X from the father and will each therefore have a 50:50 chance of being an outwardly normal carrier (X^DX^R) or a normal homozygote (X^DX^D). The sons will get a Y chromosome from the father, and will have a 50:50 chance of being X^DY (normal) or X^RY (affected) (Fig. 5-8, left).

An affected male mated to a normal female will transmit a Y chromosome to his sons, who will be unaffected, and the X chromosome carrying the mutant gene to all his daughters, who will be unaffected but carriers (Fig. 5-8, right). In the unlikely event that an affected male (X^RY) marries a carrier female (X^DX^R), the daughters will all inherit the mutant gene from their father, and will inherit from the mother either the normal allele and be car-

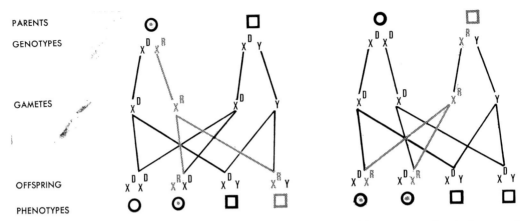

Figure 5-8. Segregation of an X-linked recessive gene in a mating of heterozygous female by normal male (left) and in a mating of affected male and normal female (right).

riers ($X^D X^R$), or the mutant allele and be affected ($X^R X^R$).

In summary, diseases showing X-linked recessive inheritance show the following pedigree characteristics, provided the gene concerned is rare:

1. The disease appears almost always in males, whose mothers are unaffected but heterozygous carriers of the mutant gene.
2. Each son of a carrier female has a 1:1 chance of being affected.
3. Affected males never transmit the gene to their sons, but transmit it to all their daughters, who will be carriers.
4. Unaffected males never transmit the gene.

Thus the gene is usually transmitted through unaffected female ancestors and appears in their male relatives. Therefore one may expect to see it in the patient's brothers, the mother's brothers, the sons of the mother's sisters, or the mother's father. Figure 5-9 is a representative pedigree. In many families, however, the disease may be sporadic—i.e., occur in only one person—either because the eligible male relatives are few and by chance have not inherited the gene, or because the patient has inherited a fresh mutation (see p. 90 for a more detailed discussion).

There are few X-linked dominant conditions. The pedigree characteristics are that these disorders are transmitted from an affected female to **half of her sons** and **half of her daughters,** and are transmitted by an affected male to **all of his daughters** and **none of his sons.** (See Chapter 9.)

Independent Segregation. Mendel was fortunate that the traits he chose to study were controlled by genes on different chromosomes and was therefore able to formulate the law of independent segregation. This states that genes (on different chromosomes) segregate independently of one another. Thus if there are two mendelian mutant genes segregating in a family, the risks for a given individual inheriting either or both diseases can be calculated from the law of independent probability. Suppose a couple has had a child with cystic fibrosis of the pancreas, so that each child has a one in four chance of inheriting this autosomal recessive disease. Suppose one parent also has neurofibromatosis, so that each child has a one in two chance of inheriting this autosomal dominant disease. Providing the mutant genes are on separate chromosomes we can say that the chance of the child inheriting both diseases is $\frac{1}{2} \times \frac{1}{4} = \frac{1}{8}$, the chance of inheriting neither disease is $\frac{1}{2} \times \frac{3}{4} = \frac{3}{8}$, the chance of inheriting only cystic fibrosis is $\frac{1}{2} \times \frac{1}{4} =$

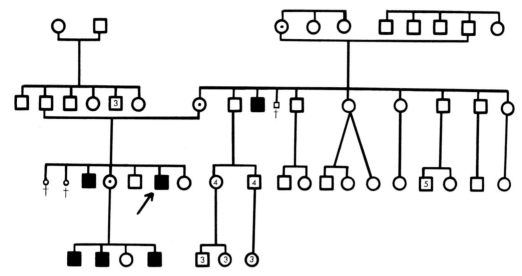

Figure 5-9. A pedigree of hemophilia illustrating the sex-linked recessive pattern of inheritance.

⅛, and the chance of inheriting only neurofibromatosis is ½ × ¾ = ⅜.

The phenomenon of linkage, by which two genes are located on the same chromosome, was discovered much later than the mendelian laws and has only recently become relevant to genetic counseling.

Linkage and Crossing-Over. If two genes occupy the same chromosome, one would expect them not to segregate independently, but to be transmitted together—that is, to be **linked.** Consider, for instance, a mother who carries on one of her X chromosomes the mutant recessive genes for colorblindness and for hemophilia, with the normal alleles for these genes on the other X. Her genotype would then be written $\frac{cb\ h}{Cb\ H}$. (When the two mutant genes are on the same chromosome they are said to be "in coupling," and when they are on homologous chromosomes they are "in repulsion.") This mother will give one X chromosome or the other to each son, who should be either colorblind and hemophiliac (cb h) or neither (Cb H). But there is one complication. At first meiotic metaphase the chromosomes may exchange strands; that is, there may be crossing-over. The farther

apart the two genes are the more often will there be crossing-over between them. We know that the genes for colorblindness and hemophilia are about 10 cross-over units apart; that is, there will have been an exchange between the two genes in 10% of the gametes formed. Thus our doubly heterozygous female will form four kinds of gametes: noncross-over gametes (45% *cb h;* 45% *Cb H*) and cross-over gametes (5% *cb H;* 5% *Cb h*). Thus we may measure how far two linked genes are from one another by counting how often they stay together and how often they cross-over during transmission from parent to child.

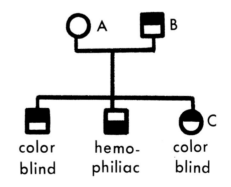

Figure 5-10. A pedigree illustrating linkage of color blindness and hemophilia.

Modern methods of searching for and calculating linkages are described elsewhere.[2]

Linkage may occasionally be useful in genetic counseling. Consider the pedigree shown in Figure 5-10. What is the probability that female C is a carrier of the gene for hemophilia? The father (B) is colorblind. The mother (A) is not colorblind but must be heterozygous for it, since she has a colorblind daughter (C). The mother has a colorblind son and a hemophiliac son, so in her the two mutant genes are in repulsion—her genotype must be $\dfrac{cb\,H}{Cb\,h}$. She will therefore produce four kinds of gametes 45% $cb\,H$; 5% $cb\,h$; 45% $Cb\,h$ and 5% $Cb\,H$.

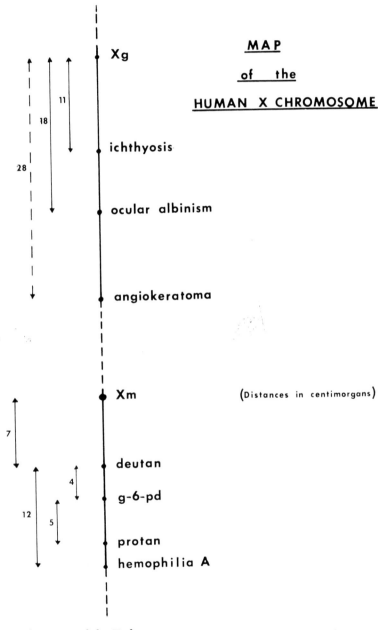

MAP

of the

HUMAN X CHROMOSOME

(Distances in centimorgans)

Figure 5-11. Linkage map of the X chromosome.

We know that the daughter, C, got either one or other of the first two, since she is colorblind and therefore got the *cb* gene from both parents. Thus the daughter has a 45/50 or 90% chance of inheriting the *cb H* chromosome from her mother and only a 5/50 or 10% chance of inheriting the *Cb h* chromosome and being a carrier. Figure 5-11 illustrates the linkage map of the X chromosome.

Irregularities in Mendelian Pedigree Patterns. Unfortunately not all mutant genes in man display the regularity of transmission and expression shown by the characters of the garden pea that Mendel chose to demonstrate his laws. Neither, as a matter of fact, did some of the other characters that Mendel studied in the pea.

Expressivity. It is well recognized that infection by the same strain of virus or bacteria can produce wide variations in severity of disease in different patients. The same is true of genes. **Variable expressivity** is the term used to refer to the variation in severity of effects produced by the same gene in different individuals For instance, the gene for multiple exostoses, which may cause large number of disfiguring osteochondromas in one person, may produce only a few small exostoses detectable only by x-ray in a near relative.

Penetrance. To carry the argument one step further, a gene that expresses itself clinically in one person may produce no detectable effect in another. This failure to reach the clinical surface is referred to as **reduced penetrance.** In statistical terms penetrance is the per cent frequency with which a dominant gene in the heterozygote or a recessive gene in the homozygote produces a detectable effect. In medical genetics, reduced penetrance is most easily detected in the case of dominant genes, where an individual who must, on genetic grounds, have carried the mutant gene does not show the mutant phenotype (Fig. 5-12).

When penetrance is close to 100%, the autosomal dominant pedigree pattern with occasional skips is easy to identify, but the lower the penetrance the more difficult it is to distinguish between dominant inheritance with reduced penetrance and more complicated modes of inheritance. The concept of reduced penetrance has sometimes

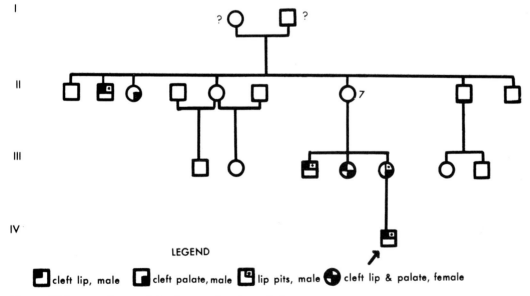

LEGEND

▮ cleft lip, male   ▐ cleft palate, male   ▐ lip pits, male   ⬤ cleft lip & palate, female

Figure 5-12. A pedigree of the dominantly inherited "lip-pit syndrome" illustrating reduced penetrance. The proband's maternal grandmother (II-7) must have carried the gene, since she has two affected sibs and three affected children, but shows no manifestation of it.

been used as an "excuse" for the fact that many familial diseases do not fit the expectation for regular mendelian behavior. Although this explanation has been misused, there is no doubt that reduced penetrance is a fact of life, which often poses problems for the counselor.

Failure of a gene to express itself phenotypically may occur for a variety of reasons. For instance, if the disease caused by the gene has a variable age of onset, a person who carried the gene might die before the disease became manifest, and would appear as a "skip" in the pedigree. In other cases the gene may involve some process with a developmental or biochemical threshold, and whether the mutant phenotype is produced depends on whether the mutant gene has an effect severe enough to prevent the individual from reaching the threshold. In this sense, variable expressivity and penetrance are closely related phenomena.

As with dominance, the degree of penetrance of a mutant gene may also depend on how hard the observer looks for signs of its presence. The sex-linked dominant gene for hypophosphatemic rickets, for instance, may produce full-blown rickets in some individuals but only a low blood phosphorus level in others. Almost nothing is known about what makes the difference. In some cases the effects of the mutant dominant gene in an unaffected carrier cannot be detected by any known means. Presumably the number of such cases will decrease as our biochemical skills increase, but will probably never disappear entirely.

CALCULATION OF RECURRENCE RISK

In estimating the genetic component of any disease, the first question likely to be asked is: "What is the frequency of the disease in the near relatives of patients?" Family histories are then collected, and the number of affected and unaffected relatives counted. However, analysis of the data must take into account certain biases inherent in the collection of such data in

man. To begin with, there are the problems of determining accurately which relatives are affected and which are not. We will not discuss these here. Secondly, the more striking the family history, the more likely it is to come to the attention of the investigator if care is not taken to avoid this bias. This is particularly true if one is using cases from the literature, but may also result from the efforts of well-meaning colleagues to refer "interesting" families. Furthermore, and quite apart from the tendency of striking families to be preferentially published or referred, if one is ascertaining families by identifying an affected individual, families with more than one affected member may be more likely to be ascertained than families with only one. We will return to the question of ascertainment bias shortly.

The basic question is this: in a group of individuals of a given relationship to an affected person, what proportion are affected? If the relation is anything other than sib the situation is reasonably straightforward. In a group of children ascertained through one affected parent, for instance, one simply counts the number of affected and unaffected children. If, on the other hand, one is interested in the *sibs* of affected persons, the situation is more complicated.

To begin with, if we are measuring the frequency of the condition in the sibs of the proband, we must *omit the proband* from the calculation since, by definition, the probability of the proband being affected is 100%. If one were measuring the risk of contracting tuberculosis in the sibs of tuberculous patients, for instance, one might ascertain 20 tuberculous patients, the probands, and find that they had a total of 60 sibs, none of whom are affected. The frequency of tuberculosis in the whole group is 20/80 = one in four, but this does not support mendelian inheritance—the recurrence risk in the sibs of the probands is 0/60, and the probands must be omitted since they were selected *because* they were affected. This seems almost too obvious to mention, but nevertheless the mistake does appear in the literature from time to time, leading to gross overestimates of recurrence risk for poliomyelitis, asthma and congenital heart disease, to cite three examples.

Ascertainment

Complete Ascertainment. Secondly, there is the question of ascertainment bias. In the case of **complete ascertainment**, every affected case in the given population is ascertained. If so, every case is a *proband*. (By definition the proband is an affected individual through whom the family is ascertained.) We wish to estimate the frequency of the disease in the sibs of probands, so for each family we omit one proband and count the family as many times as there are probands. Thus a sibship in which there were three affected and five normal children would be scored as two affected out of seven, three times, or six out of 21. This method also applies if each affected person has an equal probability of being ascertained.

Table 5-1 presents a hypothetic example in which there are five families of four siblings each. In the column headed "complete ascertainment" each family is counted as many times as there are affected individuals, omitting one affected each time. This estimates the probability of an affected sib as 8/24, or 33%. If ascertainment is in fact *not* complete, this method will overestimate the recurrence risk

Single Ascertainment. At the other extreme, **single ascertainment**, the probands are chosen in such a way that each family is ascertained only once. In this case, the more affected individuals there are in the family, the more likely it is to be ascertained, so families with more than one affected would be over-represented in the sample as compared to their frequency in the population. In single ascertainment this bias is exactly compensated for by the above procedure, that is, omitting the proband from the calculation and counting only the sibs (Table 5-1). This estimates the probability of an affected sib as 3/15 or 20%. If in fact ascertainment is not single, this method will underestimate the recurrence risk.

Incomplete Multiple Ascertainment. In practice, the situation is usually somewhere in between complete and single ascertainment. Some families with several affected sibs may be ascertained only once, the other affected sibs being identified only secondarily through the family history. Other families may be ascertained separately and independently by each affected

TABLE 5-1. *Methods of Counting the Proportion of Affected to Unaffected Sibs With Different Assumptions About the Mode of Ascertainment of Probands**

Family						Ascertainment					
						Complete Aff.	T	Single Aff.	T	Incomplete Aff.	T
1.	0	0	0	●		0	3	0	3	0	3
2.	0	●	●	0		2	6	1	3	1	3
3.	●	0	0	0		0	3	0	3	0	3
4.	●	●	●	0		6	9	2	3	4	6
5.	0	0	●	0		0	3	0	3	0	3
Ratio						8	24	3	15	5	18
% affected						33.3		20.0		27.8	

*The probands are indicated by arrows.

sib; in still others some affected sibs may be ascertained independently and others discovered only secondarily. In this case the same rule is followed: count the family once for each proband, omitting the proband each time. Table 5-1 demonstrates the procedure in the column headed "incomplete ascertainment," more properly called **incomplete multiple ascertainment.** The probability of a sib being affected is estimated by this method as 5/18 or 28%.

Sometimes, particularly with data from the literature, it is not clear which affected individuals are probands and which are secondary cases. In this case one can at least get a rough estimate by making the limiting assumptions. Calculate the frequency in sibs assuming single ascertainment, which will underestimate the real value if ascertainment is not single. Then calculate the value assuming complete ascertainment, which will over-estimate the real value if ascertainment is incomplete. The true value should lie somewhere in between.

A method that avoids the ascertainment bias is to calculate the recurrence risk only on children born after the proband, but this has the disadvantage of losing about half the data. Do *not* use children born after the first affected individual; unless ascertainment is complete this will grossly overestimate the real value (37.5% for the data in Table 5-1).

The *A Priori* Method. If the data are being tested for goodness of fit to a mendelian ratio, an *a priori* method can be used. For instance, in families of parents who are both heterozygous for an autosomal recessive gene, some will have several affected, some one affected, and some none affected, just on the basis of chance. If the families are ascertained by an affected child, the families in which there were no affected children will not be included in the data. (This is known as "truncate" selection—the normal families are "cut off.") From the binomial distribution, it is possible to calculate for any family size the expected number of families omitted because they contained no affected children, and the data can be tested to see whether, when due allowance is taken for these families, a satisfactory fit to a one in four ratio is obtained. Details can be found in many textbooks of human genetics.[2] However, the method is relatively insensitive and can be misleading unless a fairly large sample size is available. Furthermore, it cannot be used to calculate empiric recurrence risks in cases that do not fit the mendelian ratios.

Other Methods of Segregation Analysis. A number of more sophisticated methods of analyzing segregation ratios have been developed,[3] but are beyond the scope of this book. Again, they are most useful in cases where a large amount of data is available.

Mendelian Inheritance

Calculating recurrence risks is simple when the disease in question shows regular mendelian inheritance and the genotypes of the parents are known. Predictions are then made on the basis of the segregation ratios described on page 78 ff. For instance, if the disease shows autosomal dominant inheritance, the risk for any child of an affected (heterozygous) parent with a normal spouse is 1/2. For autosomal recessive diseases, the normal parents of an affected child must both be heterozygous, so the risk for each subsequent child is 1/4, and so on. It may be, however, that the genotypes of the parents are not known, but must be estimated from the family data at hand.

Dominant Inheritance. *Variable Age of onset.* Consider, for instance, a man whose father has Huntington's chorea. This disease shows autosomal dominant inheritance and has a highly variable age of onset. Our consultant is still unaffected at age 30. On the basis of the mendelian law, the probability that he inherited the gene from his father is 1/2, and the probability that he did not is 1/2. This is the *a priori* probability based only on his antecedents. But we have another source of information. He has reached the age of 30 without developing the disease. We can see intuitively that the longer he lives unaffected, the greater the probability that he did not inherit the gene. Thus his age, still unaffected, contributes additional information about the probability that he carries the gene. Previous studies have shown that about one-third of those who inherit the gene have developed signs of the disease by this age, so there is a 2/3 probability that, if he inherited the gene, he will still be unaffected at age 30. This is the *conditional* probability. What, then, is his overall (posterior) probability? There are three possible outcomes:

1. He did not inherit the gene—probability 1/2.
2. He did inherit the gene but is unaffected at age 30—probability $1/2 \times 2/3 = 1/3$.
3. He inherited the gene and is affected at age 30—probability $1/2 \times 1/3 = 1/6$.

We exclude the third outcome, since he is unaffected. So the chance that he is a carrier (1/3) compared to the chance that he is not is as 1/3 to 1/2, or 2/6 to 3/6, which is 2 to 3, or 2 out of 5 = 40%. That is, he has a 40% chance of being a carrier, rather than the 50% chance he had at birth. Risks for other ages are presented in Table 7-1.

Reduced Penetrance. A similar line of reasoning can be used in the case of a dominant gene with reduced penetrance. Suppose an affected father has an unaffected daughter who wants to know whether she may pass the gene on to her children. Assume that the gene shows 90% penetrance. There are the following possible outcomes:

1. The daughter did not inherit the gene —probability 1/2.
2. The daughter inherited the gene but does not show the phenotype—probability $1/2 \times 1/10$.
3. The daughter inherited the gene and shows the phenotype—probability $1/2 \times 9/10$.

We can exclude the third outcome; the probability of outcome 2 out of the total possible remaining outcomes is:

$$\frac{1/20}{1/20 + 1/2} = 1/11$$

Therefore the daughter has one chance in 11 of being a carrier, so the chance of her first child being affected is $1/11 \times 1/2 \times 9/10 = 9/220$, or about 4%.

Sex-linked Recessive Inheritance. *Female with Carrier Mother and Normal Sons.* This kind of reasoning is useful in cases in which a female relative of a male with a sex-linked recessive disease wants to know the chances that she is a carrier. Consider the situation in Fig. 5-13. Female A is certainly heterozygous for the gene since she transmitted it to two children.

The *a priori* probability of female B inheriting the gene is 1/2. But each normal son she has makes it less likely that she is a carrier, and she has three normal sons. The probability that she is a carrier and has three normal sons is $1/2 \times (1/2)^3 = 1/16$.

There are two possible outcomes:

1. She did not inherit the gene—probability 1/2.
2. She did inherit the gene and has three normal sons—probability 1/16.

The probability of outcome 2 is:

$$\frac{1/16}{1/16 + 1/2} = 1/9$$

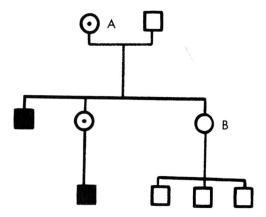

Figure 5-13. A hypothetic pedigree of a sex-linked recessive condition.

The Sporadic Case. An appreciable number of cases of X-linked recessive diseases have a negative family history. Consider, for instance, the family of a boy with Duchenne-type muscular dystrophy with no brothers, no maternal uncles and a negative family history. If he represents a fresh mutation, the risk for subsequent brothers is negligible, but if his mother is heterozygous his brothers have a 50:50 chance. What is the probability that his mother is heterozygous? We can calculate the proportion of mutant to nonmutant cases from the equation (Chapter 11):

$$m = \frac{(1-f)\,x}{3} \quad \text{or} \quad x = \frac{3m}{(1-f)}$$

when x is the frequency with which a male inherits an X chromosome bearing the mutant gene from his mother, m is the mutation rate, and f is the fitness of the gene. If there were no mutation, the probability that one of the X chromosomes carried by the mother bears the mutant gene (i.e., that she is heterozygous) would be $2x$ or $6m/(1-f)$, since she has two X chromosomes, either of which could be mutant. But each of the two X chromosomes has a probability m of acquiring the mutant gene *de novo*. If it did, the mother would not be heterozygous. So the probability that the mother is heterozygous is

$$\frac{6m}{1-f} - 2m$$

Therefore, in the case of a single affected male with no affected male maternal relatives, it may be either that:

1. The mother is heterozygous—probability $\dfrac{6m}{1-f} - 2m$

   a. and passed the mutant gene to her son—probability 1/2.

2. The mother is not heterozygous; the son received a fresh mutation—probability m.

So the posterior probability that the mother is heterozygous is

$$\frac{\frac{1}{2} \times \left(\frac{6m}{1-f} - 2m \right)}{\frac{1}{2} \times \left(\frac{6m}{1-f} - 2m \right) + m} = \frac{f+2}{3}$$

For a lethal gene, where $f = 0$, this works out to 2/3. That is, the chances are two to three that the mother is heterozygous for the gene, with a one in two risk for each subsequent male child. Thus the total risk for the brother of a sporadic case will be $2/3 \times 1/2 = 1/3$.

This risk will be modified downwards the more unaffected sons, brothers, mother's brothers, etc. there are, and upwards if the gene is not lethal and therefore more common, with proportionately fewer cases due to mutation. Since the algebra may get complex, the risks have been presented in table form (Table 5-2). For more complicated situations the reader is advised to consult a genetics counselor, who will probably refer to one of several recent expositions of the subject.[4,6]

TABLE 5-2. *Probability That the Mother of an Isolated Case of an X-linked Trait is Heterozygous (Assume $m = 1/10^5$)*

Disease Frequency	Number of Unaffected Sons					
	0	1	2	3	4	5
1/100,000	0.67	0:50	0.33	0.20	0.11	0.06
1/10,000	0.92	0.85	0.73	0.58	0.15	0.26
1/5,000	0.98	0.96	0.92	0.96	0.76	0.61
1/1,000	0.99	0.98	0.96	0.93	0.86	0.76

(Modified from Murphy, E.A., and Mutalik, G.S.: The application of Bayesian methods in genetic counselling. Hum. Hered., 19:126, 1969.)

Autosomal Recessive Inheritance. In the great majority of counseling cases in which the disease involved shows autosomal recessive inheritance, the parents have identified themselves as being heterozygous by the fact that they have had an affected child. The risk for each subsequent child is therefore one in four. Other questions may arise, however, that usually involve the question of whether near relatives of the affected person might have affected children.

Children of Near Relatives of Affected Person. For instance, the sib (B) of an affected person (A), married to an unrelated spouse (C), wants to know the risk that his children will get the disease. The risk depends on both B and C being heterozygous. The risk of B being heterozygous is 2/3. C's risk can be calculated from the Hardy-Weinberg law (Chapter 11). For cystic fibrosis of the pancreas, for instance, if the disease frequency is 1 in 2000, then

1. The frequency, q, of the *cf* gene will be 1/2000, or 1/45.
2. The frequency of the heterozygote, 2 pq, will be about 1/22.
3. The frequency that B and C will both be heterozygous is

$$\frac{2}{3} \times \frac{1}{22} = \frac{1}{33}$$

4. The probability of the first child being affected is

$$\frac{1}{4} \times \frac{1}{33} = \frac{1}{132}$$

As before, this probability would decrease with each unaffected child born to these parents, and an affected child would, of course, raise the risk to one in four.

Matings Between Affected Persons. In matings between two affected individuals who are homozygous for mutants at the same locus, all the offspring will be affected. However, the situation may be complicated by genetic heterogeneity. In a number of cases, e.g., congenital deafness

and albinism, the same phenotype can be caused by mutations at different loci. If a couple who are both congenitally deaf carry mutations at different loci, their children will be unaffected. Counseling in this situation depends on the relative frequencies of mutations at the various loci, which is usually not known for a given population. In Northern Ireland, Stevenson has shown that in two out of three matings between congenitally deaf partners (excluding those that have a known syndrome), none of the children are deaf; in one out of six matings, all the children are deaf; and in one out of six matings, some of the children are deaf and some are not. The data suggest that there must be several fairly common recessive genes leading to congenital deafness and that some of the sporadic cases (perhaps 1/2 are phenocopies.

Matings Between Consanguineous Partners. The question of marriage between cousins is one that the counselor meets from time to time, often because of the violent opposition that the prospect rouses in the family concerned. This may stem partly from the opposition of certain religions to consanguineous marriages, and partly from the popular opinion that such unions lead to deformity, insanity, idiocy, and degeneracy of all sorts. These opinions are based more on fancy than fact. The idea that cousin marriages are genetically disastrous may come from the observation that children with rare recessive diseases often have consanguineous parents, without taking into account the consanguineous parents who have children without such disease. What are the facts?

If there is a recessively inherited disease in the family, the risk of that disease occurring in the children of the cousin mating can be calculated from mendelian principles. For example, in Figure 5-14, if III-2's brother, III-3, had Tay-Sachs disease, II-2 would have a 2/3 change of being heterozygous, and the other probabilities can be calculated as shown. The chance of the first child being affected would be 1/72. If there

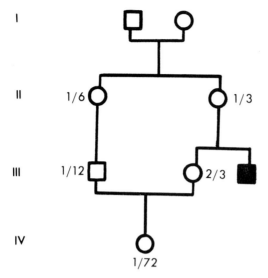

Figure 5-14. Hypothetic pedigree of an autosomal recessive condition.

than 1%.[5] This suggests that the number of genes causing recessively inherited diseases carried by the "average" person is somewhat less than one. There are also significant but small effects of inbreeding on infant mortality, I.Q., stature and other multifactorial traits,[5] but these are not large enough to be much of a deterrent to the individual couple.

For incestuous matings between first degree relatives, the theoretic risk would be considerably greater than for first-cousin matings, and the limited amount of data available suggests that this is so.[1]

In summary, the facts suggest that the genetic counseling for cousins contemplating marriage should be more optimistic than the advice they often get from their church, friends, families and, alas, some genetic counselors. Their risk of having a child with a recessively inherited disease is increased by perhaps 100-fold, but in absolute terms is still small, being of the order of 1%.

are no recessive diseases in the family, the estimate becomes much less precise. If one of the common grandparents in Figure 5-14 carried a recessive mutant gene, then II-1 and II-2 each have a one in two chance of inheriting it, III-1 and III-2 have a one in four chance, and the chance that they are both heterozygous for the gene is $1/4 \times 1/4 = 1/16$. The chance that their first child would be affected is $1/4 \times 1/16 = 1/64$. Since there are two common grandparents involved, the risk for the child is twice this, or 1/32 as is illustrated in Figure 5-8. But we do not know the probability that the grandparent carries a recessive mutant gene. The available data on offspring of consanguineous matings record a rather low frequency of diseases known to show mendelian recessive inheritance, probably less

REFERENCES

1. Adams, M. S., and Neel, J. V.: Children of incest. Pediatrics, 40:55, 1967.
2. Levitan, M., and Montague, A.: Textbook of Human Genetics. Chapter XI. London, Oxford University Press, 1971.
3. Morton, N. E.: Segregation and linkage. In Burdette, W. J. (ed.): Methodology in Human Genetics, San Francisco, Holden-Day, 1962.
4. Murphy, E. A., and Mutalik, G. S.: The application of Bayesian methods in genetic counselling. Hum. Hered., 19:126, 1969.
5. Schull, W. J., and Neel, J. V.: The Effects of Inbreeding in Japanese Children. New York, Harper and Row, 1965.
6. Stevenson, A. C., and Davison, B. C. C.: Genetic Counselling. London, Heinemann, 1970.
7. Watson, J. D.: The Molecular Biology of the Gene. 2nd ed. New York, Benjamin, 1970.

Chapter 6

BIOCHEMICAL GENETICS

It may well be that the course of metabolism along any particular path should be pictured as in continuous movement rather than as a series of distinct steps. If any one step in the process fails the intermediate product in being at the point of arrest will escape further change, just as when the film of a biograph is brought to a standstill the moving figures are left foot in air. Sir Archibald Garrod, 1908.

Genes control the structure of polypeptides and their corresponding proteins. A gene mutation in which a single nucleotide base is changed to another changes an amino acid in the corresponding protein. Depending on the nature of this amino acid substitution and where it is in the molecule, the function of the corresponding protein may be altered. Biochemical genetics deals with the biochemical changes resulting from substituting mutant for normal proteins and, by inference, with the functions of the normal proteins. Genetic defects in enzymes (which may cause "inborn errors" of metabolism or transport) and in other proteins will be considered separately.

THE INBORN ERRORS OF METABOLISM

Biochemical genetics began with the concept of **inborn errors of metabolism,** thanks to the insight of the English physician Sir Archibald Garrod. In 1909, through his studies of alkaptonuria, Garrod defined the characteristics of this group of diseases resulting from lack of a functional enzyme to carry out a particular step in a chain of metabolic reactions. The original inborn errors of metabolism were alkaptonuria, albinism, pentosuria and cystinuria (which subsequently turned out to be a transport defect instead). Thus Garrod was way ahead of his time in describing the essence of the "one gene—one enzyme" hypothesis so elegantly demonstrated experimentally by Beadle and Tatum in the breadmold, *Neurospora,* some 30 years later.

The characteristics Garrod specified were that the diseases resulting from inborn errors of metabolism had an increased frequency of parental consanguinity, tended to recur in sibs (in fact alkaptonuria was the first human trait shown to fit the expec-

TABLE 6-1. Some Genetic Metabolic Diseases Susceptible to Treatment

Disease	Treatment	Efficacy of Treatment
Amino Acid Metabolism		
Phenylketonuria	Phenylalanine-restricted diet	Good if started in first two months of life
Maple syrup urine disease	Diet restricted in leucine, isoleucine, and valine	Fair if started in neonatal period
Homocystinuria	Vitamin B₆ and cystine supplement. Diet restricted in methionine	Not yet known
Histidinemia	Histidine-restricted diet	Not yet known
Tyrosinemia	Diet restricted in phenylalanine and tyrosine	Not yet known
Cystinosis	Diet restricted in methionine and cystine; kidney transplantation (symptomatic)	Not yet known
Cystinuria	Alkali, high fluid intake, D-penicillamine	Good for prevention of urolithiasis
Diseases of the urea cycle (some forms)	Protein-restricted diet	Fair, but limited experience
Glycinemias (some forms)	Protein-restricted diet	Fair, but limited experience
Carbohydrate Metabolism		
Galactosemia	Galactose-free diet	Good if started in neonatal period
Fructosemia	Fructose-free diet	Good if started in early infancy
Malabsorption of di- and monosaccharides	Monosaccharide-free or di-saccharide-free diet	Good
Other Metabolic Pathways		
Wilson's disease	D-penicillamine, potassium sulfide, copper-restricted diet	Fair or better
Primary hemochromatosis	Removal of Fe by phlebotomy, desferrioxamine	Fair
Pyridoxine dependency	High doses of pyridoxine	Can be good if started in neonatal period
Familial hyperlipoproteinemia	Fat restriction, use of medium-chain fatty acids, cholestyramine, clofibrate	Fair
Familial defective synthesis and delivery of thyroid hormone (familial goiter)	Levothyroxine or desiccated thyroid	Good
Adrenogenital syndrome	Cortisone; mineralocorticoids in patients subject to salt loss	Good
Cystic fibrosis	Pancreatic extracts, diet, bronchial mucolytics, etc.	Short-term prognosis much improved; long-term prognosis unknown
Crigler-Najjar syndrome	Blood exchange transfusion, glucuronyl transferase stimulation by phenobarbital	Unsatisfactory long-term results
Nephrogenic diabetes insipidus	High fluid intake of low osmolarity, saluretics	Good if started in early infancy
Rickets refractory to vitamin D	Vitamin D and phosphate salts	Fair or better
Renal tubular acidosis (Butler-Albright syndrome)	Alkali therapy	Good

(From World Health Organization: Genetic Disorders: Prevention, Treatment and Rehabilitation. WHO Technical Report Series, no. 497, 1972.)

tation for a mendelian autosomal recessive gene), appeared early in life, showed marked deviations from normal, and were not subject to marked fluctuations in severity. The rapid growth of biochemical knowledge and particularly enzymology since then has led to the identification of over 60 inborn errors and to rational means of treatment for a dozen or more (Table 6-1).[13] Details of the more important of these diseases will be found elsewhere in the text. In this chapter we discuss some general principles.[3]

We have said that inborn errors of metabolism result from lack of a functional enzyme. Several mechanisms can account for this reduction in enzymatic activity. When the gene coding for a particular enzyme is changed by a mutation, this can lead to a functional deficiency of the enzyme in several ways. In homozygotes for the mutant gene, the enzyme coded for by that gene may (a) not be produced at all, or (b) be produced in an abnormal form with reduced activity. (c) The mutation may involve a gene that regulates the rate of production of the enzyme, leading to an inadequate amount of normal enzyme. So far there are no known examples of this type in man. (d) The enzyme may be degraded at an excessive rate leading to a deficiency of active enzyme, as in the case of certain types of G6PD deficiency. Finally, optimal enzyme activity may depend on association with a cofactor, and mutations that (e) interfere with absorption or biosynthesis of the cofactor, or (f) alter the binding site on the enzyme to impair binding with the cofactor, may reduce the activity of the enzyme. The vitamin-dependencies are an outstanding example of this mechanism. Thus one might expect that the activity of a particular enzyme could be reduced by mutations at several different loci and that each locus might have several different allelic mutations. This is the basis for the **genetic heterogeneity** so well recognized in many inborn errors of metabolism and elsewhere.

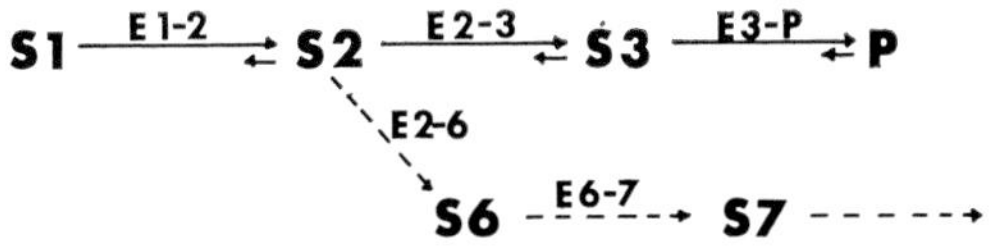

$$S1 \xrightarrow{E1\text{-}2} S2 \xrightarrow{E2\text{-}3} S3 \xrightarrow{E3\text{-}P} P$$

Figure 6-1. A hypothetic metabolic pathway converting substrate S1 to end-product P, through the successive actions of enzymes E1-2, E2-3, and E3-P. An alternative minor pathway is indicated.

One useful way of classifying the diseases resulting from inborn errors of metabolism is according to the pathologic effects of the block in the metabolic pathway. Consider a prototype metabolic pathway converting substrates 1 through a series of enzyme-catalyzed reactions to an end-product P (Fig. 6-1). Disease may result from: absence of end-product, pile-up of substrates in the pathway proximal to the block, presence of excessive amounts of metabolites, and secondary effects of the above metabolic distortions on regulatory mechanisms in the same or other pathways. Although many inborn errors show several of these results, one of them usually accounts for the major features of the child's disease. It must be admitted, however, that the precise mechanisms by which enzyme defects produce clinical defects are still a major area of ignorance.

Defects in membrane transport, although they may represent inborn errors involving enzymes of the transport process, present such special features that they will be considered separately from inborn errors of intermediary metabolism.

Diseases Resulting from Absence of End-product. One of the original inborn errors of metabolism, albinism, is a good example of a disease in which the major clinical problems result from absence of the end-product of a metabolic pathway. In our archetypal diagram, enzyme E2-3 is indicated as missing, or inactive. All substrates beyond the block are therefore absent, including P (Fig. 6-2).

In the classic type of albinism, lack of

$$S1 \xrightarrow[\rightleftharpoons]{E1\text{-}2} S2 \text{//} \text{-----} \rightarrow \quad \text{--} E3\text{-}P \text{--} \rightarrow$$

Figure 6-2. The pathway shown in Figure 6-1 blocked by the absence of enzyme E2-3.

tyrosinase in the melanocyte blocks the pathways leading from tyrosine through DOPA (3, 4-dihydroxyphenylalanine) to melanin (see Fig. 6-3, block C). Note that the mutant gene affects only melanocyte

tyrosinase and not that in the liver and elsewhere, showing that there must be at least two separate loci for this enzyme. Furthermore, genetic heterogeneity exists, since there are several other ways of blocking the pathway. In fact there are at least seven genetically different forms of albinism (Chapter 8).

Other examples of this class of disease include the various types of recessively inherited goitrous cretinism in which the

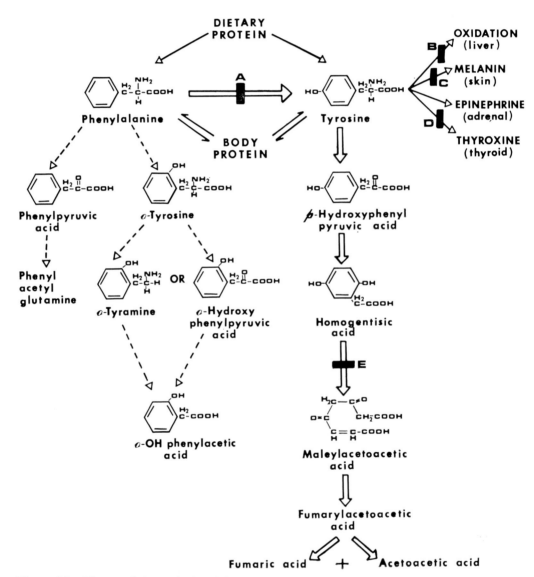

Figure 6-3. The metabolism of phenylalanine and tyrosine, illustrating the diseases produced by various enzyme deficiencies (see text).

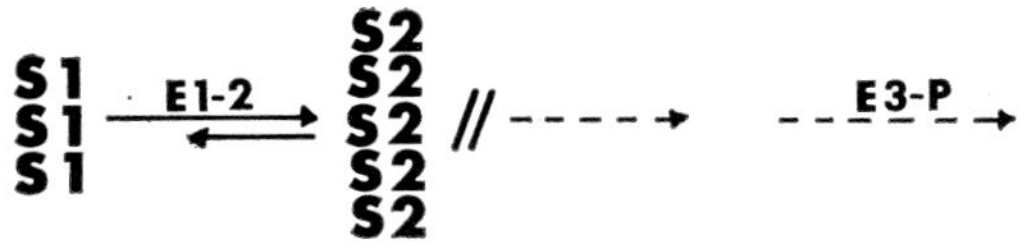

$$S1 \xrightarrow{E1\text{-}2} \begin{array}{c} S2 \\ S2 \\ S2 \\ S2 \\ S2 \end{array} \, // \, \text{---} \rightarrow \quad \text{-} \text{-} \underline{\underline{E3\text{-}P}} \rightarrow$$

Figure 6-4. The hypothetic pathway of Figure 6-1 showing pile-up of precursor S2 when enzyme E2-3 is lacking.

pathologic effects result from a lack of thyroid hormone (Fig. 6-3, block D), pitressin-sensitive diabetes insipidus in which the pituitary does not produce antidiuretic hormone, and the adrenogenital syndrome in which part of the trouble results from a deficiency of cortisol. However, the latter syndrome will be considered as an example of interference with regulatory mechanisms on page 98.

Diseases Resulting From Pile-up of Substrate(s). In some cases the substrate just before the block (in this case substrate S2), not being converted into substrate S3, will increase in concentration and may appear in abnormal quantities in blood and urine. Since most enzymatic reactions are reversible, substrate S1 may also pile up and be excreted (Fig. 6-4).

An example is galactosemia, in which the defective enzyme is galactose-1-phosphate uridyl transferase, which normally converts galactose-1-phosphate to glucose-1-phosphate (see Fig. 6-5). In the mutant homozygote this step cannot occur, and galactose-1-phosphate accumulates in the blood cells, liver and other tissues, damaging the liver, brain and kidney. Other effects will be considered in Chapter 8.

Alkaptonuria is another example; the homogentisic acid accumulates in the blood (Figure 6-3, block E) and, in polymerized form, is deposited in cartilages (ochronosis), leading to degeneration and arthritis. Some storage diseases also fit into this class, but will be considered separately (see page 98).

Diseases Resulting From Excessive Amounts of Metabolites. In this category, the damage is done not so much by the excessive amounts of precursors behind the block as by excessive amounts of metabolites produced by the breakdown of these precursors through alternate pathways that are normally used only slightly but are called upon to deal with the abnormal situation.

An example is classic phenylketonuria. Here the enzyme phenylalanine hydroxylase is inactive or missing, and phenylalanine is not converted to tyrosine. Phenylalanine therefore accumulates in the blood and is broken down to phenylpyruvic, phenylacetic and phenyllactic acids, which may be toxic substances (Fig. 6-3, block A). For instance, they may inhibit the enzyme 5-hydroxytryptophane decarboxylase, resulting in decreased synthesis of serotonin (5-hydroxytryptamine), and inhibit the melanocyte tyrosinase, accounting for the decreased pigmentation.[6] This effect could also be considered an example of diseases resulting from interference with regulatory mechanisms, illustrating that the same disease may fall into several categories.

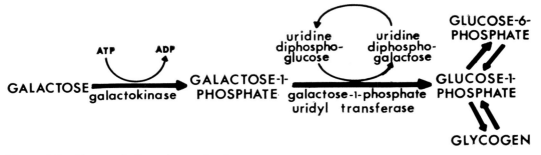

Figure 6-5. The metabolic pathway of galactose.

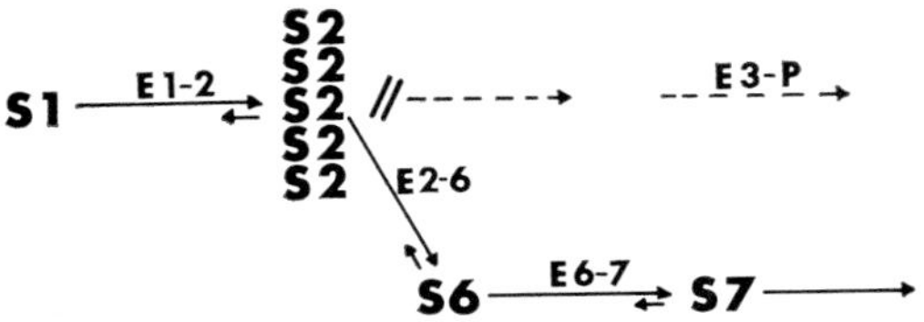

Figure 6-6. The hypothetic pathway of Figure 6-1 showing increased use of an alternate pathway.

Diseases Resulting From Interference With Regulatory Mechanisms. A fourth category of pathologic effects resulting from genetic blocks in metabolic pathways are those in which lack of the end-product or excessive amounts of a substrate interfere with feedback or other regulatory mechanisms. In the adrenogenital syndromes, for instance, there is a block in the biosynthesis of cortisol by the adrenal cortex. This deficiency stimulates excessive production of ACTH by the pituitary, since the level of cortisol normally regulates the output of ACTH by a negative feedback mechanism. The increased ACTH levels, in turn, stimulate the adrenal cortex to increase synthesis of the cortisol precursors but, of course, only as far as the block. Breakdown of the accumulated precursors by alternative pathways leads to the androgenic effects.[1]

Orotic aciduria is another example of an inborn error of metabolism affecting a regulatory mechanism. The pathway leads from aspartic acid and carbamyl phosphate through a series of steps to uridine monophosphate (UMP). In homozygotes for orotic aciduria, two enzymes, orotidylic acid pyrophosphorylase and decarboxylase, are absent, and the proximal precursor piles up and appears in the urine. (It is unlikely that this represents an operon; more probably the two enzymatic functions are carried by a multifunctional protein complex.) The end-product, UMP, is a feedback inhibitor of the first enzyme in the pathway. In its absence, the reaction appears to proceed more rapidly, leading to a great excess of orotic acid. Adding uridine to the diet inhibits the first enzyme and leads to a sharp decrease in the production of orotic acid.[11]

A further and more complicated example, the Lesch-Nyhan syndrome,[5] in which lack of a feedback inhibitor may result in excessive purine synthesis, is discussed in Chapter 9.

The Storage Diseases. In a number of inborn errors of metabolism, one of the substrates that accumulates becomes deposited in abnormal quantities in the cells and may cause damage by its simple presence. The glycogen storage diseases are classic examples.[4] Glycogen is a polymer of alpha-D-glucose, assembled into a multi-branched tree-like structure. The glycogen molecules are constantly being degraded and resynthesized to meet the varying metabolic demands of the individual; errors can occur at various steps of mobilization or synthesis. For instance, when glucose is to be mobilized, cleavage of the outer branches of the glycogen molecule is done by a phosphorylase. Absence of this enzyme in muscle cells results in accumulation of glycogen in muscle (McArdle's disease).

Many storage diseases fit into a special category only recently recognized—the **lysosomal diseases.** The lysosomes are intracellular organelles consisting of a lipid membrane enclosing a variety of acid hydrolytic enzymes. If a specific lysosomal enzyme is missing, the corresponding substrate may accumulate in the lysosome, and the cell becomes laden with the resulting storage vacuoles. The first example to be discovered was Pompe's disease, one of the glycogen storage diseases. Homozygotes are deficient in alpha-1,4 glycosidase, a lysosomal enzyme that can hydrolyse the outer chains of glycogen to give glucose. Apparently fragments of glycogen are constantly being taken up by the lysosomes and degraded. In Pompe's disease uptake goes on but degradation does not; the lysosomes become swollen with glycogen, and cell degeneration ensues. Other examples include ceramide lactoside lipidosis (Fabry's disease), fucosidosis, Gaucher's disease, glycogen storage diseases types III and IV, Gm-1 ganglisidosis, "I" cell disease, Krabbe's disease, lysosomal acid phosphatase deficiency, mannosidosis, metachromatic leukodystrophy, mucopolysaccharidosis types I-VI, Niemann-Pick disease, Sandhoff's disease and Tay-Sachs disease.[12]

Inborn Errors of Transport. Our increasing understanding of diseases resulting from genetically determined errors of membrane transport is a good example of how specific mutations can be used as tools to probe the biology of the normal organism.[10]

Inborn Errors of Amino Acid Transport. Cystinuria was first classified (erroneously) as an inborn error of metabolism of cystine, but when it was found that blood levels of cystine are not elevated in patients with the disease, Dent proposed that the condition was an inborn error of membrane transport rather than of intermediary metabolism. That is, the cystine was not being reabsorbed by the renal tubule from the glomerular filtrate, and therefore appeared in abnormal amounts in the urine. This implied a specific transport mechanism across the tubule membrane that was defective in the cystinuria patients. The discovery that not only cystine, but the structurally similar dibasic amino acids lysine, arginine and ornithine were also being excreted in abnormally large quantities, led to the idea that there was a membrane transport system that would accept all four of these amino acids but not others.

Harris demonstrated genetic heterogeneity for the disease when he showed that in some families the heterozygotes showed mild degrees of the relevant amino acidurias, while in other families they did not.[3] It was then found that some cystinuria homozygotes had the same defect in transport across the intestinal membrane, and this led to further definition of genetic heterogeneity. All homozygotes have similar urinary findings, but some (type I) have greatly impaired transport of cystine and the dibasic amino acids from the intestine into plasma; others (type II) have only

moderate impairment of intestinal membrane transport, and a third group (type III) have mild impairment. To make matters still more complicated, kinetic studies suggest that the renal system common to the four amino acids is an efflux system, and that the renal influx system has separate sites for cystine and the dibasic amino acids respectively.

Heterozygotes for the type I mutant have normal urinary amino acids; that is, the gene is "completely recessive," whereas types II and III have an excess of the relevant amino acids in the urine, somewhat more marked in type II. Matings between heterozygotes of different types produced offspring with the full blown homozygous urinary phenotype, showing that the three mutants are allelic.

The hereditary **iminoglycinurias** provide another example of genetic determination of a specific transport mechanism and of genetic heterogeneity. Homozygotes have decreased tubular resorption of proline, hydroxyproline and glycine, with normal plasma levels. This suggests a renal tubular transport mechanism specific to these substances. As with cystinuria, there is heterogeneity when intestinal transport is examined; in some homozygotes it is impaired and in others it is not. Again, family studies suggest allelism.

Hartnup disease is characterized by defective transport of the neutral amino acids (other than the imino acids and glycine), suggesting a membrane site specific to the transport of these molecules.

Finally, there are mutant genes that interfere with membrane transport of a wide variety of amino acids and other substances. The **Fanconi syndromes** I and II are well-documented examples. In some cases this may be secondary to impairment of the energy supply necessary for transport by some toxic metabolite; in others there may be a defective component in the transfer mechanism beyond the binding site. Perhaps further study of mutant phenotypes will throw more light on the nature of the transfer process, as it has on the nature of the binding sites.

Why is it that these mutant genes produce only partial defects in tubular transport of the affected amino acids? In the iminoglycinuria homozygote, for instance, about 80% of the ability to reabsorb proline, hydroxyproline and glycine is retained. Kinetic studies both *in vitro* and *in vivo* suggest that there are at least two kinds of system involved in amino acid tubular transport. One type is represented by the mutant phenotypes we have been describing. They have "group" specificity, high capacity and low affinity; they appear to operate at concentrations that exceed the usual physiologic range. Another type of transport site is characterized by low capacity, high affinity, and specificity to a particular amino acid. One would expect to find mutant phenotypes involving failure to transport specific amino acids, and this is so. Siblings have been reported with excessive amounts of cystine but not of the dibasic amino acids in the urine. There are also gene-determined hyperdibasic amino acidurias in which the transport of dibasic amino acids but not of cystine is impaired. Similarly, the "blue diaper" syndrome involves defective intestinal transport of tryptophan and there is a methionine malabsorption syndrome.

Inborn Errors of Transport of Other Than Amino Acids. Site specificity of transport is not limited to the amino acids. Genetically determined defects of membrane transport have been found for many other substances, and again, study of the disorder has often been the first evidence that there is a specific site for the transport of that particular substance. These include:

1. Renal glucosuria—failure to reabsorb glucose; harmless (except when misdiagnosed); pattern of inheritance varies from family to family.
2. Glucose-galactose malabsorption—diarrhea after ingestion of these sugars or disaccharides and polysaccharides that give rise to them; autosomal recessive.
3. Hypophosphatemic rickets—failure to reabsorb phosphate leads to loss of calcium and to rickets; X-linked dominant.
4. Renal tubular acidosis—loss of hydrogen ion; autosomal dominant.
5. Chloridorrhea, congenital — chloride lost in intestine; autosomal recessive.
6. Hereditary spherocytosis — impaired transport of sodium across the blood cell membrane; autosomal dominant.
7. Diabetes insipidus, nephrogenic—impaired tubular resorption of water; X-linked recessive.

Principles of Treatment of Inborn Errors of Metabolism. Rational methods of treating the disorders resulting from the inborn errors of metabolism depend on understanding the biochemical nature of the error and the resulting disease processes. Correction of the end results of a genetic defect has been termed "environmental engineering," as opposed to "genetic engineering" which attempts to modify the genetic material itself.[10] An impressive number of genetically determined metabolic diseases are now susceptible to treatment (Table 6-1). Part of the problem is the organization of medical resources in order to get the patient with a (usually rare) genetic disease to a source of expert diagnosis and treatment, or better still, in some cases, to get the management to the patient.[2]

Approaches to therapy are considered under the following headings.

Substrate Restriction. Diseases in which the metabolites proximal to the enzyme block interfere with development or function logically could be treated by restricting the supply of substrate. This has been quite successful when the substrate comes primarily from the diet. Thus reduction of dietary phenylalanine in phenylketonuria, of lactose and galactose in galactosemia, and of fructose in fructosemia are relatively effective in preventing the pathologic consequences of the genetic defect.

When the substrate is synthesized endogenously it may be much more difficult to control its accumulation by simple dietary restriction. Sometimes it is possible to impose a block elsewhere in the pathway, where the results may be less harmful. For instance, the accumulation of oxalate in oxalosis can be reduced by treatment with calcium carbimide, which inhibits aldehyde oxidase and thereby reduces the synthesis of glycolate and its conversion to glyoxalate and oxalate.

Removal of Toxic Products. An alternative to restricting substrate would be to remove the accumulating toxic product. This approach is taken in the treatment of Wilson's disease by removing excess copper with penicillamine, and of hemochromatosis by bloodletting and desferrioxamine. One might also place in this category the prevention of hemolytic disease of the newborn due to Rh-isoimmunization by treating Rh negative mothers of Rh positive babies with gamma globulin containing anti-Rh antibody, which neutralizes any Rh antigen the mother may have received from the baby.

Product Replacement. When the pathology results from lack of a product in the metabolic pathway distal to the block, it would seem logical to replace the product. This is the rationale for treating inherited defects of thyroid hormone synthesis with thyroxine, the adrenogenital syndromes with cortisol, orotic aciduria with uridine, hemophilia with antihemophiliac globulin, cystic fibrosis of the pancreas with pancreatic enzymes, and several other diseases. However, replacement of product may present technical difficulties, particularly if the product is intracellular, as in albinism.

In some diseases, product replacement is used together with substrate restriction. In homocystinuria, for instance, methionine is restricted but cystine must be added, since the homozygote cannot synthesize it from methionine.

Cofactor Supplementation. Diseases in which the reduced enzyme activity results from a defective or lacking coenzyme or from a change in the enzyme's capacity to bind to the coenzyme may be treated by supplying large amounts of the coenzyme. For instance, more than half of the tested cases of homocystinuria respond well to large doses of pyridoxine (vitamin B_6), a cofactor for the enzyme cystathionine synthetase, which is deficient in this disease. Vitamin B_6 is also a cofactor for cystathioninase, kynureninase, and glutamic acid decarboxylase, and is effective in the treatment of the corresponding inborn errors: cystathioninuria (one form), xanthurenicaciduria, and convulsions due to vitamin B_6 dependency. Other examples are a form of methylmalonicaciduria that responds to vitamin B_{12}, and a form of propionicacidemia that responds to biotin.

Treatment of Inborn Errors of Transport. Most hereditary transport defects of man are rather benign, and treatment is often limited to what might be called second-order clinical manifestations. For instance, cystinuria is a serious disorder only when urinary stones are formed. Keeping the urine dilute prevents stone formation (all that is needed is a glass of water and an alarm clock to awaken the patient at the appropriate hour), and solubilization of cystine with penicillamine reduces cystine excretion and causes stones to dissolve, though unfortunately there are problems with toxicity.

In nephrogenic diabetes insipidus, the logical approach is to replace the water lost by inadequate tubular resorption, and in renal tubular acidosis (Butler-Albright's disease) in which hydrogen ion clearance is inadequate, leading to excessive excretion of bicarbonate, sodium, potassium and calcium, treatment with alkali adjusts the imbalance quite well.

New Approaches. In theory the best way to treat a disease resulting from an enzyme deficiency would seem to be replacement of the enzyme, and this is already true for such diseases as congenital trypsinogen deficiency and some of the clotting disorders. This approach seems promising when the deficiency involves an extracellular enzyme, but intracellular enzymes present problems. Rapid inactivation, failure to reach the site of reaction with the substrate, and the development of antibodies to the "naked" enzyme complicate this approach. For instance, attempts to treat metachromatic leukodystrophy with arylsulfatase A infusion failed, since there was no increase in enzyme in the brain, and infusion of alpha-glucosidase in patients with type II glycogenosis led to severe immunologic intolerance. Perhaps inclusion of the enzyme in a semipermeable, inert microcapsule may avoid some of these problems, and this approach has already achieved temporary correction of the biochemical phenotype of acatalasemic mice.

One intriguing new development is the treatment of mucopolysaccharidoses. Studies of somatic cell cultures showed that when fibroblasts from a patient with Hurler syndrome were cultured with normal fibroblasts, the mutant cells stopped storing acid mucopolysaccharides. Furthermore, when cells from a patient with Hurler syndrome were cultured with cells from a patient with another form of acid mucopolysaccharidosis each type of cell corrected the metabolic defect of the other (see Chapter 8). The active factors are probably enzymatic. Application of this work to therapy led to the discovery that injection of normal serum caused striking improvement in patients with Hunter and Hurler syndromes. Injection of white cells from nonmutant donors is another approach. Time will tell whether these measures are successful.

In some cases it may be possible to induce synthesis of the missing enzymes; for example, treatment with phenobarbital induces synthesis of glucuronyl transferase and lowers the bilirubin level in the Crigler-Najjar syndrome (congenital nonhemolytic unconjugated hyperbilirubinemia). Stabilization of a defective enzyme by the addition of an appropriate compound is another, so far theoretic, possibility. Since the necessary amount of enzyme activity is often far below the normal amount, a relatively small increase in activity may be therapeutic.

Another way of correcting an enzyme deficiency would be by organ transplantation. This is complicated by the problem of graft rejection, but progress is being made. Transplantation of bone marrow and thymus is being attempted in some of the immune deficiency syndromes. Liver transplantation has been performed with short-term success in Wilson's disease and will no doubt be attempted in many other diseases involving hepatic enzymes. Renal transplantation has had some success in correcting the phenotype of Fabry disease and in correcting the uremic nephropathy in cystinosis (though not the cystine storage in other tissues).

Looking further into the future, directed gene change appears as a means of providing the missing enzyme in a mutant individual. Already it has been possible to prepare a bacteriophage that will incorporate into itself the genetic material that codes for a particular enzyme (galactose-1-phosphate uridyl transferase) and to transfer this phage to the cells of a mutant (galactosemic) individual, where it restored enzymatic activity—an example of genetic transduction. If such cells could safely be grafted back into the mutant individual, the metabolic defect would be corrected.

In this discussion of principles of treatment of the inborn errors of metabolism and transport, we have shown how an understanding of the nature of the basic error and of the mechanisms by which the error leads to the specific features of the disease leads to rational methods of treatment. We have also shown how imaginative applications of new advances in modern biology hold promise of further exciting advances in therapy. In this respect, the future looks bright.

THE GENETICS OF PROTEIN STRUCTURE

We have said that mutation of a gene results in the substitution of one amino acid for another in the corresponding polypeptide chain. This is not always true. The genetic code is redundant, and a mutation that changed one triplet to another coding for the same amino acid would not produce any change in the structure of the protein, although it might change its rate of synthesis (Chapter 12). Nevertheless, the majority of mutations in genes coding for polypeptides would be expected to result in an amino acid substitution.

The Hemoglobinopathies. Hemoglobin was the first molecule in which an association was shown between a mutant gene (for sickle cell disease) and a specific amino acid substitution. Sickle cell disease is a form of chronic hemolytic anemia characterized by the presence of elongated filiform or crescent-shaped red blood cells. Family studies in the 1940's showed (with certain exceptions that later proved the rule) that the disease fitted the segregation ratio expected for autosomal recessive inheritance. Heterozygotes showed the sickle cell trait—sickle cells were not normally present in blood smears, but when the red cells were made hypoxic by incubation or treatment with sodium metabisulfite, sickling would occur.

The disease has an extraordinarily high frequency in populations of West African origin, occurring in about 1 in 400 U.S. Negroes. In addition to the effects of chronic anemia, the patients may suffer from intravascular sickling, which results in thrombi and local infarcts in the intestine (sometimes mistaken for appendicitis), lungs, kidneys or brain.

After Pauling's discovery that the disease resulted from a physicochemical difference in the hemoglobin molecule (the first "molecular disease"), and Ingram's demonstration that sickle cell hemoglobin differed from normal hemoglobin by a single amino acid (a valine substituted for a glutamic acid), progress was rapid. The molecule, already known to be a tetramere, was shown to consist of two alpha and two beta chains. The sickle cell substitution involved the sixth amino acid from the N-terminal end. The high frequency in West Africans appears to result from an increased resistance of heterozygotes to falciparum malaria.

By electrophoretic and chromatographic procedures a large number of other "mutant" hemoglobins have been identified, almost all associated with a single amino acid substitution. By convention the normal molecule is assigned the formula $\alpha_2^A \beta_2^A$ and the mutant forms are designated according to the amino acid substitution. For instance, sickle cell hemoglobin is $\alpha_2\beta_2^{6glu-val}$, or $\alpha_2^A\beta_2^S$ for short.

One of the triumphs of molecular biology has been the use of these amino acid substitutions in specific regions of the molecule and the resulting alterations of charge and bonding to elucidate the functional properties of the molecule in physicochemical terms. The molecule is a tetramere consisting of four polypeptide chains, two alpha and two beta chains. Each chain is coiled and folded in a complex but characteristic manner, and has a pocket which contains a heme group—a porphyrin ring with an iron atom at its center which combines with oxygen (Fig. 6-7). The molecule is allosteric with respect to its affinity for oxygen; as a molecule of deoxyhemoglobin moves into a region of increasing oxygen tension, an oxygen atom binds to an iron atom in the heme group of one chain, causing the iron atom to move slightly, which results in a slight twist in the chain where the heme group is attached to it. This in turn causes a change in the conformation of the other chains in the tetramere, which increases the affinity of their heme groups for oxygen and decreases the affinity for carbon dioxide. As the next heme group combines with oxygen the affinity of the other two changes still more, and so on. Thus, when the hemoglobin arrives in the lung where the oxygen tension is high, its affinity for oxygen increases and it readily picks up oxygen, but as it moves to the periphery where the oxygen tension is low, it begins to lose oxygen and its

BETA CHAIN

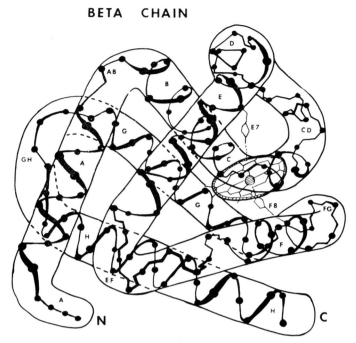

Figure 6-7. Diagram of the beta chain of hemoglobin.

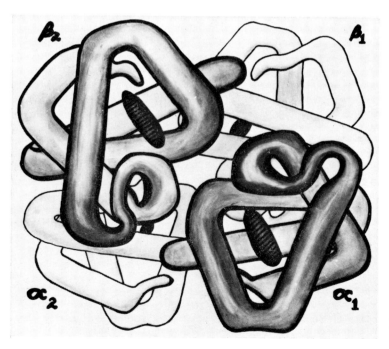

Figure 6-8. The hemoglobin molecule.

affinity decreases so that it more easily releases the oxygen where it is needed.

The alpha chain has 141 amino acids and the beta chain 146. The amino acid sequence is similar but not identical in the two chains. The sequence of amino acids is the *primary structure* of the polypeptide chain. Much of the chain is in the form of a helix, named the "alpha helix" by the protein chemists (not the same alpha as the chain), but some segments are not coiled. The helical coiling is the *secondary structure*. The (mostly) coiled chain is folded in a complex way (Fig. 6-8), forming a pocket for the heme group and surfaces for relating to the other chains of the tetramere. This is referred to as its *tertiary structure*. The tertiary structure is very similar in the two chains. Figure 6-7 indicates that there are eight helical segments, designated alphabetically, with nonhelical portions at the bends, designated by the letters of the segments they form. Specific amino acids can be numbered consecutively from the N-terminal end, or by their position in the segment. For instance, the sickle cell substitution involves amino acid 6 from the N-terminal end, or A3, since the first three amino acids are nonhelical. The advantages of the helical nomenclature is that it allows more meaningful comparisons between corresponding amino acids in different chains. Thus the histidine F8 is linked to the heme group in the alpha chain, the beta chain and myoglobin. Finally, the four chains are associated to form a more or less globular molecule, and this association is the *quaternary structure* of the molecule.

It is now clear that the primary structure of the chain determines its secondary, tertiary and quaternary substructures. It does so by means of the side chains on the amino acids, which form bonds with other side chains; the sequence of amino acids determines the positions of the bonds and thus the folding. The nature of the folding determines the external shape of the chain and thus the way in which it associates with other chains. The short side chains such as

oxygen and nitrogen tend to be polar, or hydrophilic, and the longer radicals, such as phenyl rings, tend to be nonpolar, or hydrophobic (or "greasy"). It appears that the internally situated side chains, those lining the heme pockets or binding one helical segment to another, are hydrophobic, whereas external side chains can be either hydrophilic or hydrophobic.

Amino acid substitutions cause abnormalities of the hemoglobin molecule in several ways.[8] Firstly, they may affect contact between the chain and the heme group. For instance, proline cannot form part of the alpha helix, so if it replaces an amino acid somewhere in a helix, the helix will bend (disturbing the tertiary structure) or break, and may thus lose contact with the heme group. This causes instability of the molecule and precipitation resulting in hemolysis and anemia. [Examples are hemoglobin Bibba (alpha H19 leu-pro), Genova (beta B10 leu-pro), and Santa Ana (beta F4 leu-pro).]

If the substitution involves an amino acid of different size in a part of the chain lining the heme pocket, this may allow water to enter the pocket, the heme to fall out and the molecule to precipitate. Again, a chronic hemolytic anemia may result. Examples are hemoglobins Torino (alpha CD1 phe-val), Hammersmith (beta CD1 phe-ser), Sydney (beta E11 val-ala), Kahn (beta FG5 val-met), and Zurich (beta E7 his-arg). The latter is unstable only in the presence of sulfonamide. There are no known substitutions involving amino acids with hydrophilic bonds on the walls of the heme pocket; presumably they would be too disruptive to allow survival of the molecule.

Another possible effect of an amino acid substitution is an alteration in oxygen-carrying ability; this can happen in two ways. In hemoglobins M_{Boston} and $M_{Saskatoon}$ the histidine in the E11 position (on the alpha and beta chain respectively) is changed to a tyrosine. This amino acid is adjacent to the heme group, and the tyrosine forms an ionic bond with the iron, changing it from the ferrous to the ferric state and forming methemoglobin, in which oxygen binding capacity is impaired.

Alternatively, an amino acid substitution can affect relations between the four subunits. For instance, arginine 92 (FG4) in the alpha chain forms part of the bridge from chain alpha 1 to chain beta 2. In hemoglobin Chesapeake this arginine is changed to a leucine. The resulting change in spatial relations between the chains leads to an increase in affinity for oxygen, an oxygen deficit in the peripheral tissues and a compensatory polycythemia.

Most substitutions on the external surface of the hemoglobin molecule do not seem to affect function. However, sickle cell hemoglobin may be an exception. The substitution involves the sixth amino acid in the A helix which is internal when the molecule is oxygenated but becomes exposed with the allosteric shift as the molecule loses oxygen. The sickle cell mutation causes a substitution of a nonpolar for a polar residue; it has been suggested that in the deoxygenated state the exposed nonpolar bond can attach to a similar site on another sickle cell hemoglobin molecule, and this to a third, thus leading to the formation of long chains, which is the basis for the sickling phenomenon.

The foregoing studies are an elegant example of the fruitful interaction between genetics and biochemistry. Family studies identify gene mutations affecting the molecule, and these can be used by the protein biochemist to elucidate the relation between the structure of the molecule and its function. Further examples will be found in Chapter 12, where other hemoglobin chains and mutations affecting their synthesis will be discussed.

REFERENCES

1. Bongiovanni, A. M.: Disorders of adrenocortical steroid biogenesis (the adrenogenital syndrome associated with congenital adrenal hyperplasia). In Stanbury et al., op. cit.
2. Clow, C. L., Fraser, F. C., Laberge, C., and Scriver, C. R.: On the application of knowledge to the patient with genetic diseases. In Steinberg, A. G., and Bearn, A. (eds.): Progress in Medical Genetics. vol. 9. New York, Grune & Stratton, 1973.
3. Harris, H.: The principles of human biochemical genetics. In Neuberger, A., and Tatum, E. L. (eds.): Frontiers of Biology. vol. 19. New York, American Elsevier, 1970.
4. Howell, R. R.: The glycogen storage diseases. In Stanbury et al., op. cit.
5. Kelley, W. N., and Wyngaarden, J. B.: The Lesch-Nyhan syndrome. In Stanbury et al., op. cit.
6. Knox, W. E.: Phenylketonuria. In Stanbury, et al., op. cit.
7. Lehmann, H., and Carrell, R. W.: Variations in the structure of human haemoglobin. Brit. Med. Bull., 25:14-23, 1969.
8. Lehmann, H., and Huntsman, R. G.: The hemoglobinopathies. In Stanbury, et al., op. cit.
9. Scriver, C. R.: Treatment of inherited disease: realized and potential. Med. Clin. N. Amer., 53: 941-963, 1969.
10. Scriver, C. R., and Hechtman, P.: Human genetics of membrane transport, with emphasis on amino acids. In Hirschhorn, K., and Harris, H. (eds.): Advances in Human Genetics. vol. 1. New York, Plenum Press, 1970. pp. 211-274.
11. Smith, L. H., Huguley, C. M., and Bain, J. A.: Hereditary orotic aciduria. In Stanbury et al., op. cit.
12. Stanbury, J. B., Wyngaarden, J. B., and Fredrickson, D. S. (eds.): The Metabolic Basis of Inherited Disease. 3rd ed. New York, McGraw-Hill, 1972.
13. World Health Organization: Genetic Disorders: Prevention, Treatment and Rehabilitation. WHO Technical Report Series, no. 497, 1972.

Chapter 7

AUTOSOMAL DOMINANT DISEASES

Homo sum; humani nil a me alienum puto. Terence

In this and the two following chapters a number of disease entities produced by single mutant genes are presented. The selection of these diseases, as the selection of the chromosomal disorders, reflects the experience of the authors. For the most part the diseases chosen were considered to be important for one or more reasons: the frequency with which they are encountered; the diagnostic problems that they present; or fundamental points that they illustrate. Sometimes they have been selected mainly because the authors find them interesting.

In Chapter 5 the principles of dominant inheritance were discussed. A dominant disease is one that is expressed in the heterozygote; that is, only a single dose of a mutant gene is required to produce the disease. Every affected individual has an affected parent unless the disease has arisen as a fresh mutation. Each offspring of an affected parent has a 50:50 chance of having the disease, but unaffected relatives of affected persons will *not* have affected children. Because these diseases are rare, it is

highly unusual in a random-mating population for more than one parent to have the disease. These points will be illustrated with a clinical example, a family with Marfan syndrome. The diagnostic features of the Marfan syndrome are detailed later in the chapter.

Clinical Example. The proband in this family (Fig. 7-1) was a four-year-old girl with classic Marfan stigmata who had severe congestive failure of sudden onset. She had a loud mitral insufficiency murmur that had not been previously detected and the diagnosis of ruptured mitral chordae

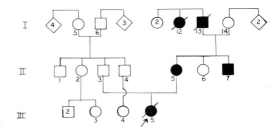

Figure 7-1. Pedigree of family with Marfan syndrome presented in case history.

107

tendineae was made. The girl expired before she could be taken to surgery where an effort to replace the mitral valve would have been made.

The mother (II-5) also had classic stigmata of the Marfan syndrome, an apical ejection click and a grade 2 mitral insufficiency murmur. After the initial shock of this tragedy had dissipated, and with the full knowledge that a similar fate may be awaiting her, this mother wanted to know the risks of future pregnancies. She was told that there was a 50:50 chance that her next child would also have Marfan syndrome, that amniocentesis could not at this time predict the outcome of the next pregnancy, and that her own mitral disease provided sufficient medical grounds for avoiding pregnancy.

The aunt of the proband (II-6), who had recently married, was also deeply concerned about future pregnancies. A careful physical examination failed to disclose any stigmata of the Marfan syndrome. Therefore, we counseled this young woman that we could be reasonably confident that her offspring would not have Marfan syndrome.

The 19-year-old uncle (II-7) of the proband was a biology major and a basketball player at the same college at which his father had starred in basketball. He had already read extensively about Marfan syndrome, knowing that his father had died suddenly in his early thirties and his aunt in her teens of the disease, which also afflicted him. Even before his niece died, he had decided never to marry. The counseling session with this young man was unusual. He did not want to know the nature of his disease or the risk to future offspring; this knowledge he already possessed. What he wanted was some reasonable prediction of his life expectancy because he wanted to go to medical school, yet he did not want to deprive someone else of a place in a medical school class if he were not going to live long enough to use his medical training. Needless to say, we were moved by this young man. Since we were unable to

detect any evidence of cardiovascular disease, we encouraged him to continue with his plans to go to medical school.

In the following list of diseases, space does not permit clinical descriptions in the detail needed for precise diagnosis. We offer, rather, a guide, indicating the kinds of diagnostic and prognostic problems and some of the genetic pitfalls of which the counselor must be aware.

ACHONDROPLASIA[1]

History. True achondroplasia has emerged as a distinct entity from the broader category of dysplastic dwarfs which has been recognized throughout medical history. The designation "achondroplasia," which had previously been loosely assigned to a variety of disorders, should be reserved for patients with the clinical findings enumerated below (Fig. 7-2).

Diagnostic Features. *General.* Equal sex distribution. Severely dwarfed. Early motor progress may be slow but intelligence is normal.

Head. Large head, prominent forehead, saddle-nose with midfacial hypoplasia, small foramen magnum (occasionally producing hydrocephalus).

Vertebrae. Lumbar lordosis with anterior beaking of upper lumbar vertebrae; progressive narrowing of lumbar interpeduncular spaces, small cuboid vertebral bodies with short pedicles.

Extremities. Short tubular bones with epiphyseal ossification centers inserted into metaphyseal ends of bones, producing ball-and-socket appearance; short trident-shaped hand.

Pelvis. Small iliac wings and reduced sacroiliac curve with narrow greater sciatic notch.

Prevalence. 1:10,000, as high as 90% being fresh mutations—these show an increased mean paternal age.

Clinical Course. Hydrocephalus may occur because of the narrow foramen magnum. Spinal cord compression is not un-

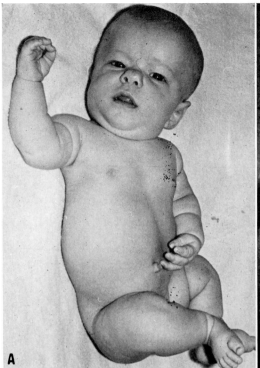
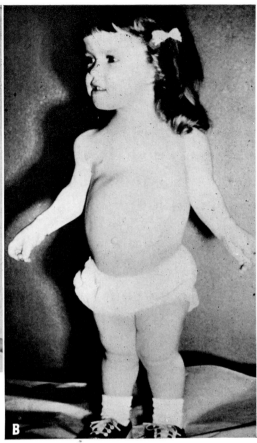

Figure 7-2. (A) Infant and (B) child with achondroplasia. Note short extremities, large head, saddle-nose.

common, especially in the second and third decades, due to bony impingement or herniated intervertebral discs; neurologic disabilities, such as paraplegia, may result.

Treatment. Symptomatic and supportive; relief of spinal cord compression, should it occur.

Differential Diagnosis.

1. *Spondyloepiphyseal dysplasia*, pseudoachondroplastic form.
2. *Metaphyseal dysostosis* (Schmid type).
3. *Cartilage-hair hypoplasia.* (See under recessive inheritance, Chapter 8.)
4. *Diastrophic dwarfism.* (See under recessive inheritance, Chapter 8.)

ACROCEPHALOSYNDACTYLY (APERT SYNDROME)[2]

History. Apert receives the credit for describing this syndrome in 1906, although Wheaton reported similar patients in 1894. A comprehensive series was presented by Blank in 1960.

Diagnostic Features. *General.* Severe mental deficiency may or may not occur. Some shortness of stature.

Head. High forehead, flat occiput, short anteroposterior diameter, irregular craniosynostosis, midfacial hypoplasia, hypertelorism, antimongoloid slant, strabismus (Fig. 7-3).

Ears. Often low-set.

Mouth. Narrow, high-arched palate, occasional cleft palate.

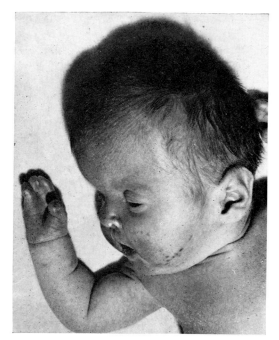

Figure 7-3. Characteristic appearance of head and hands in Apert syndrome.

Skeleton. Osseous and/or cutaneous syndactyly of hands and feet, most often involving digits 2 to 4 or "mitten-hand" (Figs. 7-4, 7-5). Variable fusion of nails. Syndactyly of all toes. Occasional limitation of joint mobility, radioulnar synostosis, fused vertebrae.

Cardiovascular. Rare congenital lesions, including coarctation of the aorta.

Gastrointestinal. Occasional esophageal atresia, pyloric stenosis.

Genitourinary. Occasional polycystic kidney, hydronephrosis.

X-ray. Osseous syndactyly; occasional radioulnar synostosis, vertebral fusion, and diastasis of the symphysis pubis.

Prevalence. 1:160,000, with the majority of patients representing fresh mutations.

Clinical Course. Intellectual impairment may progress with increased intracranial pressure. Evaluation (and treatment) of the many possible associated anomalies must be considered.

Treatment. Early surgical relief of the craniosynostosis if accompanied by in-

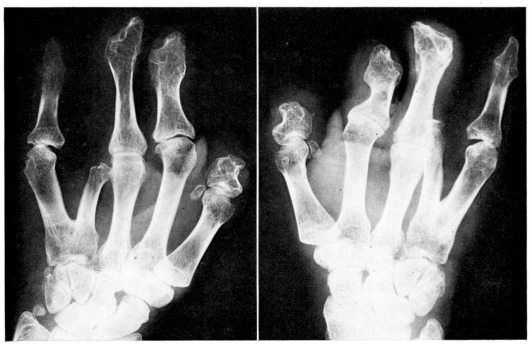

Figure 7-4. X-ray view of "mitten hand" in Apert syndrome.

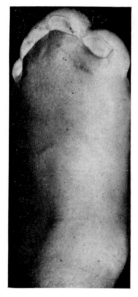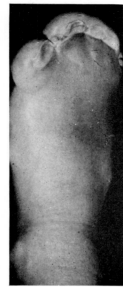

Figure 7-5. Syndactyly of the foot in Apert syndrome.

tracranial pressure. Surgical mobilization of the thumb (when indicated) and separation of cutaneous syndactyly. Surgical intervention in congenital cardiovascular and genitourinary malformations. Special schooling for the retarded.

Differential Diagnosis. A number of genetically determined disorders have craniosynostosis as a feature, most of which are inherited as autosomal dominants and most of which have syndactyly as an associated abnormality. Among these are the following:

1. *Crouzon craniofacial dysostosis* is not associated with syndactyly.
2. *Acrocephalopolysyndactyly Type I (Noack syndrome).* (See next section.)
3. *Acrocephalopolysyndactyly Type II (Carpenter syndrome)* is similar to Noack syndrome except that it shows autosomal recessive inheritance. Obesity may be quite pronounced and retardation is common.
4. Other autosomal dominant acrocephalosyndactylies, such as those of Waardenburg, Pfeiffer and Vogt, may be distinguished by certain features of the hand malformation. They may well be clinical variants of the same mutant gene, but until treatment allows propagation and family studies, the question remains open.

ACROCEPHALOPOLYSYNDACTYLY, TYPE I (NOACK SYNDROME)[3]

This condition resembles acrocephalosyndactyly, with the addition of preaxial polydactyly. Retardation has not been a feature.

BRACHYDACTYLY[4]

Brachydactyly occurs as a feature of several syndromes or by itself (Fig. 7-6). The following are among those forms that show autosomal dominant inheritance. They are described in detail to illustrate how specific the developmental effects of a gene can be.

1. *Brachydactyly, Type A-1, Farabee Type.* This was the first example of mendelian dominant inheritance demonstrated in man (by Farabee, in 1903). In Type A brachydactylies, the shortening is confined to the middle phalanges. In Type A-1 all of the digits are involved; the middle phalanges are rudimentary and often fused with the terminal phalanges.
2. *Brachydactyly, Type A-2, Mohr-Wriedt Type.* The shortening of the middle phalanges affects only the index finger and the second toe.
3. *Brachydactyly, Type A-3.* Shortening involves the middle phalanx of the fifth finger and produces clinodactyly.
4. *Brachydactyly, Type A-4.* The second and fifth digits are involved.
5. *Brachydactyly, Type B.* The terminal phalanges as well as the middle phalanges are shortened or rudimentary. Some syndactyly may also be present.
6. *Brachydactyly, Type C.* There is shortening of the middle and proximal phalanges of the second and third fingers.
7. *Brachydactyly, Type D.* The terminal

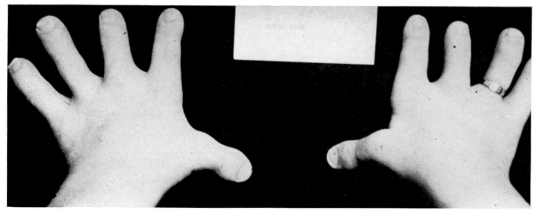

Figure 7-6. Brachydactyly.

phalanges of the thumbs and big toes are short and broad ("stub thumb").

8. *Brachydactyly, Type E.* There are short metacarpals and metatarsals, especially the third and fifth metacarpals, and moderate shortness of stature, as in Albright's hereditary osteodystrophy, but without ectopic calcifications, cataracts and mental retardation.

9. *Biemond syndrome.* Brachydactyly with short fourth metacarpal and third metatarsal, accompanies nystagmus and cerebellar ataxia.

CARDIAC ARRHYTHMIA, PROLONGED Q-T INTERVAL (ROMANO-WARD SYNDROME)[5]

The affected patient may be first recognized because of a syncopal episode during exertion. The electrocardiogram reveals a prolonged Q-T interval and exercise may elicit an episode of ventricular fibrillation (Fig. 7-7). (A provocative exercise test is not advised unless one is prepared to apply immediate electrical defibrillation.) This disorder is distinct from the Jervell and Lange-Nielsen syndrome, which is recessively inherited and in which deafness is a cardinal feature. Treatment is maintenance propranalol for the affected family members.

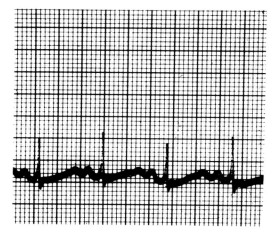

Figure 7-7. Prolonged Q-T interval (0.41 sec. at rate of 110/min.) in Romano-Ward syndrome.

CLEFT LIP WITH LIP PITS[6]

This dominantly inherited disorder has, as its sentinel lesion, pits in the vermilion of the lower lip that are the openings of accessory glands (Fig. 7-8). Mucous discharge from these pits may be distressing enough to warrant excision of the fistulas. From the point of view of genetic counseling, the more important consideration is that over half of patients with familial lip pits have a cleft lip and/or palate. Therefore, when counseling for cleft lip or cleft palate, the physician should look carefully

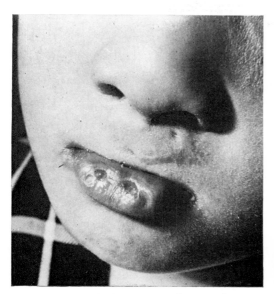

Figure 7-8. Cleft lip (repaired) with lip pits.

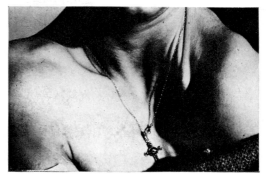

Figure 7-9. Ability to appose shoulders in cleidocranial dysostosis.

at the lips of the patient (and of the parents) before giving the usual low recurrence risk. If lip pits are present in a parent, the child's risk for lip pits is 50% and for cleft lip and/or palate about 25%.

CLEIDOCRANIAL DYSOSTOSIS[7]

History. Marie and Sainton reported the first clinical observation of this disorder in a father and son. The antiquity of this malformation is illustrated by the fact that it has been observed in a Neanderthal skull by Grieg.

Diagnostic Features. *General.* Normal intelligence. Equal sex distribution. Moderately reduced stature. Variable severity.

Head. Open cranial sutures or late mineralization with bulging calvarium and frontal and parietal bossing.

Mouth. High-arched palate, late dentition, abnormal dysplastic teeth.

Thorax. Partial to complete aplasia of clavicles, which allows the patient to appose the shoulders (Fig. 7-9).

Hands. Asymmetric length of fingers (short middle phalanx, fifth finger; long second metacarpal).

Skeletal. In addition to skull and clavicle

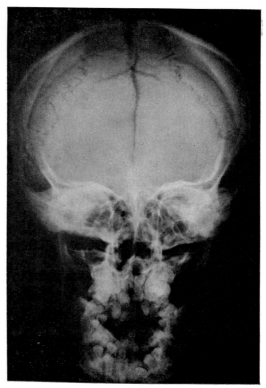

Figure 7-10. X-ray evidence of open sagittal suture in an adult with cleidocranial dysostosis.

defects, a wide symphysis pubis, vertebral malformations.

X-ray. Late mineralization of cranial sutures and pubic rami, absent or hypoplastic clavicles, pseudoepiphyses of metacarpals (Figs. 7-10, 7-11).

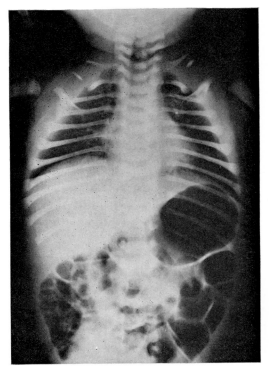

Figure 7-11. X-ray showing hypoplastic clavicles in an infant with cleidocranial dysostosis.

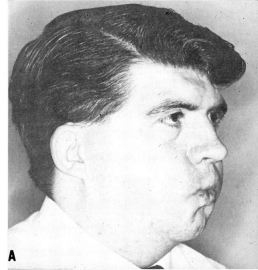

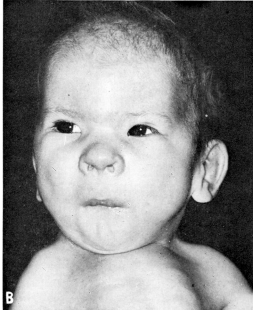

Clinical Course. Closure of the cranial sutures may be delayed for many years. The eruption of permanent teeth may also be significantly delayed, and when they appear they are usually abnormal—enamel hypoplasia, retention cysts, supernumerary teeth and malformed roots (which complicate extraction). The narrow pelvis in the female may make normal delivery impossible.

Treatment. Supportive.

CRANIO-CARPO-TARSAL DYSPLASIA (WHISTLING FACE SYNDROME)[8]

The particularly apt term, "whistling face syndrome," describes the facial appearance produced by microstomia and the shape of the chin and cheeks (Fig. 7-12). Ulnar deviation of the hand and finger contractures with thickening of the skin and subcutaneous tissues over the flexor surface of the

Figure 7-12. Characteristic facies of cranio-carpo-tarsal dysplasia in father and son. (From Fraser, F.C., *et al.*: JAMA, 211:1374, 1970. Copyright 1970, American Medical Association.)

hands constitute the "carpo" part of the disorder (Fig. 7-13), and clubbing and varus deformity of the feet represent the "tarsal" component. It is also referred to as the Freeman-Sheldon syndrome.

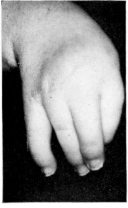 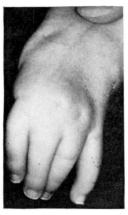

Figure 7-13. Ulnar deviation and finger contractures with thickening of tissue over flexor surface of hands in craniocarpo-tarsal dysplasia. (From Fraser, F.C., *et al.*: JAMA, 211:1374, 1970. Copyright 1970, American Medical Association.)

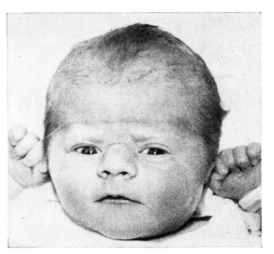

Figure 7-14. Newborn with Crouzon craniofacial dysostosis. Note that the hands are normal (as contrasted with Apert syndrome).

At birth the patients have the features described above and other stigmata, including microglossia, high-arched palate, deepset eyes with hypertelorism, dolicocephaly, a small nose with characteristically notched alae, a short neck and thoracic scoliosis. The small mouth may make feeding exceedingly difficult during infancy and dental work challenging at all ages.

As the patients get older the hand deformities improve greatly and orthopedic correction is required for the foot abnormalities. Eventual height attainment is diminished but intelligence is not. Respiratory function may be impaired and may be life-threatening in the first few years.

CRANIOFACIAL DYSOSTOSIS (CROUZON DISEASE)[9]

This characteristic facies is associated with premature synostosis of the cranial sutures of varying degree and age of onset (Fig. 7-14). There may be acro- or brachydactyly, shallow orbits leading to exophthalmos and liability to optic nerve damage, hypertelorism, hypoplasia of the maxilla, beaked nose, short upper lip, high-arched short palate, malocclusion. Mental retarda-

tion is an occasional feature, as are coarctation of the aorta and aortic stenosis.

Progressive visual impairment occurs in many patients and neurosurgery may be indicated.

DEAFNESS, DOMINANT FORMS[10]

A number of genetically determined forms of deafness, with and without other associated abnormalities, follow an autosomal dominant mode of inheritance. The following list is extracted from the useful review by Konigsmark. These include syndromes discussed in this presentation (Leopard, Waardenburg and Treacher Collins syndromes), as well as:

A. Deafness without associated anomalies:
   1. Congenital severe deafness.
   2. Progressive nerve deafness, childhood onset.
   3. Unilateral deafness.
   4. Low frequency hearing loss.
   5. Midfrequency hearing loss.
   6. Otosclerosis (penetrance of 25 to 40%).
B. Deafness with external ear malformations:

7. Deafness with preauricular pits.
8. Incudostapedial abnormality, thickened ears.
9. Conductive hearing loss and deformed ears.

C. Deafness with defects of the integument:
10. Waardenburg syndrome (see p. 138).
11. Congenital deafness with albinism.
12. Leopard syndrome (see text).
13. Progressive hearing loss with anhidrosis.
14. Deafness with keratopachyderma, digital constrictions.
15. Hearing loss with knuckle pads, leuconychia.

D. Deafness with eye defect:
16. Hearing loss, myopia, cataract, saddle-nose.
17. Hearing loss, myopia, neuropathy, joint stiffness.

E. Deafness with nervous system disease:
18. Acoustic neurinomas.
19. Sensory radicular neuropathy.

F. Deafness with skeletal defects:
20. Hearing loss, proximal symphalangism.
21. Craniofacial dysostosis (see p. 115).
22. Mandibulofacial dysostosis (see p. 122).
23. Osteogenesis imperfecta (see p. 129).
24. Deafness, bony fusions, shortness, mitral insufficiency, freckles (Forney syndrome).

DEAFNESS, CARDIAC DISEASE, FRECKLES (LEOPARD SYNDROME)[11]

The clinical features of this syndrome may be summarized as follows:

Lentigenes, multiple.
Electrocardiographic conduction defects.
Ocular hypertelorism.
Pulmonary valve stenosis.
Abnormalities of genitalia.
Retardation of growth.
Deafness, sensorineural.

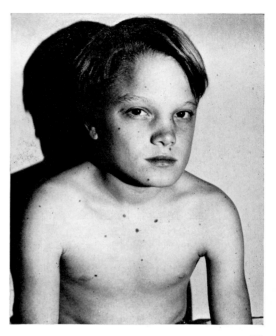

Figure 7-15. Skin lesions in Leopard syndrome.

This mnemonic device, suggested by Gorlin and colleagues, which may or may not be useful to individual clinicians, does distinguish this syndrome from other cardiocutaneous syndromes. The lentigenes are usually freckle-sized and darkly pigmented (Fig. 7-15). The electrocardiographic abnormality is most often left axis deviation; undescended testes in the male constitutes the genital abnormality.

The amount of overlap between this syndrome and the Forney syndrome, the Klippel-Feil syndrome, neurofibromatosis and the Ullrich-Noonan syndrome is readily apparent. On clinical grounds it is useful to distinguish between these syndromes. On etiologic grounds it may be useful to study the similarities.

ECTODERMAL DYSPLASIA

Ectodermal dysplasia exists in several forms, which may show autosomal dominant, autosomal recessive or X-linked inheritance.

Ectodermal Dysplasia, Hidrotic (Clouston Type)[12]

These patients have alopecia that is often total, severe dystrophy of the nails, hyperpigmentation of the skin, especially over joints, and palmar dyskeratosis (Figs. 7-16 to 7-18). Cataracts, mental subnormality and shortness of stature have occasionally been described. In this syndrome the teeth, sweat and sebaceous glands are normal. Clouston reported a pedigree of 119 individuals in a French-Canadian family.

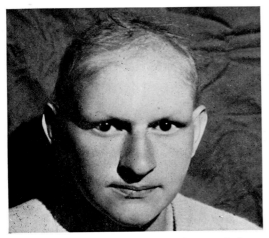

Figure 7-16. Ectodermal dysplasia, hidrotic (Clouston type). Mother of children in Figure 7-18.

Ectodermal Dysplasia (Robinson Type)[13]

This syndrome is characterized by dystrophic nails, peg-shaped teeth, partial anodontia, moderate sensorineural deafness. Syndactyly and polydactyly occasionally occur. Some patients have elevated sweat electrolytes.

ELLIPTOCYTOSIS[14]

Patients with this autosomal dominant disorder have 50% or more oval, elliptic, sausage-shaped, elongated and rod-shaped red cells circulating in the peripheral blood, appearing at three to four months of age (Fig. 7-19). The abnormality of red cell shape is first seen at the reticulocyte stage. There must be two different loci that each produce the condition, since in some families there is linkage to the Rh blood group gene and in others there is not. This condition is usually asymptomatic, but may exist with varying degrees of hemolysis, including a severe hemolytic form associated with aplastic crises. In those patients with associated hemolytic anemia, splenomegaly may be present and splenectomy may prolong the life span of the red cells. Differential diagnosis includes thalassemia minor and sickle cell trait.

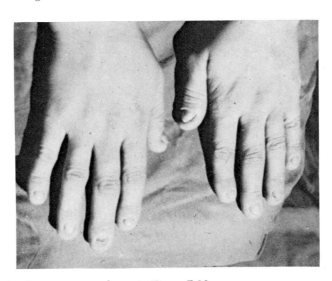

Figure 7-17. Nail dysplasia in patient shown in Figure 7-16.

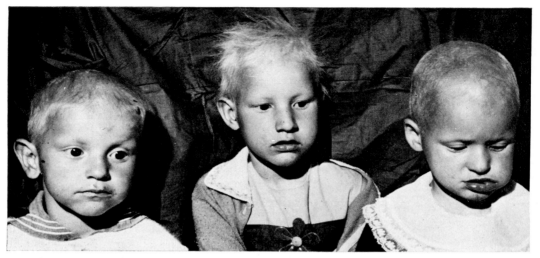

Figure 7-18. Siblings with hidrotic ectodermal dysplasia.

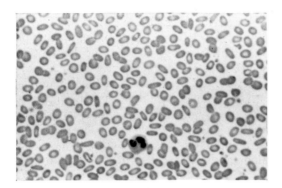

Figure 7-19. Elliptocytosis.

EPIDERMOLYSIS BULLOSA[15]

There are several (perhaps five) forms of this disease. The common forms are dominant and the uncommon and more debilitating forms, which may be lethal, are recessive. The *simple* dominant form may be observed at birth as superficial blisters (Fig. 7-20), or may not be noted until produced by mild trauma, such as that associated with crawling. The lesions are intraepidermal and are not followed by scarring. The *dystrophic* dominant form may lead to scarring and contractures. Ankles and fingers are particularly vulnerable.

FIBRODYSPLASIA OSSIFICANS PROGRESSIVA (MYOSITIS OSSIFICANS CONGENITA)[16]

Usually in childhood, localized swellings that may be attached to deep fascia appear in the back, neck and limbs. Initially the swellings come and go, but eventually fascia, tendons and ligaments are replaced by bone. The spine may become rigid as well as the proximal portions of the extremities, making it impossible for patients to sit and often difficult for them to walk. There is microdactyly of the great toe and thumbs. Intelligence is normal. Life expectancy, even in severe cases, may not be significantly reduced. A dominant mode of inheritance of the microdactyly has been observed, but since patients with fibrodysplasia seldom reproduce, the majority of cases appear to be sporadic, presumably representing fresh mutations. A variety of therapeutic approaches aimed at arresting the progressive course of the disease have been tried, including EDTA, x-ray therapy, beryllium and adrenocorticosteroids, all without obvious benefit.

HEART AND HAND SYNDROME (HOLT-ORAM)[17]

In this syndrome a cardiac anomaly, commonly atrial septal defect or ventricular

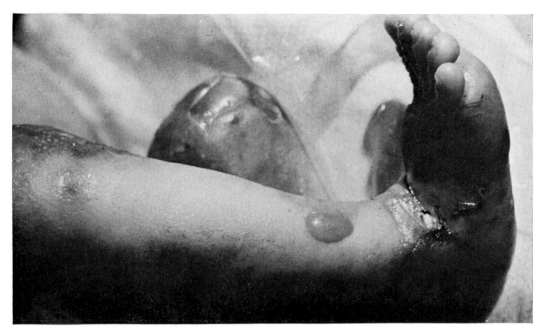

Figure 7-20. Epidermolysis bullosa in newborn infant.

septal defect, is associated with a skeletal malformation involving the radial aspect of the upper limb (Figs. 7-21, 7-22). Most often the thumb is finger-like (digitalization of the thumb) but it may be hypoplastic or absent. The radius and the forearm are variably involved and, in the severest forms, phocomelia may occur. The clinician should be alert to the possibility of coexisting gastrointestinal anomalies such as tracheoesophageal fistula in patients with thumb abnormalities or radial dysplasia with or without cardiac involvement. Anal atresia is also occasionally encountered in patients with limb and cardiac anomalies (see VACTERL association, p. 285).

HEMOGLOBIN M DISEASE[18]

Methemoglobin is formed when hemoglobin is oxidized to the ferric form. Normally there is only a small amount in the blood, since it is reduced again by the enzyme DPNH methemoglobin reductase. In hemoglobin M disease, an amino acid substitution changes the relationship to the heme group so that the iron is permanently

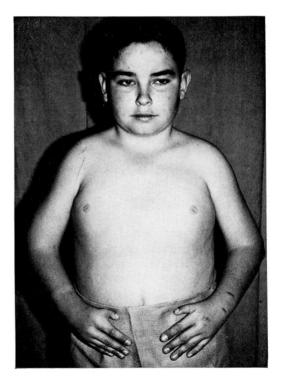

Figure 7-21. Patient with Holt-Oram syndrome (with VSD and ASD). Note severe dysplasia of thumbs.

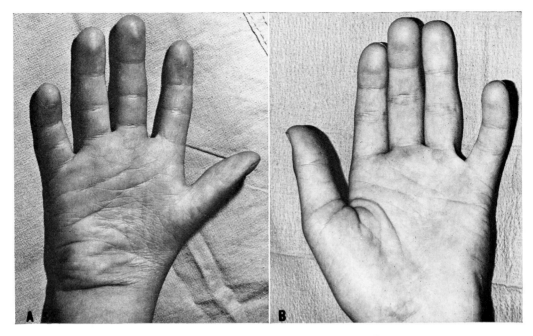

Figure 7-22. Lesser degrees of dysplasia of thumbs in Holt-Oram syndrome.

in the ferric state (see Chapter 6, p. 105); thus there is methemoglobinemia with cyanosis and hypoxia. Several hemoglobin M diseases have been described. In Hgb M_{Boston}, tyrosine replaces histidine in position 58 on the alpha chain, which is a component of fetal as well as adult hemoglobin. These patients will be cyanotic from birth. Hemoglobin M_{Iwate} is also an alpha chain abnormality. In Hgb $M_{Saskatoon}$, tyrosine replaces the homologous histidine in position 63, and in Hgb $M_{Milwaukee}$, glutamic acid replaces valine in position 67 of the beta chain. Since fetal hemoglobin is not affected, the cyanosis appears gradually as adult replaces fetal hemoglobin. Only heterozygotes have been identified in this dominantly inherited condition; presumably the homozygous condition would be fatal. The only symptom is cyanosis that is not relieved by ascorbic acid or methylene blue, unlike recessive methemoglobinemia, which results from a deficiency of the enzyme DPNH methemoglobin reductase (diaphorase).

HUNTINGTON'S CHOREA[19]

This syndrome may become manifest in childhood, but is usually recognized in the third or fourth decades. The initial manifestation is often emotional disturbance followed by choreic movements, seizures and progressive dementia. Death usually results between four and 20 years after the onset of symptoms. Huntington's chorea is an example of a serious and disabling autosomal dominant disease that continues to be transmitted through successive generations because its late onset results in a relatively small reduction in reproductive fitness. The late onset of the disease also makes genetic counseling difficult. The counseling situation often involves an unaffected grandchild of an affected grandparent and a parent who is, as yet, unaffected. The parent had a risk of 50% of inheriting the mutant gene, and if he (or she) carries the gene, the risk to the grandchild is also 50% at conception. However, if the parent does not carry the gene, there is no risk to the grandchild. The longer the

TABLE 7-1. Risk of Developing Huntington's Chorea for a Child Whose Father's Father is Affected and Father is Normal. A *priori* Risk for Father is 50%

Age of Father	Plus Ogive	Risk for Father Becoming Affected (%)	Risk for Young Child (%)
20-24	20	44	22
25-29	31	40	20
30-34	50	33	16.5
35-39	66	25	12.25
40-44	80	14	7
45-49	90	9	4.5

parent remains unaffected the less likely he is to have inherited the abnormal gene, and the probability can be estimated from the age of onset curve (see Chapter 5). Table 7-1 lists the risk for a grandchild whose parent is still free of findings of Huntington's chorea as of certain ages.

HYPERBILIRUBINEMIA I (GILBERT DISEASE, NONHEMOLYTIC JAUNDICE)[20]

This dominantly inherited condition has elevation of indirect bilirubin with clinical jaundice, but is a relatively mild disease. The bilirubin levels are not high enough to cause kernicterus. Whether this represents a single specific entity or not is subject to discussion. The uptake of bilirubin into the liver cell and a defect in glucuronide transformation have been proposed as mechanisms.

HYPERELASTOSIS CUTIS (EHLERS-DANLOS SYNDROME)[21]

History. Ehlers in 1901 and Danlos in 1908 described features of this syndrome. However, many observers prior to the twentieth century had also provided clinical descriptions, perhaps the earliest of which was the case of van Meekeren, reported in 1682.

Diagnostic Features. *General.* Normal intelligence and growth. Equal sex distribution. Variable in severity.

Skin. Strikingly hyperextensible, velvety, fragile and prone to laceration from minor trauma (Figs. 7-23, 7-24, 7-25). "Cigarette-paper" scars and mulluscoid pseudotumors at pressure points. Subcutaneous bleeding. Increase in number of elastic fibers, but no pathologic features by EM or light microscopy.

Eyes. Epicanthic folds, blue sclerae, strabismus, keratoconus, retinal detachment and subluxation of the lens.

Ears. Hypermobile, tendency to "lop ears."

Musculoskeletal. Hyperextensibility of joints with tendency to dislocation, kypho-

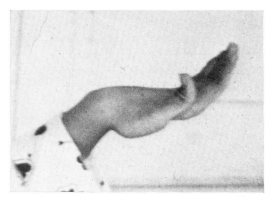

Figure 7-23. Joint laxity in hyperelastosis cutis (Ehlers-Danlos syndrome).

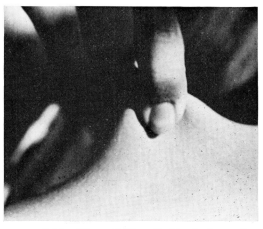

Figure 7-24. Distensibility of skin in hyperelastosis cutis.

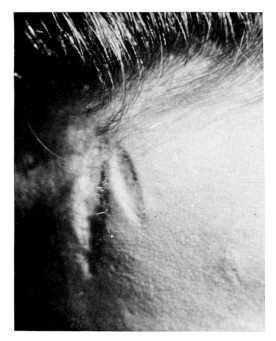

Figure 7-25. Scarring of laceration-prone skin in Ehlers-Danlos syndrome.

scoliosis and inguinal and diaphragmatic hernias.

Cardiovascular. Risk of cystic medial necrosis and dissection of medium-sized arteries (e.g., subclavian, renal) and occasionally dissecting aneurysm of the aorta. Atrioventricular valve regurgitation.

Lungs. Risk of rupture of lung, mediastinal emphysema and pneumothorax.

Abdomen. Risk of gastrointestinal diverticulae and friability of the bowel with spontaneous rupture.

Clinical Course. Patients with this disorder, like those with the Marfan syndrome, may lead a reasonably normal life or may be seriously debilitated. They are at risk for vascular accidents and sudden death. Ruptured aneurysms of the cerebral arteries, dissection and rupture of subclavian, carotid, femoral and other medium-sized arteries, as well as dissecting aneurysms of the aorta, can all lead rapidly to death in children and adults. Also rupture of lungs and abdominal viscera have been reported to

produce fatalities in this syndrome. Unfortunately, the magnitude of the risk is not known. Frequent lacerations from minor injuries, which are not easily sutured because of the fragility of the skin, result in excessive scarring and skin ulcerations.

Treatment. Symptomatic and supportive. Surgical intervention for vascular and visceral accidents.

LYMPHEDEMA, HEREDITARY (MILROY AND MEIGE TYPES)[22,23]

Congenital lymphedema is generally referred to as Milroy disease (Fig. 7-26). Most cases are sporadic. Lymphedema developing at puberty (also dominantly inherited) is sometimes referred to as the Meige type. The disease may be quite debilitating, with enormous swelling of the legs, as well as being cosmetically distressing. Surgical intervention, while relieving the swelling, produces exorbitant scarring.

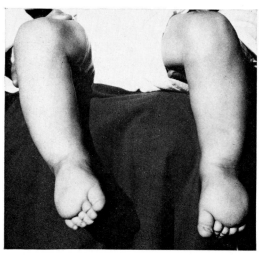

Figure 7-26. Congenital lymphedema (Milroy) in young child.

MANDIBULOFACIAL DYSOSTOSIS (TREACHER COLLINS SYNDROME; FRANCESCHETTI-KLEIN SYNDROME)[24]

History. In 1900 Treacher Collins reported a patient with this pattern of anomalies and has since been accorded the eponym. A more extensive treatment of the problem was presented by Franceschetti and Klein in 1949, who called the condition mandibulofacial dysostosis; they are also sometimes credited with the eponym.

Diagnostic Features. *General.* Usually normal intelligence. Equal sex distribution.

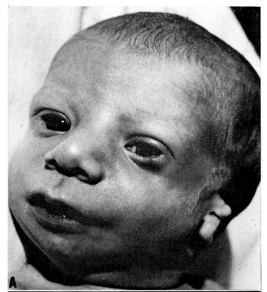

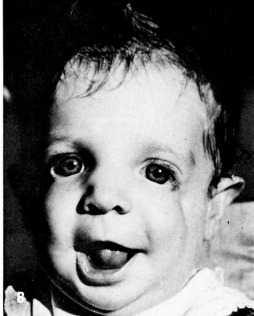

Figure 7-27. Mandibulofacial dysostosis in infant and young child. Note eye and ear anomalies.

Normal growth in stature. Features of the syndrome are very variable, and may be minimal; there is reduced penetrance.

Head. Mandibular and malar hypoplasia, depression of the temple, extension of scalp hair to cheeks, occasional skin tags and fistulas between ear and mouth, occasional cleft palate.

Eyes. Antimongoloid slant, notches at junction of outer and middle third of lower lids, absence of eyelashes (partial or complete), occasional microphthalmia (Fig. 7-27).

Ears. Malformed auricles and defects of the external ear canal; conductive deafness.

Nose. Occasional choanal atresia.

Skeletal. Occasional cervical vertebral anomalies.

Cardiovascular. Occasional congenital heart disease.

Genitourinary. Occasional cryptorchism.

Prevalence. Figure unavailable. The disorder is relatively common for a single mutant gene syndrome. About 60% of patients do not have affected parents, but it may be impossible to distinguish between fresh mutation and reduced penetrance in a particular case, making counseling difficult.

Clinical Course. The growth of the facial bones in childhood, especially during adolescence, produces considerable cosmetic improvement. An awareness of the high frequency of hearing deficit is necessary to ensure prompt recognition and treatment.

Treatment. Plastic surgery and hearing aids as indicated.

Differential Diagnosis. 1. *Robin syndrome.* Mandibular hypoplasia, glossoptosis and posterior cleft palate. Although familial cases have been seen they are rare, and this syndrome does not fit a simple mendelian pattern.

2. *Goldenhar syndrome* (oculo-auriculo-vertebral dysplasia) shares many features of mandibulofacial dysostosis, but in addition there are epibulbar dermoids, and there is notching (usually unilateral) of the upper rather than the lower lid. A few familial

cases have been reported. *Hemifacial microsomia* (unilateral microtia, macrostomia and failure of formation of the mandibular ramus and condyles) may be a variant of the same syndrome.

MARFAN SYNDROME (ARACHNODACTYLY, DOLICHOSTENOMELIA)[25]

History. Antoine Marfan, a professor of pediatrics in Paris, reported the skeletal manifestations of this syndrome in 1896. He originally called the condition dolichostenomelia (long, thin extremities). Achard renamed the disorder arachnodactyly (spider fingers) in 1902. It was not until 1931

that the inheritance of the syndrome, as a dominant trait, was demonstrated by Weve.

Diagnostic Features. The diagnostic features are not invariable, and carriers of the gene may have anything from virtually no signs of the disease to the full-blown syndrome (see Figs. 7-28, 7-29).

General. Taller than unaffected sibs. Normal intelligence. Equal sex distribution. Variable expressivity and reduced penetrance complicate the diagnosis and counseling.

Head. Dolichocephaly (long head).

Eyes. Superior-temporal subluxation of lens and iridodonesis, myopia, spontaneous retinal detachment, blue sclerae.

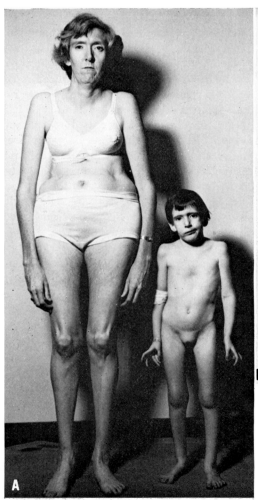

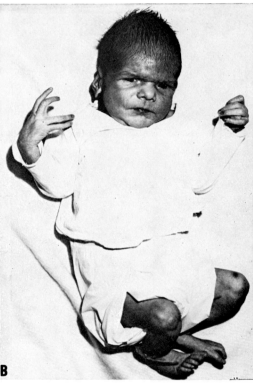

Figure 7-28. (A) Marfan syndrome in mother and daughter. (B). Marfan syndrome in infancy. Note long fingers and toes as early expression of the syndrome.

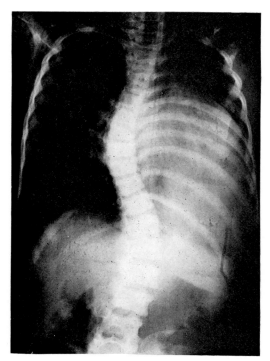

Figure 7-29. Prominent scoliosis in four-year-old girl with Marfan syndrome.

Musculoskeletal. Frequent hypotonia and muscular underdevelopment. Long, thin extremities, kyphoscoliosis and joint laxity. Pectus excavatum or carinatum. Ratio of upper segment (vertex to pubis) to lower segment (pubis to sole) less than normal for age (e.g., 0.85 instead of 0.93 in white adult males). Arm span is greater than height. Hand-height ratio greater than 11%; foot-height ratio greater than 15%. Increased metacarpal index (length/width). Frequent inguinal and femoral hernias.

Cardiovascular. Aortic cystic medial necrosis with dissecting aneurysm; aortic dilatation with aortic valvular insufficiency; aneurysms (with rupture) of sinuses of Valsalva. Mitral insufficiency secondary to redundancy or rupture of chordae tendineae. Medial degeneration of pulmonary arteries with dissection. Progressive dilatation of pulmonary arteries.

Laboratory. The presence of metachromatic granules in fibroblast cultures in some familial cases and the absence of granules in other familial cases and sporadic cases suggest the possibility of subdividing the Marfan syndrome on clinical and laboratory grounds. Those with metachromatic granules apparently have a higher proportion of hyaluronic acid in cultured cells. Unfortunately, the absence of metachromatic granules in cells cultured from amniotic fluid does not rule out this disease.

Prevalence. 1:60,000.

Clinical Course. As with some other single mutant gene syndromes the Marfan syndrome may be regarded as an **abiotrophy.** That is, many of the features may not be present at birth, but may become manifest over a period of years. This is particularly true of the cardiovascular abnormalities, which are usually responsible for the premature deaths of these patients. Death may occur in infancy or childhood, or in early or later adult life, depending on the rate of progression of the cardiovascular disease. Feared complications often responsible for rapid deterioration are dissecting aneurysms of the aorta, ruptured sinus of Valsalva and ruptured mitral chordae tendineae. More gradual deterioration may be found in patients who have progressive aortic or mitral regurgitation. It is interesting to note that the cardiovascular complication tends to be the same within a given family.

Treatment. Symptomatic and supportive. Surgical intervention for aortic aneurysm and aortic and mitral valvular disease.

Differential Diagnosis. *Homocystinuria.* Differentiating points found in homocystinuria are: presence of homocystine in the urine, the high frequency of mental retardation, inferior nasal subluxation of the lens, thrombosis of medium-sized arteries, and osteoporosis.

METAPHYSEAL DYSOSTOSIS (SCHMID TYPE)[26]

The most common form of metaphyseal dysostosis is the dominantly inherited Schmid type, although there are other types, the inheritance of which are not clearly es-

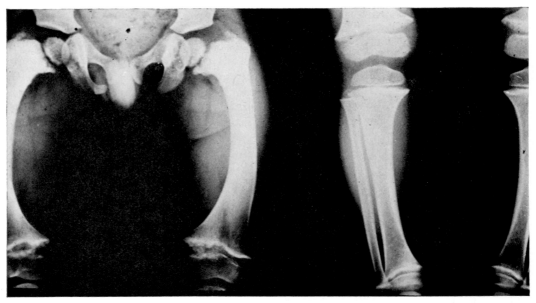

Figure 7-30. Radiographic findings in metaphyseal dysostosis (Schmid type). Note bowing and irregularities at metaphyseal ends of long bones.

tablished (some with dominant pedigrees and some with recessive). The most striking clinical feature is the bowing of the legs (Fig. 7-30). Lower tibial bowing, coxa vara and waddling gait become noticeable when the patient starts to stand and walk, but spontaneous improvement during childhood may be expected. Irregularities of the metaphyseal ends of the long bones are demonstrable radiologically. As points of differentiation from achrondroplasia, the skull is not affected and the radiographic changes in the spine and pelvis are not present.

MYOTONIA

Two myotonic disorders that are inherited as autosomal dominant diseases deserve mention. Only one of these, myotonic dystrophy, is progressive and severely disabling.

Myotonic Dystrophy (Steinert Disease)[27]

This illness may occur in childhood, but is more likely to be recognized in early adult life. There is difficulty in relaxing con-

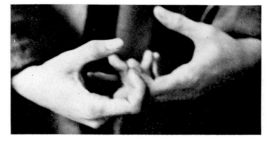

Figure 7-31. Difficulty in relaxing contracted muscles of hands in myotonic dystrophy.

tracted muscles, often first noticed in the jaw or hand (Fig. 7-31). Muscle wasting and weakness follows. Involvement of the facial muscles produces the expressionless facies of myotonia dystrophica. Cataracts develop, which may be detected initially as iridescent flecks. Frontal baldness is characteristic in males. This disorder, which affects males and females equally, produces hypogonadism in both sexes. The male has testicular atrophy and the female has amenorrhea, dysmenorrhea and ovarian cysts. Cardiac arrhythmias, conduction defects and congestive heart failure are common. Mental deterioration is also a feature. Death occurs in the fourth, fifth or sixth decades and is often related to pneumonia or congestive heart failure. Corticosteroids, quinine and procaine amide have been suggested to provide symptomatic improvement. Linkage with the secretor locus will provide opportunity for prenatal diagnosis.

Myotonia Congenita (Thomsen Disease)[28]

This disorder is more of an annoyance than a serious disability. Symptoms (difficulty in relaxing contracted muscles) begin in childhood. The voluntary muscles, especially of the limbs and trunk, hypertrophy. The myotonia, which is most severe on the first contraction, diminishes after a period of "warming up." The affected individual learns to avoid sudden movements, fatigue, chills and excitement, which exacerbate the myotonia. The disease may be distinguished from myotonic dystrophy by its lack of progression, absence of cataracts, hypogonadism, mental deterioration, frontal baldness, and the presence of muscle hypertrophy. Life expectancy is normal. Symptomatic improvement has been gained by treatment with corticosteroids, chlorthiazides (potassium depletion), quinine and procaine amide.

NAIL-PATELLA SYNDROME[29]

The nails, especially on the thumb, are hypoplastic or sometimes absent; the patellae are hypoplastic or absent. There may be hypoplasia of the fibular head, lateral condyle, elbows and scapulae. Iliac spurs are common. Cloverleaf pigmentation of the inner iris margin occurs in about half the cases; occasionally keratoconus, cataracts and ptosis occur. Nephropathy, resulting in proteinuria or in overt renal disease (30%) with glomerulonephritic pathology may be fatal. The major disability is the limitation in joint mobility and the complicating osteoarthritis. The nail-patella locus is linked to the ABO blood group locus with a recombination frequency of about 10%.

NEPHROPATHY WITH DEAFNESS (ALPORT SYNDROME)[30]

The progressive renal disease ranges from acute glomerulonephritis to interstitial pyelonephritis; there may be early onset nerve deafness, and occasionally defects of the anterior chamber of the eye or cataract. It is usually more severe in males than females, who are often asymptomatic. There are unusual features of the genetic segregation. Risk of developing overt renal disease approaches one in two for offspring of affected females and daughters of affected males, but is much lower (about one in eight) for sons of affected males. If the gene carrier is asymptomatic the risk is lower.

NEUROFIBROMATOSIS (VON RECKLINGHAUSEN DISEASE)[31,32]

This disorder, first recognized and reported by von Recklinghausen in 1882, is one of the most common diseases produced by single mutant genes.

Diagnostic Features. *General.* Variable manifestations. Intellectual impairment in 10%. Equal sex distribution. Occasional excessive limb growth.

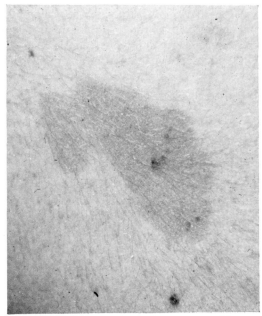

Figure 7-32. Café-au-lait spot in neurofibromatosis.

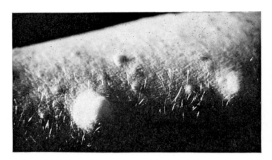

Figure 7-33. Skin tumors in neurofibromatosis.

Skin. Café-au-lait spots; 75% of patients have six or more spots more than 1.5 cm. across (Fig. 7-32). Neurofibromatous tumors occur subcutaneously along nerves; molluscum fibrosum; axillary freckles; occasionally lipomata, angiomata (Fig. 7-33).

Eyes. Rarely tumors of the eyelid, optic disc, retinal detachment, buphthalmos, exophthalmos, glaucoma, corneal opacity.

C.N.S. Tumors of brain, cranial nerves, and spinal cord—gliomas and cysts. Seizures in 12%.

Skeletal. Subperiosteal cysts (Fig. 7-34), scoliosis, bowing of lower leg, rib fusion, local overgrowth.

Cardiovascular. Rarely, hypertension secondary to pheochromocytoma; neurofibroma of heart and pulmonic stenosis.

Other. Occasional neurofibroma of kidney, stomach, tongue; acromegaly; sexual precocity.

X-ray. Subperiosteal cysts, scoliosis, scalloping of vertebral bodies, rib fusion.

Prevalence. 1:3,000. About 50% of patients represent fresh mutations.

Clinical Course. Café-au-lait spots are frequently the first clue to the presence of this disorder. Subcutaneous tumors may be noted later. Almost half of the patients will eventually experience neurologic problems. Nerve compression involving the optic nerve may lead to blindness.

Treatment. Surgical relief of tumor compression, excision of pheochromocytoma and general supportive care.

Differential Diagnosis. Disorders in

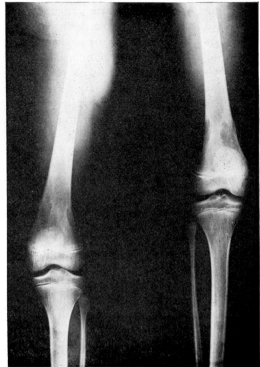

Figure 7-34. Lesions of long bones in neurofibromatosis.

which café-au-lait spots and neurologic deficits occur, such as tuberous sclerosis, must be distinguished from patients having neurofibromatosis. See also multiple mucosal neuromas.

NEUROMAS, MULTIPLE MUCOSAL[33]

In this rare condition a characteristic facies is associated with mucosal neuromas or neurofibromas and a high risk of developing pheochromocytoma or carcinoma of the thyroid. Sometimes the build is marfanoid. The face is acromegaloid with thick, protuberant lips, with neuromas scattered over the mucosal surface of lips, buccal mucosa, anterior tongue, nostril and conjunctiva (Figs. 7-35, 7-36). The upper eyelid margin tends to be everted. It is probably distinct from neurofibromatosis. Most cases are sporadic but dominant transmission occurs.

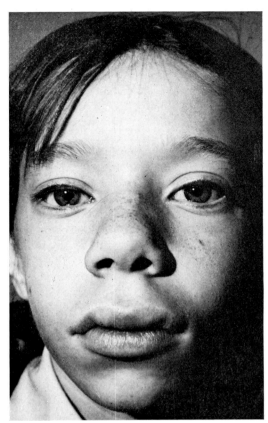

Figure 7-35. Acromegaloid facies and protuberant lips of multiple mucosal neuromas.

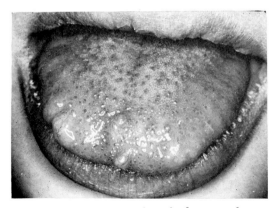

Figure 7-36. Tongue with multiple mucosal neuromas.

OCULODENTODIGITAL (ODD) SYNDROME[34]

As the name for this rare syndrome implies, there are abnormalities of the eyes (microphthalmos, microcornea, occasionally small palpebral fissures, epicanthic folds), teeth (enamel hypoplasia, occasional micro- or anodontia), and digits (camptodactyly of the fifth digits, hypoplasia or absence of the midphalanx of the second through fifth toes, syndactyly of the fourth and fifth fingers and the third and fourth toes). The alae nasae are thin and the nares small; the tubular bones are broad and the mandible has a wide alveolar ridge. Glaucoma, conductive hearing loss and cleft lip and palate are occasionally present. Mental retardation is not a feature.

OSTEOGENESIS IMPERFECTA[35]

History. In 1788, Ekman reported the occurrence of brittle bones in three generations. Since then, numerous reports stressing various aspects of the syndrome—brittle bones, blue sclerae and deafness—have cluttered the literature with many alternative eponyms and descriptive names.

Diagnostic Features. *General.* Normal intelligence. Equal sex distribution. Stature short to severely malformed and dwarfed. Increased metabolic rate, hyperthermia, excessive sweating.

Head. Thin, bulging calvarium, open fontanelles, overhanging occiput and temporal areas (helmet-head). Multiple wormian bones. Translucent teeth, predisposition to caries.

Eyes. Blue sclerae, occasional keratoconus, megalocornea, embryotoxon.

Ears. Deafness, otosclerotic, usually not beginning until adulthood.

Musculoskeletal. Frequent fractures with normal healing rate, leading to bowing of the legs, pseudoarthroses, "hourglass" vertebrae, kyphoscoliosis (Figs. 7-37, 7-38). Pectus excavatum and carinatum, hyperextensible joints. Long bones have thin cortex, slender shaft, abrupt widening at epiphyses, osteoporosis.

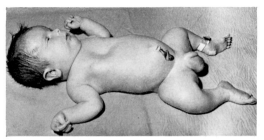

Figure 7-37. Newborn with osteogenesis imperfecta and deformities of multiple fractures at birth.

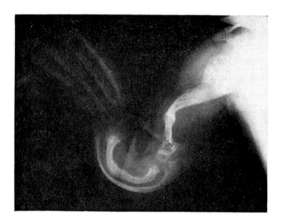

Figure 7-38. Fracture deformities of arm of newborn with osteogenesis imperfecta.

Cardiovascular. Premature arteriosclerosis. Mucoid, valvular changes.

Skin. Thin, translucent; capillary fragility.

Prevalence: 1:60,000.

Clinical Course. In **osteogenesis imperfecta tarda,** fractures may be present at birth or begin in infancy or childhood. The patient may have had dozens of fractures by puberty, when there is a trend to improvement. Frequent fractures (and the basic connective tissue disturbance?) may result in severe dwarfing. Some carriers of the gene may have only blue sclerae, and some may have no signs (incomplete penetrance). There may be a variant without blue sclerae (Lobstein's osteopsathyrosis), also dominant; whether this is a different allele or a different locus is not known.

Osteogenesis imperfecta congenita lethalis of Vrolik is much more severe than the tarda type, involving numerous fractures *in utero,* deformed long bones and a skull that crackles on pressure. In at least some cases there is recessive inheritance. Counseling of a sporadic case of osteogenesis imperfecta is therefore difficult. If there are fractures at birth, one must decide between an early onset tarda type or the true congenita type. If it is the tarda type, it may be a fresh mutation (low recurrence risk) or there may be reduced penetrance in a parent. We counsel a fairly low but not negligible risk if there are no other cases of blue sclerae or bone fragility in the family. If the baby has the congenita type, the likelihood of recessive inheritance must be considered. More data are needed.

Treatment. Symptomatic and supportive. The beneficial effects of large doses of magnesium on the postulated metabolic error are being studied.

Differential Diagnosis. The most difficult disorder to distinguish from osteogenesis imperfecta is pycnodysostosis. However, the absence of blue sclerae, the recessive inheritance and the severe micrognathia favor the diagnosis of pycnodysostosis. On the basis of these differences, Maroteaux and Lamy have suggested that Toulouse-Lautrec suffered from pycnodysostosis rather than osteogenesis imperfecta.

PARAMYOTONIA CONGENITA (EULENBURG DISEASE)[36]

This is a rare disease in which symptoms are present from infancy. Exposure to cold triggers the myotonia, especially of the face and limbs. Prolonged exposure to cold produces progression through myotonia to flaccid weakness. Even cold food may cause slurring of speech. The frequency and severity of the episodes appear to diminish with age. Normal life expectancy and normal functioning is the rule. Avoidance of chilling is the major consideration in prophylactic management.

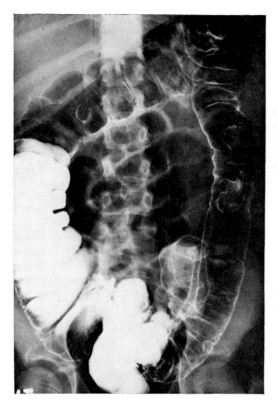

Figure 7-39. Radiographic evidence of polyps in colon of patient with polyposis I.

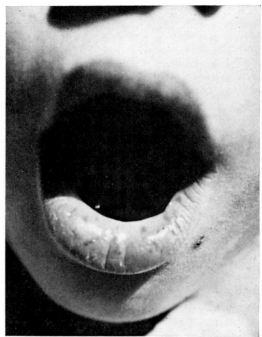

Figure 7-40. Pigmented spots on lips of child with polyposis II (Peutz-Jeghers syndrome).

POLYPOSIS OF THE COLON (INTESTINAL POLYPOSIS I)[37]

In this disorder the manifestations are restricted to the colon (Fig. 7-39). Malignant change may occur as early as the second decade. Gastrointestinal bleeding and diarrhea may be presenting complaints. Colectomy is required. First degree relatives of affected individuals should have regular examinations.

POLYPOSIS, JEJUNAL (PEUTZ-JEGHERS SYNDROME; INTESTINAL POLYPOSIS II)[38]

Pigmented spots (blue-gray or brown) appear in infancy or early childhood and have a tendency to fade in the adult. These spots, which are located on the lips, perioral area, buccal mucous membranes and fingers, serve as sentinel signs of the syndrome (Fig. 7-40). Benign polyps are located mainly in the jejunum but occasionally elsewhere in the intestine, bladder and respiratory tract. Colicky abdominal pain, gastrointestinal bleeding and intussusception are complications of the disease, which usually appear in childhood, but malignant transformation of the polyps is rare.

POLYPOSIS WITH OSTEOMATA AND SKIN TUMORS (GARDNER SYNDROME; INTESTINAL POLYPOSIS III)[39]

Sebaceous and epidermal inclusion cysts of the face, scalp and back and osteomata of face, jaw and calvarium are the lesions associated with intestinal polyps in this syndrome. The adenomatous polyps are usually present in the colon or rectum but may occasionally be found in the stomach or small intestine. Carcinoma develops in almost half of the individuals with this syndrome,

PORPHYRIAS, HEPATIC[40]

In **acute intermittent porphyria** (known as the "Swedish type," but not restricted to Swedes), there are no skin lesions. Acute colicky abdominal pain and neuropathic attacks occur, which may be precipitated by barbiturates. Porphobilinogen is always present in the urine and uroporphyrin may appear later in the attack, turning the urine burgundy red. In **porphyria variegata** (the "South African type," but worldwide in distribution), in addition to the acute visceral and neurologic attacks, there is photosensitivity with cutaneous lesions developing on exposure to the sun. In **porphyria cutanea tarda**, the visceral complaints are much milder than in porphyria variegata. These three types almost always become symptomatic after puberty. **Hereditary coproporphyria** resembles acute intermittent porphyria except that symptoms may begin in childhood and coproporphyrin III is present in large amounts in the feces.

Avoidance of precipitating factors such as barbiturates, alcohol and sunlight is an important aspect of the treatment. The acute episode may terminate fatally with neurologic damage and water and electrolyte imbalance. Personality changes, "hysteria" and "neurosis," are described in patients having visceral attacks. Needless to say, the diagnosis must be made correctly to avoid the disaster of sedating such a "hysterical" patient with barbiturates.

SICKLE CELL TRAIT[41]

Sickle cell trait, the heterozygous manifestation of the gene for sickle cell disease, is inherited as a dominant and produces relatively little disability when compared with the homozygous form. The trait is present in about one of 11 North American blacks, most of whom are asymptomatic but may exhibit a mild chronic anemia. Certain stress situations may be fatal, however, as illustrated by the death of four black heterozygote army recruits at Fort Bliss, Texas, in 1970. Under lowered oxygen tension, as experienced in unpressurized aircraft or parachute drops, heterozygotes may develop symptoms similar to homozygotes or even infarction of the spleen. Sickledex and dithionite tests appear to be useful for screening and confirmation is made by hemoglobin electrophoresis. Some sickle cell disease researchers feel that sickle cell screening tests should be legally required premaritally, so that heterozygous couples could be advised of their high risk of having children with sickle cell disease.

SPHEROCYTOSIS, CONGENITAL[42]

Congenital spherocytosis is a chronic hemolytic anemia in which the red blood cells are spheroid in shape and have increased osmotic fragility (Fig. 7-41). The disorder is highly variable, appearing clinically shortly after birth in some individuals and not until adulthood, if at all, in others. Splenomegaly is usually present. Infections can lead to crises associated with more severe anemia, weakness, pallor and other symptoms, depending upon the degree of anemia. These crises result from temporary bone marrow aplasia with no new red blood cell production. Diagnosis depends on demonstration of spherocytes in the peripheral blood and increased osmotic fragility, sometimes demonstrable only after incubation at 37° C for 24 hours. Treatment consists of splenectomy, which is beneficial only because it lengthens the red cell life span but carries the risk of increased susceptibility to infection. Spherocytosis and increased osmotic fragility persist following splenec-

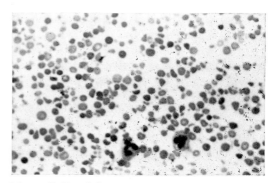

Figure 7-41. Spherocytosis.

tomy. The counseling is complicated by reduced penetrance; carriers may be detected only by special tests, such as autohemolysis, or sometimes not at all. About 20% of cases are sporadic, presumably representing fresh mutations.

SPONDYLOEPIPHYSEAL DYSPLASIA, PSEUDOACHONDROPLASTIC FORM[43,44]

These patients appear to be normal at birth. The prominent forehead and scooped-out nose of classic achondroplasia is not present. As the patient reaches the age when walking begins, a peculiar waddling gait is observed. Growth is slow and the eventual height attainment is of the order of three feet. Lumbar lordosis, scoliosis, bowing of the lower extremities, short tubular bones and a limitation in joint mobility is found; at this stage they may be misdiagnosed as having Morquio disease. The patients have normal intelligence.

Radiographic findings include flattened, irregular vertebral bodies, mushroomed metaphyses with "ball-in-socket" epiphyses and spatulate ribs. The characteristic facies of achondroplasia and the cystic masses in the auricles of the ears of diastrophic dwarfs help to differentiate these syndromes from spondyloepiphyseal dysplasia.

TELANGIECTASIA, OSLER HEREDITARY[45]

Telangiectases are the characteristic feature, most commonly occurring on nasal mucosa, face, conjunctiva, nailbeds, and fingertips; occasionally they affect the brain, lungs, liver and gastrointestinal tract. Bleeding may occur from any of the sites of vascular abnormality, but most often comes from the nose.

THALASSEMIA MINOR

The heterozygous form of thalassemia major is usually an asymptomatic disorder and detected either through family studies or some other problem. A few patients have moderate anemia. Morphologic changes of the red cells on peripheral blood smears are usually disproportionate to the hemoglobin level. No treatment is indicated.

TUBEROUS SCLEROSIS[46]

This disorder of skin, brain and bones, sometimes incorrectly referred to as adenoma sebaceum, has been recognized in the world literature for approximately 100 years.

Diagnostic Features. *General.* Mild to severe intellectual impairment. Equal sex distribution. Normal growth. Seizures beginning in childhood. The signs and symptoms are highly variable, and the condition often goes unrecognized.

Skin. Adenoma sebaceum in a "butterfly" distribution on the face (Fig. 7-42). Shagreen (granular, untanned leather) patches on trunk, depigmented patches (Fig. 7-43), café-au-lait spots, hemangiomas, fibromas.

Eyes. Retinal lesions, nodular, cystic or phacomatous; unequal pupils may be associated with CNS lesions in some patients.

C.N.S. Intracranial mineralization; cortical gliomas and angiomas.

Skeletal. Bone cysts, especially in hands.

Visceral. Rhabdomyomas of the heart or kidney; tumors or hemangiomas of kidney, liver, spleen or lung.

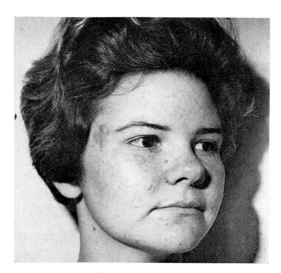

Figure 7-42. Adenoma sebaceum of face in patient with tuberous sclerosis.

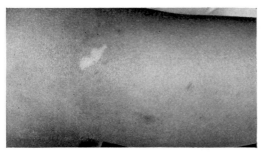

Figure 7-43. Depigmented area on leg as first sign of tuberous sclerosis presenting in the child of the patient in Figure 7-42.

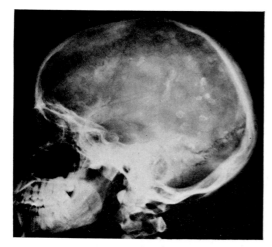

Figure 7-44. Intracranial calcifications in tuberous sclerosis.

X-ray. Intracranial calcifications (Fig. 7-44), bone cysts of the hand, abnormal IVP. A pneumogram may reveal the characteristic tumors.

Laboratory. Abnormal EEG.

Clinical Course. The earliest manifestation of this disorder may be convulsions. In the infant having seizures there may not yet be adenoma sebaceum, fibrous nodules of the face or shagreen skin, but small depigmented patches of the skin should alert the physician to this diagnosis. Examination with a Woods light is useful in detecting the depigmented areas. Screening of any patient with mental retardation or seizures of unknown cause, and the parents, is rec-

ommended. Intracranial calcification may also take years to become evident by x-ray. The seizures may become progressively harder to control and behavioral problems and intellectual deficiencies declare themselves with increasing involvement of the brain. Over one-third of the patients function at a satisfactory level in adult life maintaining homes and jobs, although requiring anticonvulsant therapy.

Cardiac arrhythmias and obstruction secondary to the rhabdomyomas of the heart present a threat to life, although not as frequent a threat as status epilepticus. Tumors of the kidney are found in many patients and space-occupying intracranial tumors in a small percentage of individuals with this disorder.

Treatment. Anticonvulsant therapy. Anti-arrhythmic therapy (for cardiac arrhythmias); surgical excision of operable tumors; custodial care for the severely affected patients.

Differential Diagnosis. This condition should be considered in cases of unexplained mental retardation or seizures. Other disorders associated with convulsions, skin lesions and intracranial calcifications, such as Sturge-Weber syndrome, von Hippel-Lindau syndrome, Maffucci syndrome and neurofibromatosis are readily distinguishable on clinical and radiologic grounds.

THE ULLRICH-NOONAN SYNDROME (XX AND XY TURNER PHENOTYPE, ULLRICH, BONNEVIE-ULLRICH, PTERYGIUM COLLI SYNDROME)[47]

This syndrome shares many features of the XO Turner syndrome, but whether there is any etiologic relationship is debatable. For the purposes of genetic counseling it is treated as an autosomal dominant disease, although there is much that is unexplained. Ullrich-Noonan syndrome is estimated to be at least twice as common as the XO Turner syndrome and may have a population frequency between 1:1,000 and 1:2,500.

The majority of the findings are the same in the Turner and Ullrich-Noonan syndromes (see Table 7-2). Those features

TABLE 7-2. Features of the Ullrich-Noonan Syndrome*

Area	Findings
General	Female or male. Normal life expectancy except as modified by cardiovascular disease. Small stature not invariable; **chromatin-positive female.**
Neurologic	Intellectual development is fair to good but usually below that of siblings; occasional hearing loss.
Head	Characteristic facies; narrow maxilla, small mandible.
Eyes	Frequent epicanthic folds, **ptosis and hypertelorism.**
Ears	Usually prominent, fleshy, posteriorly rotated and low-set.
Neck	Webbed in about 50% of patients; low posterior hairline.
Chest	Shield-shaped; widely spaced hypoplastic nipples; breast development variable in females.
Cardiovascular	Anomalies in approximately 35%; **pulmonic stenosis** is most common; coarctation of aorta rarely occurs. **IHHS and pulmonary branch stenosis** frequently found.
Extremities	Cubitus valgus; lymphedema of dorsum of hands and feet in infancy; dystrophic nails; short fifth finger with clinodactyly.
Urogenital	Variable fertility. Ovarian dysgenesis and infertility in some females, **normal fertility in others.** Cryptorchism in the usually infertile male.
Skeletal	Pectus excavatum frequent; scoliosis, kyphosis in about 20%, sometimes Klippel-Feil syndrome.
Skin and Nails	Pigmented nevi frequent; marked **tendency to keloid formation** (beware if correcting webs or ptosis); nails dystrophic, short, wide, not convex.
Dermatoglyphics	Distal axial triradius; ridge count not increased.
Incidence	Undetermined but estimated to be between 1:1,000 and 1:2,500.

* Many findings are similar or identical to those observed in the XO Turner syndrome. Features that help to distinguish between the syndromes are in **bold face.**

that are useful in distinguishing the syndromes will be emphasized. First, female patients with the Ullrich-Noonan syndrome are chromatin-positive, but this does not rule out Turner syndrome resulting from mosaicism or structural anomalies of the X chromosome (discussed in Chapter 4).

Small stature, characteristic facial features, webbing of the neck, cubitus valgus, lymphedema and other classic Turner stigmata are found in the Ullrich-Noonan syndrome (see Figs. 7-45 to 7-48). Some female patients having Ullrich-Noonan may be over 60 inches tall, but they are often significantly shorter than their sibs. The males are often between 66 and 70 inches in height, but again they are usually significantly shorter than their male sibs. Ptosis and ocular hypertelorism are perhaps more common in the Ullrich-Noonan than in the Turner syndrome.

The cardiovascular anomalies are useful differentiating findings. The Ullrich-Noonan patient has pulmonic stenosis and rarely coarctation of the aorta, which is just the opposite of the XO Turner syndrome. However, XO Turner mosaics may have pulmonic stenosis. A number of other heart lesions may be found in either type of patient, but there is almost no overlap with respect to pulmonic stenosis and coarctation of the aorta. One important heart lesion recently recognized in Ullrich-Noonan patients is idiopathic hypertrophic subaortic stenosis (IHSS), which may be missed because it is obscured by pulmonic stenosis. A clue to the presence of IHSS is the electrocardiographic finding of left axis deviation. Pulmonary artery branch stenosis is also common in Ullrich-Noonan syndrome.

Although some patients with Ullrich-

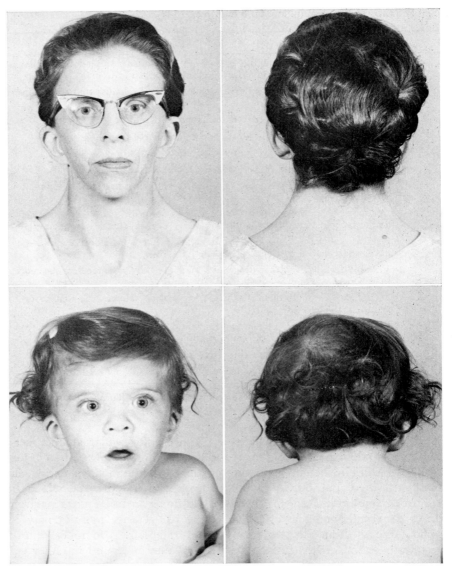

Figure 7-45. Characteristic facial features of Ullrich-Noonan syndrome in mother and daughter. (From Nora, J.J. and Sinha, A.K.: Amer. J. Dis. Child., 116:345, 1968. Copyright 1968, American Medical Association.)

Noonan syndrome may have a lower than average ridge count, and the Turner patients an increase, there is so much overlap in the distributions that the difference is not useful for discriminating the individual case.

In regard to fertility, although some female patients with Ullrich-Noonan syndrome have streak gonads, many do not. They may develop secondary sexual characteristics and reproduce. The authors have personally seen 13 female patients who have given birth to a total of 29 children, 13 of whom had Turner stigmata (eight girls and five boys). Cryptorchism is a characteristic finding in the males, most of whom are infertile. The authors have now seen two males with many stigmata of the Ullrich-

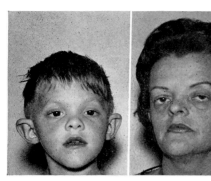

Figure 7-46. Ullrich-Noonan syndrome in mother and son. (From Nora, J. J. and Sinha, A. K.: Birth Defects: Original Article Series 5(No. 5):29, 1969. The National Foundation, New York.)

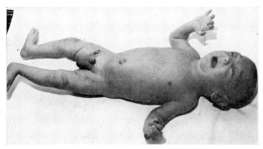

Figure 7-47. Full length view of male infant with Ullrich-Noonan syndrome.

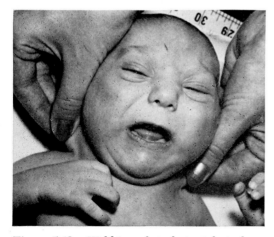

Figure 7-48. Webbing of neck in infant shown in Figure 7-47.

Noonan syndrome who have transmitted these features—one to a male offspring and one to a male and a female offspring. Orchiopexy has been attempted in a number of males with this syndrome and has been almost entirely unsuccessful. The infertility of the male, however, is not associated with lack of virilization. Many of these males are heavily muscled.

Intellectual achievement in patients with the Ullrich-Noonan syndrome is variable as it is in the Turner syndrome, in both cases being compatible with high intelligence or moderate mental retardation. We have the clinical impression that the usual patient with Ullrich-Noonan syndrome falls slightly to moderately below the midparent I.Q.

The clinical course is influenced to a great extent by the presence or absence of cardiovascular disease. In its absence normal life expectancy can be predicted. The counseling of individuals with Ullrich-Noonan syndrome must approach the questions of fertility and transmission of the disease. For the female, the probability that she is fertile appears to be reasonably good. The male is most likely to be infertile. The findings of direct transmission from male to male and female of many features of the syndrome in two families favors autosomal dominant inheritance. However, the possibility of homologous loci on the X and Y chromosomes exists; if so, a mutant gene or submicroscopic deletion in this region could be the explanation.

VON HIPPEL-LINDAU SYNDROME[48]

This disorder, affecting mainly the eye and cerebellum, is not usually manifest in childhood. Retinal angiomata may be discovered in the third decade, at which time cerebellar signs may also become apparent. Hemangioblastoma is most commonly found in the cerebellum, but also occurs in the spinal cord. Cyst formation and calcification are not uncommon. Hemangiomata also arise in the adrenal, lung, liver, kidney, and face. Pheochromocytoma is an occasional lesion, which sometimes leads to the combination of hypertension with intracranial angiomata, producing subarachnoid hemorrhage.

VON WILLEBRAND DISEASE[49]

Von Willebrand disease (vascular hemophilia) is characterized by a capillary defect and an absence of factor VIII (the antihemophiliac globulin). Platelets may exhibit decreased adhesiveness. Clinical features include nosebleeds, bruising and bleeding following trauma. The bleeding time is prolonged and the tourniquet test is usually positive. Fresh plasma or cryoprecipitate may be useful in controlling bleeding at times when surgery may be indicated.

WAARDENBURG SYNDROME[50]

This pattern of anomalies was first reported by Waardenburg in 1951.

Diagnostic Features. *General.* Normal intelligence. Equal sex distribution. Normal growth. The features of the syndrome may not all be present in each patient.

Skin. Occasional patches of vitiligo.

Head. White forelock, premature graying of hair in about one third of patients; medial overgrowth of eyebrows.

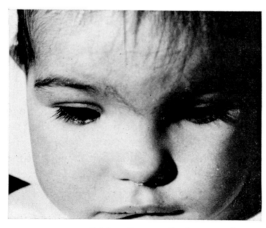

Figure 7-49. Child with Waardenburg syndrome. Note lateral displacement of median canthi, medial overgrowth of eyebrows and broad nasal bridge.

Eyes. Lateral displacement of median canthi, pale irises or heterochromia of irises (e.g., one blue eye and one brown eye).

Nose. Broad, high nasal bridge.

C.N.S. Congenital deafness.

Prevalence. 1:42,000 (in Holland).

Clinical Course. Only about 20% of patients have congenital deafness. The white forelock may appear early in childhood or not until adult life, and may even become pigmented after having been white. About one third of Waardenburg's original probands did not have affected parents and presumably represented fresh mutations.

Treatment. Hearing aids may benefit selected patients.

REFERENCES

Achondroplasia
1. Mörch, E. T.: Chondrodystrophic dwarfs in Denmark. Copenhagen, E. Munksgaard, 1941.

Acrocephalosyndactyly (Apert Syndrome)
2. Blank, C. E.: Apert's syndrome (a type of acrocephalosyndactyly). Observations on British series of thirty-nine cases. Ann. Hum. Genet., 24:151, 1960.

Acrocephalopolysyndactyly, Type I (Noack Syndrome)
3. Noack, M.: Ein beitrag zum krankheitsbild der akrozephalosyndaktylie (Apert). Arch. Kinderheilk., 160:168, 1959.

Brachydactyly
4. Bell, J.: On brachydactyly and symphalangism. *In* Treasury of Human Inheritance. vol. 5. London, Cambridge University Press, 1951.

Cardiac Arrhythmia (Romano-Ward Syndrome)
5. Garza, L. A., *et al.*: Heritable QT prolongation without deafness. Circulation, 41:39, 1970.

Cleft Lip with Lip Pits
6. Bowers, D. G.: Congenital lower lip sinuses with cleft palate. Plast. Reconstr. Surg., 45:151, 1970.

Cleidocranial Dysostosis
7. Lasker, G. W.: The inheritance of cleidocranial dysostosis. Hum. Biol., 18:103, 1946.

Cranio-Carpo-Tarsal Dysplasia
8. Fraser, F. C., Pashayan, H., and Kadish, M. E.: Cranio-carpo-tarsal dysplasia. JAMA, 211:1374, 1970.

Craniofacial Dysostosis (Crouzon Disease)
9. Vulliamy, D. G., and Normandale, P. A.: Craniofacial dysostosis in a Dorset family. Arch. Dis. Child., 41:375, 1966.

Deafness, Dominant Forms
10. Konigsmark, B. W.: Hereditary deafness in man. New Eng. J. Med., 281:713, 774, 827, 1969.

Deafness, Cardiac Disease, Freckles, (Leopard Syndrome)
11. Gorlin, R. J., Anderson, R. C. and Blaw, M.: Multiple lentigenes syndrome. Complex comprising multiple lentigenes, electrocardiographic conduction abnormalities, ocular hypertelorism, pulmonary stenosis, abnormalities of genitalia, retardation of growth, sensorineural deafness and autosomal dominant hereditary pattern. Amer. J. Dis. Child., 117:652, 1969.

Ectodermal Dysplasia, Hidrotic (Clouston Type)
12. Williams, M., and Fraser, F. C.: Hidrotic ectodermal dysplasia—Clouston's family revisited. Canad. Med. Assoc. J., 96:36, 1967.

Ectodermal Dysplasia (Robinson Type)
13. Robinson, G. C., Miller, J. R., and Bensimon, J. R.: Familial ectodermal dysplasia with sensorineural deafness and other anomalies. Pediatrics, 30:797, 1962.

Elliptocytosis
14. Geerdink, R. A., Nijenhuis, L. E. and Huizinga, J.: Hereditary elliptocytosis, linkage data in man. Ann. Hum. Genet., 30:363, 1967.

Epidermolysis Bullosa
15. Davison, B. C. C.: Epidermolysis bullosa. J. Med. Genet., 2:233, 1965.

Fibrodysplasia Ossificans Progressiva
16. McKusick, V. A.: Heritable Disorders of Connective Tissue. 3rd ed. St. Louis, C.V. Mosby, 1966.

Heart and Hand Syndrome (Holt-Oram)
17. Holt, M. and Oram, S.: Familial heart disease with skeletal malformations. Brit. Heart J., 22:236, 1960.

Hemoglobin M Disease
18. Gerald, P. S., and Efrom, M. L.: Chemical studies of several varieties of HbM. Proc. Nat. Acad. Sci., 47:1758, 1961.

Huntington's Chorea
19. Myrianthopoulos, N. C.: Huntington's chorea. J. Med. Genet., 3: 298, 1966.

Hyperbilirubinemia I (Gilbert Disease)
20. Powell, L. W., et al.: Idiopathic unconjugated hyperbilirubinemia (Gilbert's syndrome). A study of 42 families. New Eng. J. Med., 277:1108, 1967.

Hyperelastosis Cutis (Ehlers-Danlos Syndrome)
21. Barabas, A. P.: Heterogeneity of the Ehlers-Danlos syndrome: description of three clinical types and a hypothesis to explain the basic defect(s). Brit. Med. J., 1:612, 1967.

Lymphedema, Hereditary (Milroy and Meige Types)
22. Esterly, J. R.: Congenital hereditary lymphoedema. J. Med. Genet., 2:93, 1965.
23. Goodman, R. M.: Familial lymphedema of the Meige's type. Amer. J. Med. Genet., 32:651, 1962.

Mandibulofacial Dysostosis (Treacher Collins Syndrome)
24. Rovin, S., et al.: Mandibulo-facial dysostosis, a familial study of five generations. J. Pediat., 65:215, 1964.

Marfan Syndrome (Arachnodactyly)
25. McKusick, V. A.: Heritable Disorders of Connective Tissue. 3rd ed. St. Louis, C.V. Mosby, 1966.

Metaphyseal Dysostosis (Schmid Type)
26. Rosenbloom, A. L. and Smith, D. W.: The natural history of metaphyseal dysostosis. J. Pediat., 66:857, 1965.

Myotonic Dystrophy (Steinert Disease)
27. Caughey, J. E., and Myrianthopoulos, N. C.: Dystrophia Myotonica and Related Disorders. Springfield, Ill., Charles C Thomas, 1963.

Myotonia Congenita (Thomsen Disease)
28. Thomasen, E.: Myotonia, Thomsen's disease: paramyotonia, and dystrophia myotonica. Op. Ex. Domo Biol. Hered. Hum. U. Hafniensis, 17:11, 1948.

Nail-Patella Syndrome
29. Lucas, G. L. and Opitz, J. M.: The nail-patella syndrome. Clinical and genetic aspects of 5 kindreds with 38 affected family members. J. Pediat., 68:273, 1966.

Nephropathy with Deafness (Alport Syndrome)
30. Preus, M., and Fraser, F. C.: Genetics of hereditary nephropathy with deafness (Alport disease). Clin. Genet., 2:331, 1971.

Neurofibromatosis (von Recklinghausen Disease)
31. Canale, D., Bebin, J., and Knighton, R. S.: Neurologic manifestations of von Recklinghausen's disease of the nervous system. Confin. Neurol., 24:359, 1964.
32. Rosenquist, G. C., et al.: Acquired right ventricular outflow obstruction in a child with neurofibromatosis. Amer. Heart J., 79:103, 1970.

Neuromas, Multiple Mucosal
33. Williams, E. D., and Pollock, D. J.: Multiple mucosal neuromata with endocrine tumors. A syndrome allied to von Recklinghausen's disease. J. Path. Bact., 91:71, 1966.

Oculodentodigital (ODD) Syndrome
34. Gorlin, R. J., Meskin, L. H., and St. Geme, J. W. Oculodentodigital dysplasia. J. Pediat, 63:69, 1963.

Osteogenesis Imperfecta

35. McKusick, V. A.: Heritable Disorders of Connective Tissue. 3rd ed. St. Louis, C.V. Mosby, 1966.

Paramyotonia Congenita (Eulenberg Disease)

36. Drager, G. A., Hammill, J. F., and Shy, G. M.: Paramyotonia congenita. Arch. Neurol. Psychiat., 80:1, 1958.

Polyposis of the Colon (Intestinal Polyposis I)

37. McKusick, V. A.: Genetic factors in intestinal polyposis. JAMA, 182:271, 1962.

Polyposis II (Peutz-Jeghers Syndrome)

38. **Andre, R.,** *et al.*: Syndrome de Peutz-Jeghers avec polypose disophagienne. Bull. Soc. Med. Hop. Paris, 117:505, 1966.

Polyposis III (Gardner Syndrome)

39. Gardner, E. J.: Follow-up study of a family group exhibiting dominant inheritance for a syndrome including intestinal, polyps, osteomas, fibromas and epidermal cysts. Amer. J. Hum. Genet., 14:376, 1962.

Porphyrias, Hepatic

40. Dean, G.: The porphyrias. Brit. Med. Bull., 25:48, 1969.

Sickle Cell Trait

41. Ingram, V. M.: Abnormal human haemoglobin. III. The chemical difference between normal and sickle cell haemoglobins. Biochim. Biophys. Acta, 36:402, 1959.

Spherocytosis, Congenital

42. Morton, N. E., *et al.*: Genetics of spherocytosis. Amer. J. Hum. Genet., 14:170, 1962.

Spondyloepiphyseal Dysplasia

43. **Maroteaux, P., and Lamy, M.: Les Formes** pseudo-achrondroplasiques des dysplasies spondylo-epiphysaires. Presse Med., 67:383, 1959.

44. Lindseth, R. E., *et al.*: Spondylo-epiphyseal dysplasia (pseudoachondroplastic type). Case report with pathologic and metabolic investigations. Amer. J. Dis. Child., 113:721, 1967.

Telangiectasia, Osler Hereditary

45. Bird, R. M., *et al.*: Family reunion: study of hereditary hemorrhagic telangiectasia. New Eng. J. Med., 257:105, 1957.

Tuberous Sclerosis

46. Lagos, J. C., and Gomez, M. R.: Tuberous sclerosis: reappraisal of a clinical entity. Mayo Clin. Proc., 42:26, 1967.

Ullrich-Noonan Syndrome

47. Nora, J. J., and Sinha, A. K.: Direct familial transmission of the Turner phenotype. Amer. J. Dis. Child., 116:343, 1968.

Von Hippel-Lindau Syndrome

48. Christoferson, L. A., Gustafson, M. B., and Peterson, A. G.: Von Hippel-Lindau's disease. JAMA, 178:280, 1961.

Von Willebrand Disease

49. Weiss, H. J.: Von Willebrand's disease—diagnostic criteria. Blood, 32:668, 1968.

Waardenburg Syndrome

50. Di George, A. M., Olmsted, R. W., and Harley, R. D.: Waardenburg's syndrome. J. Pediat., 57:649, 1960.

Chapter 8

AUTOSOMAL RECESSIVE DISEASES

Diseases produced by single mutant genes, whether they are transmitted as dominants or recessives, autosomal or X-linked, are uncommon disorders. The dividing line between common and uncommon diseases is generally taken as 1:1,000. No mendelian disease in the white North American population is more common than 1:1,000, with cystic fibrosis being the closest to this incidence. Sickle-cell disease in black North Americans, which generally exceeds the 1:1,000 incidence and thus qualifies as a common disease, is recognized as a special case as it offers a heterozygote advantage in resistance to malaria.

An autosomal recessive disease is manifested clinically only in the homozygote. In the usual random-mating situation both parents are free of the disease but are heterozygous for the mutant gene. The affected child often appears to be a sporadic case, because it is unlikely that the mutant gene will become homozygous in the parental relatives (unless there is inbreeding), and with the small size of most human families, the one in four risk of recurrence is often not realized.

At the molecular level the mutant gene results in an abnormal or deficient enzyme. This may be illustrated by the disease phenylketonuria. A patient with this disease is homozygous for a mutant form of the gene that specifies phenylalanine hydroxylase and has little or none of this enzyme, which is necessary to maintain a key metabolic pathway. This allows the toxic accumulation of metabolites that damage the central nervous system. The heterozygous parents of the patient each have only about half as much of this enzyme as normals, but this half-dose is sufficient to perform the necessary functions, so they are clinically unaffected.

A typical clinical experience with a patient having an autosomal recessive disorder is the following case of a child with Hurler syndrome.

Clinical Example. These young parents admitted their 18-month-old son for evaluation of his failure to develop normally. His three-year-old sister had walked at 11 months and the patient, who had been able to pull himself to a stand at 12 months, was still not walking without support. The father attributed this to the large protuberant abdomen and the mother thought that arthritis was responsible. Both parents felt that the child did not hear well and commented on the coarsening of his facial appearance. Many classic findings of a mucopolysac-

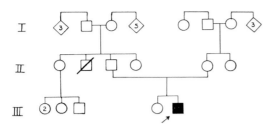

Figure 8-1. Pedigree of patient with Hurler syndrome discussed in case history.

charidosis were apparent, including a "gargoyle" facies, rhinitis, corneal clouding, thoracolumbar gibbus, clawhands, stiffness of knees and hepatosplenomegaly. X-rays revealed beaking of lumbar vertebrae, spatulate ribs and a shoe-shaped sella. A urinary screening test was positive for mucopolysaccharides and a more definitive urinary analysis disclosed both chondroitin sulfate B and heparitin sulfate.

The diagnosis of Hurler syndrome, with its genetic and prognostic implications, was initially difficult for the parents to accept because there was no other family member known to be affected (Fig. 8-1) and because the child had appeared to be normal for so many months. The first concern was to have the patient's older sister examined to be sure she was not developing findings of Hurler syndrome; she was not. The next concern was about the possibility of having another affected child. The risk to the next offspring was presented as being one in four. The parents wanted to accept this risk even before knowing about the possibility of identifying an affected fetus by amniocentesis.

The mother has not yet conceived, but when she does, an amniocentesis will be done at about 16 weeks of gestation to search for the appropriate enzyme deficiency in fetal cells. If this is found, a therapeutic abortion would be recommended. If not, she should be reasonably confident of carrying to term a baby who would not have Hurler syndrome.

The following list of selected, recessively

inherited diseases is intended to inform the reader of the main features and modes of treatment as an indication of what these diseases mean from the counselor's point of view. This discussion should not be regarded as a complete clinical guide to diagnosis and therapy.

ADRENAL CORTICAL HYPERFUNCTION, INHERITED[1]

Excess Androgen Secretion (Adrenogenital Syndrome)

Defect of 21-Hydroxylase. This is by far the most common type of adrenal cortical hyperfunction (about 90% of cases). The defect leads to lack of hydrocortisone, resulting in overproduction of pituitary corticotropin, which leads to adrenocortical hypoplasia with overproduction of metabolites behind the block and of androgens. This results in pseudohermaphroditism in females (Fig. 8-2) and premature virilization in males. In some cases (about 2%) the block is not quite complete and enough hydrocortisone is produced to maintain electrolyte balance. In the others there is loss of sodium with anorexia, vomiting, diarrhea and dehydration. The two types are family-specific. The myocardial effects of

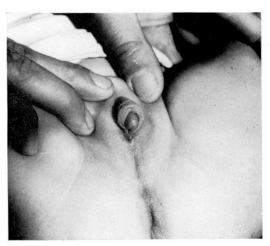

Figure 8-2. Virilization in patient with adrenal cortical hyperfunction (female pseudohermaphrodite).

TABLE 8-1. Inherited Adrenal Cortical Hyperfunction Syndromes

Enzyme	Virilization	Salt	Hypertension
21-hydroxylase	Excess	K retention Na loss in 1/3	No
11-hydroxylase	Excess	Na retention K loss	Yes
3-beta-hydroxysteroid hydrogenase	Incomplete in male	K retention Severe Na loss in all patients	No
17-hydroxylase	No	Na retention K loss	Yes

hyperkalemia are particularly life-threatening, and may be misdiagnosed as congenital heart disease until the electrocardiogram reveals the hyperkalemic changes.

Defect of 11-Hydroxylase. In this much less common form of adrenogenital syndrome, the block results in a pile-up of the hydrocortisone precursor, compound S and desoxycortisone. The latter results in hypertension. Virilization occurs as in the common type of adrenogenital syndrome.

Defect in 3-Beta Hydroxysteroid Dehydrogenase. This is a rare defect in which the patients are salt-losers and males are incompletely virilized because the testicular hormones are not synthesized. Males have hypospadias with or without cryptorchism, and salt-loss is severe, usually leading to death in infancy. Treatment includes hydration, hydrocortisone and, for the salt-losers, desoxycortisone acetate.

Lipoid Adrenal Hyperplasia

Another rare defect results from a deficiency of one of the enzymes involved in the synthesis of progesterone from cholesterol. Lipids and cholesterol accumulate in the adrenal cortex. Patients are salt-losers, and males are feminized.

Excess Mineralocorticoid Secretion

Partial Defect of 17-Hydroxylase. Although the genetics of this condition are not clear, it is mentioned here for convenience. It causes hypertension, hypokalemia and lack of sexual maturation in the few cases (all female) reported.

AGAMMAGLOBULINEMIA, SWISS TYPE[2]

In this disease the usual pattern of inheritance is autosomal recessive. However, there are X-linked recessive pedigrees of a disorder (Bruton type) that is clinically distinguishable from the autosomal recessive, Swiss type agammaglobulinemia.

Diagnostic Features and Clinical Course. In this disease both humoral and cellular immunity are deficient. Patients do not have tonsils or adenoids and have a vestigial or dysplastic thymus. Viral and fungal infections, as well as the bacterial infections encountered in Bruton's disease, threaten the life of the patient. The capacity to reject allografts is lost. Patients are also at risk from fatal graft versus host reactions (GVH) from blood transfusions that include lymphocytes. A smallpox vaccination may result in a fatal progressive vaccinia. Laboratory studies reveal an absence or marked decrease in IgG, IgM and IgA. There is a gross deficiency in lymphocytes and plasma cells.

This disease has been invariably fatal. Death usually occurs before one year of age in the autosomal recessive form, and within the first two years in the X-linked recessive patients. Persistent infections of the lungs, chronic diarrhea, wasting and runting precede a fatal infection.

Treatment. Bone marrow transplantation from carefully matched, histocompatible, related donors has recently been therapeutically effective in providing the patient with immune competence without producing a fatal GVH reaction.

Differential Diagnosis. There are autosomal and X-linked forms of the Swiss type disease which may sometimes be distinguished by pedigree analysis. The differentiating features of this disorder from some of the other immunologic deficiency states are presented in Table 20-5.

ALBINISM[3]

Albinism is a hereditary defect in the metabolism of melanin resulting in an absence or major decrease of this pigment in the skin, mucosa, hair and eyes. Generalized "classic" oculocutaneous albinism was one of Garrod's original four inborn errors of metabolism. There are at least six genetically different types of generalized albinism.

Indirect evidence for genetic heterogeneity came from the observation that the frequency of albinism was higher (one in 20,000) than would be expected on the basis of the observed frequency of parental consanguineous matings (about 20% first cousin marriages). More direct proof came from the observation of matings between two albino parents that resulted in nonalbino offspring.

Tyrosinase-negative Oculocutaneous Albinism

This is the "classic type" in which the hair bulb does not develop pigment when incubated with tyrosine, indicating an absence of tyrosinase activity. Melanocytes are present and contain protein structures (premelanosomes) on which melanin is normally deposited, but no melanin granules are present. The skin and hair are milk white and the iris color is red or, in oblique light, translucent gray to blue (Fig. 8-3). The retina has no visible pigment, and there is severe photophobia and nystagmus.

The frequency is about one in 35,000 persons, though it may be higher in certain

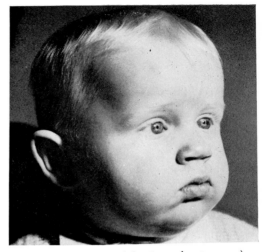

Figure 8-3. Albinism (classic oculocutaneous).

populations (perhaps 1:15,000 for Northern Ireland, for instance). The heterozygote, if lightly pigmented, may have a translucent iris.

Albinism With Hemorrhagic Diathesis (Hermansky-Pudlak Syndrome)

These albinos resemble the classic type and have a negative tyrosine-incubation test. Possibly they lack melanocytes in hair and skin. They also have bleeding tendencies, manifested by bruising, repeated nosebleeds and prolonged bleeding after tooth extraction. The reticuloendothelial cells in blood vessels, spleen, liver, lymph nodes and bone marrow are packed with a black to greenish-blue pigment, possibly a ceroid. The coagulation defect may reside in the platelets.

Tyrosinase-positive Oculocutaneous Albinism

In this type the affected child may be very blond in infancy but may gradually accumulate pigment with age, so the hair changes from white to cream, tan, yellow or light brown or red, particularly in members of dark-skinned races. Photophobia and nystagmus are less severe than in the classic type. The frequency is about one in

14,000 in U.S. Negroes and one in 40,000 Caucasians, but reaches 1.2% in the Brandywine isolate of Maryland. The biochemical defect is not known, but the tyrosine-incubation test is positive.

Albinism With Giant Granules in Leucocytes (Chediak-Higashi Syndrome)

In this fatal disease of childhood there is hypopigmentation, photophobia, anemia, leukopenia, thrombocytopenia, a marked susceptibility to infection, peripheral neuropathy and frequently a lymphoma. Instead of the normal granulations, the granulocytes have a few peroxidase-positive giant granules that stain like the normal granulations for that cell type. The lymphocytes and monocytes have one or two azurophilic inclusions. They may be absent at birth but have been observed as early as two weeks of age.

Hypopigmentation-microphthalmia-oligophrenia (Cross Syndrome)

In a consanguineous Amish family two brothers and a sister were described with white hair, microphthalmia, severe mental and physical retardation, spasticity and athetoid movements. The tyrosine-incubation test was weakly positive. There is a similar mutant in the mouse, microphthalmia-white.

The Yellow-type Albino

In some albinos the hair is white at birth but develops a bright yellow cast by the age of about one year. The tyrosine-incubation test is equivocal. Photophobia and nystagmus are less severe than in the tyrosine-positive type. The basis for the pigment defect is unclear. The condition is frequent in Amerindians, particularly the Jemez (one in 140) and the Tuke Cuna of the Honduras.

ALPHA-1-ANTITRYPSIN DEFICIENCY (LIVER AND LUNG DISEASE)[4,5]

This recently recognized familial disorder may be one of the most common diseases determined by single mutant genes. Current estimates place the frequency of the homozygote at about one in 1,500. The discovery of the deficiency on serum electrophoresis survey was traced back to adult patients with emphysema. Further surveys revealed the presence of familial cirrhosis of the liver in children with the same deficiency. The liver disease in young children and the lung disease in adults are relentlessly progressive. Recently lung disease has also been recognized in children. Genetic studies have revealed a number of alleles that may be considered codominant and are collectively known as the Pi system. Not all patients with genetically determined alpha-1-antitrypsin deficiency develop liver or lung disease, suggesting that important interactions might be involved in the eventual expression of the disorder. At present, from the point of view of genetic counseling, it is best to counsel parents of a homozygous child with cirrhosis and alpha-1-antitrypsin deficiency that the risk of homozygous recurrence is 25% and the heterozygous state 50%. There also appears to be an increased risk of lung disease in the heterozygote, which is exacerbated by cigarette smoking. If so, population screening for heterozygotes, who have a frequency of about one in 20, and warning them of their increased risk from smoking, would be a worthwhile application of preventive medicine.

AMINO ACID METABOLISM, INBORN ERRORS[6,7]

This group of diseases is not only important as a fertile field for contemporary investigation, but has great historic interest. Sir Archibald Garrod, in 1902, consulting with Bateson, discovered the first disease in man that followed a recessive mendelian pattern of inheritance, alkaptonuria. From this disease he developed the concept of inborn errors of metabolism and suggested that the cause could be the absence of a special enzyme, thus anticipating by decades the idea of one gene—one enzyme. Through the technology of modern biochemistry, the yield from this field is approaching bumper-crop proportions. No effort will be made to list completely the known errors (and variants) in the metabolism of amino acids. Rather, a selection of disorders that have fundamental, clinical or historic importance will be presented. These diseases are summarized together with additional related disorders in Table 8-2.

Alkaptonuria[8]

Alkaptonuria is a rare disorder with an estimated incidence in the population of about 1:200,000. The basic defect in the activity of an enzyme (which Garrod predicted in 1908) was eventually demonstrated by La Du and coworkers in 1958 to be an absence of homogentisic acid oxidase. An arrest occurs in the catabolism of tyrosine and large quantities of homogen-

TABLE 8-2. Selected Inborn Errors of Amino Acid Metabolism

Amino Acid	Enzyme	Disease	Clinical Manifestations
Cystine	Defects in renal and GI transport	Cystinuria	Three types, all with progressive renal colic and GU obstruction.
Cystine	?	Cystinosis	Three types, deposition of cystine crystals in reticuloendothelial system, kidney and eye; growth retardation, rickets, renal failure; death in first decade.
Histidine	Histidase	Histidinemia	Impaired speech, some mental retardation.
Methionine	Cystathionine synthesis	Homocystinuria	Ectopia lentis and occasionally other Marfan-like features, coronary artery disease, frequent mental retardation.
Phenylalanine	Phenylalanine hydroxylase	Phenylketonuria	Mental retardation, schizoid behavior, eczematous rash, light pigmentation, convulsions.
Tryptophan	Defect in GI transport of tryptophan	Hartnup disease	Cutaneous photosensitivity with rash, cerebellar ataxia, pyramidal tract signs.
Tryptophan	Defect in GI transport of tryptophan	Blue diaper syndrome	Indicanuria (causing blue diaper), hypercalcemia, nephrocalcinosis.
Tyrosine	Homogentisic acid oxidase	Alkaptonuria	Black urine, black cartilage; blue ears, nose, cheeks, sclerae; arthritis.
Tyrosine	Tyrosinase	Albinism	Two recessive types; fair skin, ocular problems, nystagmus, refractive errors.
Tyrosine	P-OH-phenylpyruvate oxidase?	Tyrosinemia	Failure to thrive, hepatic cirrhosis, renal tubular defects with hypophosphatemic rickets. Tyrosyluria.
Tyrosine	1. ? Iodine Peroxidase 2. ? Coupling Enzyme 3. Diodinase	Three types of goitrous cretinism	Dwarfism, mental retardation, characteristic facies, umbilical hernia.
Valine, leucine, isoleucine	Defect in decarboxylation of ketoacids	Maple syrup urine disease	Maple syrup odor to urine; mental and neurologic deterioration; death in infancy.

tisic acid are excreted in the urine (see Fig. 6-3). The urine of affected patients turns black on standing and alkalinization from a polymerized product of homogentisic acid, permitting diagnosis in infancy by black staining of the diaper (if left long enough). The reducing properties of the urine distinguish it from the black urine of phenol poisoning or melanotic tumors. The accumulation of the homogentisic acid polymer in mesenchymal tissue such as cartilage is responsible for the bluish-black discoloration of the ears, nose, cheeks and sclerae. Arthritis, occurring in about half of the older patients, results from degeneration of pigmented cartilage. The patient is otherwise symptom-free.

Cystinuria[9]

This disorder, or rather group of disorders (there are at least three types) is also of historic interest. It is another of Garrod's four original inborn errors of metabolism. The family-specific clinical differences and the discovery of doubly heterozygous individuals may be explained by allelism of at least three genes at one locus. The clinical findings in the homozygotes of all three types include the formation of cystine stones in the kidney, renal colic and urinary tract obstruction. In cystinuria I the homozygote excretes large amounts of amino acids (cystine, ornithine, arginine and lysine) and the heterozygote has no abnormal aminoaciduria. In cystinuria II the heterozygote has moderate aminoaciduria and may occasionally form stones. In cystinuria III the heterozygote does not excrete abnormal amino acids while the homozygote excretes only a moderate excess of cystine. Specific enzyme abnormalities have not been discovered, although the problem seems to be localized to renal and gastrointestinal transport. For further details, see Chapter 6.

Histidinemia[10]

This disorder was described in 1961 by Ghadimi and co-workers. Delay and defect in speech without mental retardation was the characteristic finding in the early patients. However, some subsequent patients have been retarded. The urine reacts with ferric chloride to give a green color as in phenylketonuria, so that the diagnosis rests on demonstrating elevated plasma levels of histidine. The enzyme defect is an absence of histidase. The prevalence and life expectancy have not been determined.

Homocystinuria[11]

History. This disorder was first recognized independently in 1962 by Carson and Neill in Ireland and by Gerritsen and colleagues in Wisconsin. The absence of cystathionine synthetase was demonstrated to be the basic defect by Mudd and colleagues in 1964. The original patients were ascertained through surveys of mentally retarded populations. Other affected individuals have been recognized as having the Marfan syndrome.

Diagnostic Features. *General.* Frequent mental retardation. Equal sex distribution. Height varies from normal to tall.

Skin. Malar flush.

Eyes. Subluxation of lens (inferior-nasal), myopia, cataracts.

Skeletal. Some patients resemble Marfan syndrome: tall, slender, long fingers and toes, pectus excavatum or carinatum, genu valgum, kyphoscoliosis, joint laxity, US/LS ratio less than normal (Figs. 8-3, 8-4).

Cardiovascular. Arterial thromboses of coronary, renal, carotid, cerebral, and other medium-sized vessels, leading to myocardial infarction, renal hypertension and stroke. Venous thromboses and pulmonary infarction.

Gastrointestinal. Bleeding secondary to vascular disease and infarction.

C.N.S. Abnormal EEG, seizures.

X-ray. Osteoporosis.

Laboratory. Homocystine in urine by the nitroprusside test, electrophoresis or column chromatography.

Clinical Course. The disease may be well-tolerated for several decades or be fatal in the first decade depending, in large measure, on the vascular complications. Cerebral vascular disease may be responsible for early or late death. Myocardial infarction is more likely to occur after age

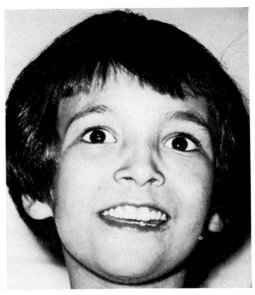

Figure 8-5.   Inferonasal subluxation of lens may be seen best in right eye of this patient with homocystinuria.

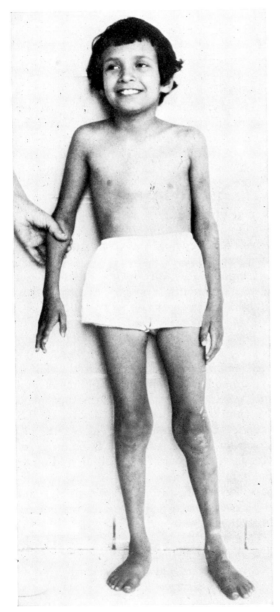

Figure 8-4.   Full body view of child with homocystinuria. The habitus is slim but barely suggestive of Marfan syndrome. The fingers and toes are not excessively long nor is the US/LS ratio abnormal.

20. Although over half of the patients are retarded, some may attend college. The visual impairment may be particularly disabling.

Treatment. Restrict methionine. Supplement with vitamin B_6 and cystine.

Differential Diagnosis. The most important diagnostic alternative is the *Marfan syndrome*, which may be distinguished by dominant inheritance, a negative nitroprusside test, superior-temporal subluxation of the lens, vascular disease of the great vessels, and absence of mental retardation and malar flush. In addition, the Marfan syndrome has more striking arachnodactyly and joint laxity.

Maple Syrup Urine Disease (Branched Chain Ketonuria)[12,13]

Menkes and co-workers described, in 1954, a family in which four of six infants died in the first weeks of life with vomiting, hypertonicity and a maple syrup odor to the urine. In 1957, Westall, Dancis and Miller found an elevation in the urine and blood of the branched chain amino acids, valine, leucine, and isoleucine. The frequency is estimated as three per million births. The biochemical defect seems to be in oxidative decarboxylation of ketoacids, a deficiency in branched chain ketoacid decarboxylase. Death usually occurs during the first year following progressive neurologic deterioration in untreated patients. Arrest of neurologic damage has been achieved by dietary management through the exclusion of valine, leucine and isoleucine from the diet. A special preparation lacking these amino acids is used to reduce the quantity of excess branched chain amino acids. Then gradually foods containing these amino acids are restarted in the diet and maintained at a low level to meet requirements for growth.

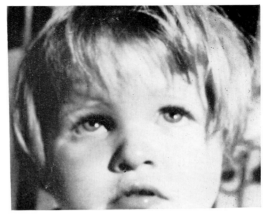

Figure 8-6. Fair skin and hair and blue eyes are common in patients with PKU (as in this example) but far from invariable.

Phenylketonuria[14]

Phenylketonuria was first discovered by Følling in 1934. Jervis then demonstrated the autosomal inheritance of the disease, the inability to oxidize phenylalanine to tyrosine, and the absence of liver phenylalanine hydroxylase in these patients. The incidence in Caucasian populations is about seven per 100,000, though considerably higher than this in Eire, low among Ashkenazi Jews and American Negroes, and very low in Finland. Because the harmful effects of the mutant can be prevented by early treatment, screening of newborns for PKU is compulsory in many areas.

Diagnostic Features and Clinical Course. Affected children appear perfectly normal at birth but, if not treated, the developmental milestones may be delayed within the first few months, and the delay becomes progressively more severe, including a precipitous loss of I.Q. in the first year. Seizures may begin at six to 12 months, and the majority have abnormal EEG's even if they have no seizures. The skin is dry and rough, and the hair and eyes tend to be lighter than expected from the family background (Fig. 8-6). They are hyperactive, irritable children, with an increased muscle tone and awkward gait, who show voluntary, purposeless, repetitive motions. The biochemical findings are discussed in Chapter 6.

The classic diagnostic test is the ferric chloride test or the Phenistix test (Ames Co.), but this may not become positive for several days. Routine screening procedures make use of the Guthrie test (a bacterial inhibition assay), paper chromatography or fluorimetric methods. The diagnosis should always be confirmed by a quantitative measurement of plasma phenylalanine.

An unexpected example of maternal-fetal interaction was the discovery that children of phenylketonuric mothers may be brain-damaged, have microcephaly, and may have major malformations, particularly of C.N.S. and heart. This will be an increasing problem as treated PKU mothers reach the age of reproduction.

Treatment. Treatment consists of a low phenylalanine diet instituted as soon as possible. Some phenylalanine must be added to prevent depletion of the body's proteins. Phenylalanine levels must be monitored frequently, as the requirements decrease in the first few years. If the biochemical abnormalities are corrected, convulsions cease and growth is normal. There is some disagreement about whether damage to the intelligence can be prevented altogether, but recent studies have shown that this is possible with careful monitoring and control of the phenylalanine intake.

Heterozygote Detection. The detection of individuals heterozygous for the PKU gene would be of value in some counseling situations, and more so as the frequency of successfully treated adults increases. Quite good discrimination is achieved by giving intravenous phenylalanine and following the kinetics of its disappearance from the blood, using the phenylalanine/tyrosine ratio. In spite of claims to the contrary there do not seem to be any deleterious effects of the heterozygous gene.

Hyperphenylalaninemia. Screening programs for phenylketonuria are complicated by the presence of an occasional case of hyperphenylalaninemia without the characteristic findings of phenylketonuria. These must be distinguished, since these children will not benefit and, indeed, may suffer when put on a low phenylalanine diet. Although the situation is still unclear, there appears to be one type in which the liver phenylalanine hydroxise is late-maturing, and which will revert to normal within a few months. Another type produces a mild hyperphenylalaninemia, usually without neurologic damage. A third type may result from a defective binding site of the cofactor.

Tyrosinemia[15]

The predominant clinical findings in the infant are severe or fatal liver failure, and in the older patients, chronic hepatic cirrhosis and renal tubular failure. The hypoglycemia, hepatomegaly and ascites are prominent clinical manifestations. Tyrosinemia is defined as a plasma level greater than 0.70 μmol/ml, and can be detected by current screening methods for aminoacidopathies. There is a deficiency of p-hydroxyphenylpyruvic acid oxidase, but there is still some doubt as to whether this is the primary defect.

Treatment consisting of dietary limitation of tyrosine and phenylalanine through special formulas has been successful in producing improved liver function, reduction of ascites and satisfactory weight gain.

Hereditary tyrosinemia must be distinguished from acquired neonatal tyrosinemia in which an apoenzyme that can be activated is present (steroids and folic acid benefit these patients).

ANEMIA

Constitutional Aplastic Anemia (Fanconi Pancytopenia)[16]

This disease is characterized by pancytopenia, bone marrow hypoplasia and characteristic congenital anomalies, most commonly abnormalities of the thumb, absent radii, microcephaly, a patchy dark skin pigmentation and shortness of stature. Associated anomalies may include abnormalities of the eye, heart, kidney and skeleton as well as mental retardation and deafness (Fig. 8-7).

The pancytopenia generally does not develop until three to 12 years of age. The bone marrow is hypocellular with increased fat content. Hemoglobin electrophoresis reveals an increase in Hgb F to 5 to 15%. Chromosomal studies show increased chromatid breaks along with unusual chromosomal alignments. A high incidence of leukemia has been reported in patients with

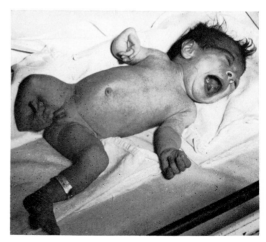

Figure 8-7. Skeletal anomalies in newborn with Fanconi pancytopenia.

constitutional aplastic anemia and their families.

Clinical complications include bleeding, infections and anemia, which require symptomatic treatment with platelets, antibiotics and red cells. Other therapy consists of combined corticosteroids and androgens. Patients may show hematologic response in two to four months, at which time the corticosteroids and androgens may be reduced but usually are not withdrawn completely without relapse.

Confusion in nomenclature results from the fact that at least three disorders bear the eponym Fanconi: Fanconi pancytopenia with multiple anomalies, and Fanconi syndromes I and II, which are also autosomal recessive. Fanconi syndrome I is a disorder characterized by vitamin D-resistant rickets, osteomalacia, chronic acidosis, glycosuria and aminoaciduria without cystinosis, which becomes manifest in infancy and childhood. Fanconi syndrome II presents in adults in the fourth and fifth decades of life with findings similar to (though less severe than) Fanconi I.

Hemoglobin C Disease[17]

Hemoglobin C disease is the homozygous manifestation of a beta chain abnormality that produces moderately severe hemolytic anemia. The molecular basis of the disorder is the replacement of glutamic acid by lysine in residue 6 of the beta chain. The disease is relatively common and the usually asymptomatic heterozygote is estimated to represent about 2% of the American Negro population. Because of the high gene frequencies involved, heterozygotes with hemoglobin S and hemoglobin C are not uncommon and the compound heterozygote has a hemolytic anemia that is difficult to distinguish clinically from sickle cell disease. A clinical clue to the presence of hemoglobin C disease is the presence of target cells (frequently more than 50% of the red cells, Fig. 8-8). Electrophoresis will confirm the diagnosis.

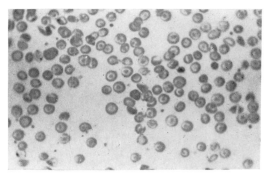

Figure 8-8. Target cells characteristic of hemoglobin C disease.

Hemoglobin S Disease (Sickle Cell Anemia)[17]

This disorder occupies a most important position in the development of medical genetics. In 1949, Neel demontrated its mendelian basis, and Pauling and co-workers attributed the sickling phenomenon to an abnormal hemoglobin and suggested that this was a molecular disease. In 1956, Ingram characterized the hemoglobin molecule and demonstrated that one gene caused the substitution of one amino acid for another at a particular point in a protein (valine for glutamic acid at the sixth position from the N-terminal of the beta chain), producing hemoglobin S.

Sickle cell disease is transmitted as an autosomal recessive disorder, and sickle cell trait, which is generally benign under normal conditions (see Chapter 7), is inherited as an autosomal dominant. Sickle cell disease is characterized by chronic anemia and intravascular sickling resulting from lowered oxygen tension (Fig. 8-9). The sickling of the red blood cells results in increased blood viscosity, which produces capillary stasis, vascular occlusion and thrombi and infarction. Infection often instigates the above cycle, which is referred to as a crisis and is associated with pain. The bone marrow may temporarily cease to function during this period, resulting in more severe anemia. The homozygote usually does not survive childhood, although

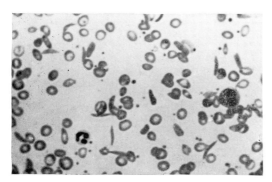

Figure 8-9. Sickle cells in hemoglobin S disease.

affected adults are encountered. Growth and development are poor.

The diagnosis is made by demonstration of the sickling phenomenon on peripheral blood smear and confirmed by hemoglobin electrophoresis, which reveals hemoglobin S. Mass screening tests are currently being emphasized, such as the Sickledex and dithionite tests.

Treatment consists of avoiding low oxygen tension situations (such as nonpressurized aircraft) and prompt attention to infections. Crises are treated symptomatically depending on the severity. The individual should be kept well hydrated during an episode. If the hemoglobin level drops to low levels, blood transfusion may be necessary. However, indiscriminate blood transfusions should be avoided in these patients. For the patient in crisis, other therapeutic recourses in various stages of clinical trial and acceptance include urea and invert sugar, cyanate and injections of testosterone.

Pyruvate Kinase Deficiency[18]

This chronic hemolytic anemia is highly variable in its severity. Diagnosis is by enzyme assay, which is also capable of detecting the asymptomatic heterozygote. Conservative management with transfusions is recommended. Splenectomy sometimes helps by decreasing transfusion requirements, but is not curative.

The Thalassemias[19]

The thalassemias have been observed in most racial groups, but have a particularly high incidence in the Mediterranean region, the Middle East and the Orient. The anemia of thalassemia results essentially from reduced production of hemoglobin alpha chains or beta chains. Thus there are two groups of thalassemias: the alpha thalassemias and the beta thalassemias. Their genetics are very complex.

The Beta Thalassemias. Remember that the loci for beta and delta chains are closely linked. The beta and delta chains combine with alpha chains to form hemoglobin A and A_2 respectively. The genes for gamma chains and for alpha chains are not linked. Alpha and gamma chains form fetal hemoglobin. The gene for beta thalassemia is closely linked to the beta and delta structural loci. There are two main types of beta thalassemia gene: beta thalassemia$^+$ in which suppression is only partial, and beta thalassemia^0 in which suppression is complete.

"True" beta thalassemia, or Cooley's anemia, occurs in homozygotes during the first few months of life, with severe anemia, frequent infections, stunting of growth, bossing of the skull and maxillary overgrowth, hepatosplenomegaly and, if the patient survives long enough, hemochromatosis. The blood smear shows anisopoikilocytosis, hypochromia, target cells and basophilic stippling. Fetal hemoglobin is increased, and A_2 levels are low, normal or high, but almost always high if expressed as a proportion of hemoglobin A.

The heterozygous gene varies in expression from almost as severe as the homozygous form (thalassemia intermedia) to mild (thalassemia minor) to virtually normal (thalassemia minima). Hemoglobin A_2 is elevated and small amounts of hemoglobin F are present.

A rare *delta-beta thalassemia* is milder than Cooley's anemia. Only hemoglobin F is present in the homozygote. The heterozygote resembles thalassemia minor, with a higher level of hemoglobin F.

Hemoglobin Lepore appears to have arisen by unequal crossing-over between the genes for the delta and beta chains, having a delta sequence at the N terminal and a beta sequence at the C terminal. Since the composite delta-beta chain is formed at a reduced rate, the gene behaves like a thalassemia gene.

The gene for *hereditary persistence of fetal hemoglobin* has a total deficiency of beta and delta chains from the genes on the chromosome upon which it is located (the cis position), but the gamma gene is normal so the homozygote continues to produce hemoglobin F and there is no clinical abnormality.

The beta thalassemia genes interact with the beta chain structural mutants and are thus called "interacting" types. For instance a patient with a hemoglobin S gene on one chromosome and a beta thalassemia⁰ allele on the other has a disease similar to sickle cell disease, since the majority of the hemoglobin produced is hemoglobin S.

The Alpha Thalassemias. Mutants at the alpha thalassemia locus suppress alpha chain production to varying degrees. The severe type, alpha thalassemia-1, is fatal in the homozygote, causing severe hydrops fetalis or early postnatal death with edema and hepatosplenomegaly. The hemoglobin present is Barts, or gamma-4. The heterozygote has a mild thalassemia with normal levels of F and A₂, and a decreased alpha chain production demonstrable by isotope incorporation studies.

Hemoglobin H disease appears to result from a combination of the alpha thalassemia-1 gene with a milder variant, the alpha thalassemia-2 gene. Patients have a course similar to that of thalassemia major or a milder one, depending on the allele involved. There are varying levels of hemoglobin H (beta-4).

The alpha thalassemia genes in the heterozygote produce mild abnormalities, if any.

Therapy is entirely supportive, including transfusions, folic acid, and intensive treatment of infections. Splenectomy is indicated only if there are indications of hypersplenism and preferably after five years of age because of the increased risk of infection.

ATAXIA, FRIEDREICH[20]

This degenerative disease is characterized by cerebellar ataxia, pes cavus (Fig. 8-10), loss of deep tendon reflexes and scoliosis beginning in preadolescence. Clinical manifestations of the spinocerebellar disorder are incoordination of limb movements, dysarthria and nystagmus. Average duration of life is about 15 years from the time of onset. Heart disease, an unusual myocardiopathy, frequently is responsible for death of the patient in congestive heart failure or cardiac arrhythmia.

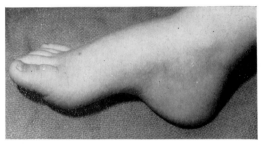

Figure 8-10. Pes cavus in Friedreich ataxia—a sentinel feature.

ATAXIA TELANGIECTASIA (LOUIS-BAR SYNDROME)[21]

The cardinal features of this disorder are ataxia, telangiectases, and an immunologic deficiency of both cellular and humoral immunity. The first manifestations, progressing from infancy, are usually related to the ataxia: incoordination, often severe enough to prevent ambulation; choreoathetosis; nystagmus; dysarthric speech and drooling.

The child has frequent infections and failure to thrive; later, respiratory infections involving the sinuses and the lungs predominate, which fail to respond to antimicrobial therapy. This may be related to the absence of IgA, the secretory immunoglobulin that protects the mucous mem-

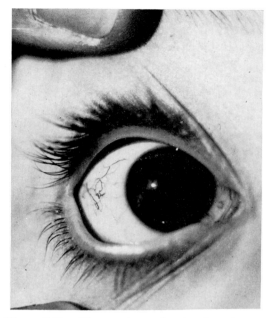

Figure 8-11. The eye in ataxia telangiectasia.

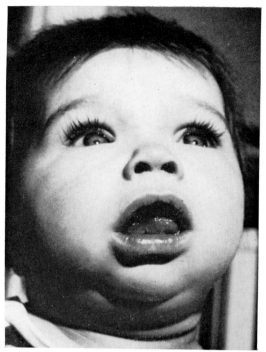

Figure 8-12. Characteristic coarse facies and thick protuberant tongue of cretinism.

branes. In addition to the humoral immune deficit there is a cellular immune deficiency with the characteristic findings of lymphopenia and diminished delayed hypersensitivity and capacity for allograft rejection. The thymus is small and dysplastic at postmortem.

Because the telangiectases may not be readily apparent until later in the course, some patients may be misdiagnosed as having Friedreich ataxia. When telangiectases appear, they are most evident in the bulbar conjuctivae (Fig. 8-11).

COLOR BLINDNESS, TOTAL[22]

This autosomal recessive form of color blindness is due to absence of the cones. The vision of affected individuals is better at night. The more common forms of color blindness are X-linked and the general problem of color blindness and biologic variability is discussed in Chapter 10.

CRETINISM[23]

There are at least five or six distinct biochemical defects in thyroid hormone pro-

duction that are mendelizing. The two points to be emphasized here are that these disorders are autosomal recessive and that the resulting cretinism must be recognized and differentiated from other genetically determined disorders such as 21 trisomy, the mucopolysaccharidoses and glycogen storage diseases. Too often an infant is followed by a physician who makes a suspected diagnosis of, say, 21 trisomy and discovers that cretinism is the diagnosis when it is too late to prevent brain damage.

The familiar physical findings in infancy are: sluggishness; cool extremities with mild peripheral cyanosis; myxedema with thick protruding tongue, hoarse cry, increased subcutaneous tissue and muscle mass; slow growth and maturation with delayed radiographic bone age and epiphyseal dysgenesis; large fontanelles; umbilical hernia; and progressively more obvious signs of mental retardation. Permanent impairment of development of the central nervous system results if prompt treatment with thyroid hormone is not instituted. In some instances the intrauterine deprivation of thyroid hormone may be so severe that a degree of mental retardation will occur even in those treated early.

The laboratory confirmation of the clinical diagnosis of thyroid disease utilizes such findings as protein-bound iodine, butyl-extractable iodine and the uptake of radioactive iodine.

Treatment consists of oral thyroid hormone replacement in the forms of desiccated thyroid, sodium L-thyroxine or triiodothyronine. Serum levels of protein-bound iodine may be used to monitor the adequacy of treatment of the first two medications but are of no value with triiodothyronine.

CUTIS LAXA SYNDROME[24]

This rare autosomal recessive syndrome of generalized elastolysis should not be confused with the autosomal dominant Ehlers-Danlos syndrome (cutis hyperelastica). The skin in cutis laxa may give a young child a very elderly appearance with a drooping jowl, blood-hound facies and unwrinkled, sagging folds of skin on the trunk and extremities, causing extreme cosmetic problems. Important associated abnormalities are pulmonary emphysema with hypertension, pulmonary artery branch stenosis, inguinal umbilical and diaphragmatic hernias, diverticula of the gastrointestinal tract and bladder, congenital dislocation of the hips, and a deep voice. In contrast with Ehlers-Danlos, there is no fragility or difficulty in healing of the skin and biopsy reveals absence of elastic fibers. The cardiopulmonary complications are a significant cause of morbidity and mortality.

CYSTIC FIBROSIS (MUCOVISCIDOSIS)[25]

This is the most common disease caused by a single mutant gene in Caucasian children. Estimates of the incidence of cystic fibrosis in the American population range from 1:1,000 to 1:3,700, but it is rarely encountered in Negroes and Orientals. The first comprehensive clinical and pathologic description of the disease was presented by Andersen in 1938, and the mode of transmission was demonstrated by Lowe and coworkers in 1949. The recent discovery by Rao and Nadler[26] of a trypsin-like substance in the saliva, possibly a kallikrein, which is reduced in the saliva of affected patients, may be an important lead to the basic defect.

Cystic fibrosis may present as an acute surgical emergency of the newborn as meconium ileus, or become evident in early childhood as chronic pulmonary disease and steatorrhea. Other possible clinical findings include cirrhosis of the liver, cor pulmonale, prolapse of the rectum, glycosuria, ocular lesions, and massive salt loss with dehydration, coma and even death from high environmental temperatures. The disease may be diagnosed by an elevated sweat chloride (> 60 mEq/L) and absence of pancreatic enzymes.

Treatment is directed at the control of the pulmonary infections, dietary management, and prevention and replacement of abnormal salt loss. Even with the latest therapeutic advances half of the children with this disease die before ten years of age, and 80% before 20 years of age. Males are sterile due to testicular tubule degeneration; a few female patients have reproduced. The question has not been satisfactorily answered as to how the high incidence of such a lethal mutant gene can be maintained in the population. Heterozygote advantage and genetic heterogeneity are possible explanations.

Detection of Carriers. Numerous methods to detect the presence of the gene in the heterozygote have met with little success, including elevated sweat chlorides, inhibition of cilia from rabbit trachea or oysters, the presence of metachromatic granules in cultured fibroblasts, and reduced salivary tryptic activity of carriers.

Antenatal Diagnosis. High hopes that the accumulation of metachromatic granules in cultured fibroblasts might be a useful diagnosis were dashed by the fact that the phenomenon is not sufficiently specific and occurs also in heterozygotes. At present there is no satisfactory method of antenatal diagnosis.

DEAFNESS[27,28]

Congenital deafness is often a difficult problem for the counselor who, in the sporadic case, has to decide between an environmental cause such as kernicterus, rubella or meningitis, or a dominant gene, either as a fresh mutation or showing reduced penetrance, or a recessive gene. It can be roughly estimated that 75% of cases result from recessive genes, of which there are several different kinds, 20% are due to environmental causes, 3% to autosomal dominant genes, and 2% to X-linked genes.

Empiric risk rates for profound childhood deafness not associated with a syndrome have been provided by Stevenson[28] (see Table 8-3). Of course these risks are approximate and will change according to the number of normal or abnormal children born.

In addition, deafness is a part of a number of syndromes. Those showing recessive inheritance are listed below:

A. Deafness with no associated anomalies:
    1. Congenital severe deafness.

TABLE 8-3.   Risk for Sib or Child of Person With Congenital Deafness

Family Situation		Risk For:
Parents consanguineous	sib	1/4
Two or more deaf sibs	sib	1/4
Nonconsanguineous parents, sporadic case	sib	1/6
One parent deaf, sporadic case	child	1/30
Parent deaf, with deaf relatives	child	1/10
Deaf parents, deaf child	sib	1/2
Both parents deaf, one with deaf relatives	child	1/7
Both parents deaf, with deaf relatives	child	1/3

    2. Early onset neural deafness.
    3. Congenital moderate hearing loss.

B. Deafness with external ear malformations:
    1. Conductive hearing loss with low-set malformed ears.

C. Deafness with integumentary system disease:
    1. Neural hearing loss with atopic dermatitis.
    2. Hearing loss with pili torti.
    3. Onychodystrophy and deafness.

D. Deafness associated with eye disease:
    1. Hearing loss with myopia and mild mental retardation.
    2. Congenital deafness with retinitis pigmentosa.
    3. Hearing loss with retinal degeneration and diabetes mellitus (Alström-Hallgren syndrome).
    4. Deafness, retinal changes, muscular wasting and mental retardation.
    5. Hearing loss, optic atrophy and juvenile diabetes.
    6. Hearing loss with polyneuropathy and optic atrophy.

E. Deafness with nervous system disease:
    1. Deafness with mental deficiency, ataxia and hypogonadism (Richards-Rundel syndrome).

F. Deafness associated with skeletal disease:
    1. Conductive hearing loss, cleft palate, characteristic facies and bone dysplasia (oto-palato-digital syndrome).
    2. Deafness with tibial absence.
    3. Deafness with split hand and foot.
    4. Deafness with splayed long bones (Pyle disease).

G. Deafness with other abnormalities:
    1. Deafness with goiter (Pendred syndrome). This may account for as much as 10% of hereditary deafness. Patients may be euthyroid.
    2. Neural hearing loss with goiter, high PBI and stippled epiphyses.

3. Deafness, prolonged Q-T interval and sudden death (Jervell and Lange-Nielsen syndrome). The patient is at risk for sudden death from ventricular fibrillation. Maintenance doses of propranolol may prevent the arrhythmia.

DIPLEGIA, ICHTHYOSIS, MENTAL RETARDATION (SJÖGREN-LARSSON SYNDROME)[29]

The syndrome of ichthyosis, spasticity of the lower extremities, mental retardation and shortness of stature was first recognized in Sweden and traced back through 600 years to a common ancestor. The disorder has since been described in North America. Additional abnormalities may include retinal degeneration, hypertelorism, hypoplasia of teeth and seizures.

DYSAUTONOMIA (RILEY-DAY SYNDROME)[30]

In these infants and children, first described by Riley, Day and co-workers in 1949, there is central dysfunction of the autonomic nervous system associated with degeneration of cells in the autonomic ganglia and demyelination in the medulla. This disorder affects mainly Ashkenazi Jews and is characterized in infancy by failure to thrive, lack of tearing, swallowing difficulty, aspiration and cyclic vomiting, diarrhea, and absence of papillae on the tongue. Other findings that become apparent are emotional lability, mental retardation, paroxysmal hypertension, increased sweating, blotching of the skin, poor coordination and unstable temperature with bouts of unexplained fever. Almost half of the patients fail to survive to adult life, with aspiration pneumonia being a common cause of death.

DWARFISM

Many genetic and chromosomal diseases are accompanied by short stature. This section refers to a selected number that do not obviously fall into any other category, such as Down syndrome or Morquio disease.

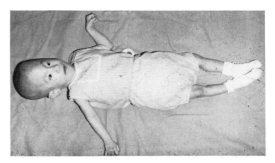

Figure 8-13. Extreme dwarfism (length 25″ at 37 months of age). Patient has microcephaly, a prominent nose, strabismus, 11 ribs, cryptorchism and severe mental retardation. The clinical diagnosis was felt to be most consistent with Seckel syndrome.

Bird-Headed Dwarfism (Seckel Syndrome)[31]

These are among the most severely dwarfed of all patients. Eventual height attainment is rarely over 42 inches. Mental retardation, a small head and a prominent nose (contributing to the bird-like facies) are consistent features (Fig. 8-13). Skeletal anomalies include dislocation of joints and the presence of only 11 ribs. Cryptorchism is usual in the male.

Bloom Syndrome[32]

This relatively rare disorder is characterized by short stature, a telangiectatic erythema of the face resembling lupus erythematosus and malar hypoplasia. Sunlight exacerbates the butterfly facial lesions, and telangiectases may be found in the hands and arms. Chromosomal breakage and terminal malignancy, most often leukemia, are important features.

Cartilage-Hair Hypoplasia[33,34]

This disorder was recognized by McKusick and colleagues in the inbred Old Order Amish religious isolate and has since been observed in other groups. The clinical features are short-limbed dwarfism, metaphyseal dysostosis (by x-ray), cartilage hypoplasia (by biopsy) and fine sparse hair. Intestinal malabsorption, which improves with age, may be the presenting complaint in infancy. Anemia, Hirschsprung disease and severe or fatal response to chickenpox are additional findings.

Chondrodystrophia Calcificans Congenita (Conradi Disease)[35]

This disorder, reported by Conradi in 1914, has only recently received wide recognition. The most characteristic finding is the radiographic demonstration of *multiple stippled epiphyses*. However something must prompt the physician to obtain x-rays of the skeleton and this is usually the recognition of short limbs and flexion contractures of the elbows, knees and hips (Fig. 8-14). The low nasal bridge with the short limbs may bring to mind the diagnosis of achondroplasia. Cataracts, club feet, congenital heart disease, skin and hair problems, dislocation of the hip and craniosynostosis may be encountered. The diagnostic finding is the punctate areas of mineralization in developing cartilage (Fig. 8-15). Respiratory infections are a particular problem and death from pneumonia is common. About 50% of these patients have some degree of mental retardation. There is also a dominant, much less severe form.

Chondroectodermal Dysplasia (Ellis-van Creveld Syndrome)[36,37]

History. This clinical entity was recognized by Ellis and van Creveld in 1940. The pattern of inheritance was shown to be autosomal recessive by Metrakos and Fraser in 1954. McKusick, in 1964, reported a number of patients from an inbred Amish population that approximately equaled the

number of all previously reported cases in the world literature (which illustrates the deleterious effects of inbreeding in making manifest the effects of autosomal recessive single mutant genes).

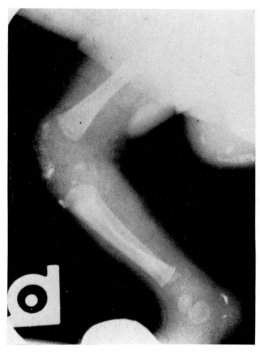

Figure 8-15. Punctate calcific deposits in Conradi syndrome.

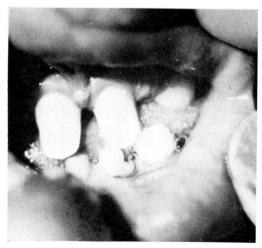

Figure 8-16. Dental dysplasia and frenulum binding short upper lip to alveolar ridge in Ellis-van Creveld syndrome.

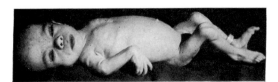

Figure 8-14. Note short proximal long bones (especially humerus), flexion contractures and saddle nose in patient with Conradi syndrome.

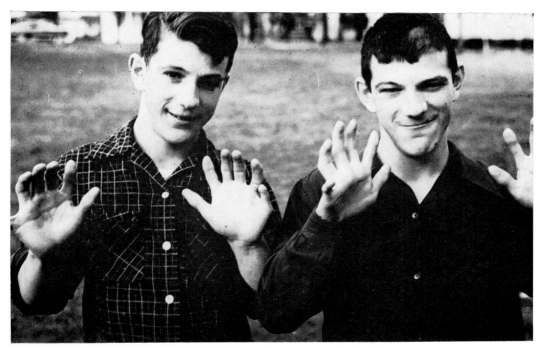

Figure 8-17. Brothers with Ellis-van Creveld syndrome. Note polydactyly.

Diagnostic Features. *General.* Intelligence is usually normal. Equal sex distribution. Moderately to severely dwarfed.

Head. Abnormalities of mouth; short upper lip bound by frenula to alveolar ridge; dental problems (dysplastic teeth, delayed eruption) (Fig. 8-16).

Musculoskeletal. Polydactyly, ulnar (Fig. 8-17); short extremities, more extreme distally; spondylolisthesis; fusion of hamate and capitate, inability to make a fist.

Cardiovascular. Congenital heart lesions in about 50% of patients, commonly single atrium.

Clinical Course. In the past many of these patients have died in infancy as a consequence of their congenital heart lesions. Those without heart disease or with mild or treated cardiac lesions will survive into adult life with the major handicaps being shortness of stature and, in some, the limitation of hand function.

Treatment. Symptomatic and supportive, especially for the congenital heart defects.

Differential Diagnosis. Other disorders causing dwarfism, polydactyly, and congenital heart disease; in particular, asphyxiating thoracic dystrophy.

Diastrophic Dwarfism[38]

Patients with this disorder may look like achondroplastic dwarfs at birth because of the shortness of their limbs (Figs. 8-18, 8-19). However there are classic stigmata

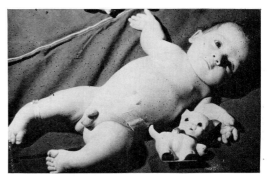

Figure 8-18. Infant with diastrophic dwarfism. Club feet help to distinguish this disorder from achondroplasia.

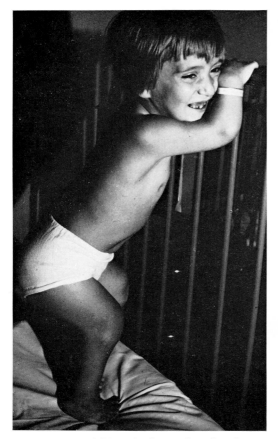

Figure 8-19.   Child with diastrophic dwarfism.

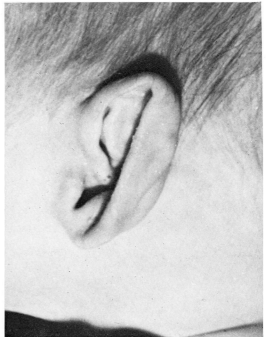

Figure 8-20.   Cystic swelling of external ear, a differentiating feature of diastrophic dwarfism.

that distinguish diastrophic dwarfism from other forms of dwarfism detectable at birth. One is the cystic swelling of the external ear, much in appearance like the "cauliflower ear" of the wrestler or boxer, followed by calcification of the lesion (Fig. 8-20). Other differentiating features are club feet (varus deformity) and short first metacarpals associated with small proximally placed thumbs. Intelligence and overall general health are satisfactory. Orthopedic correction of the foot deformity and the progressive scoliosis have not proved to be entirely satisfactory.

Thoracic Dystrophy, Asphyxiating (Jeune Syndrome)[39,40]

This disease usually terminates fatally in infancy. The thoracic cage is greatly con-

stricted by shortened ribs, which impedes respiratory excursions and produces asphyxiation (Figs. 8-21, 8-22). There are relatively short limbs, hypoplastic iliac wings and irregular epiphyses and metaphyses. Polydactyly may be present and the overall picture of skeletal anomalies has led some observers to consider this disease to be a variant of the Ellis-van Creveld syndrome. Those patients who survive infancy have improvement in the relative growth of the rib cage and satisfactory respiration, but progressive renal disease becomes manifest.

GALACTOSEMIA[41]

This disease, first reported by Goppert (1917) as galactosuria, results from the absence of a specific enzyme, galactose-1-phosphate (Gal 1-P) uridyl transferase. Diagnosis is by the finding of nutritional failure, mental retardation, cataracts and hepatosplenomegaly with cirrhosis. Urinalysis for reducing substances with Benedict's

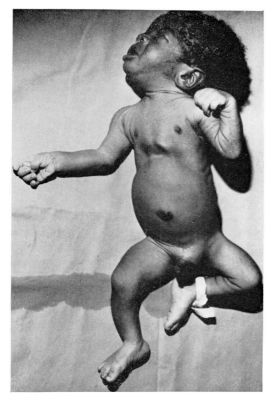

Figure 8-21. Constricted thoracic cage impeding respiration in Jeune syndrome.

solution is positive, but with Clinistix (glucose oxidase) is negative, indicating that the reducing sugar is not glucose. Galactose may be identified in the urine by chemical and chromatographic means, along with other amino acids and albumin. Blood galactose is elevated; there is an abnormal galactose tolerance test (beware of insulin shock) and a deficiency of Gal 1-P uridyl transferase in the erythrocytes.

Vomiting, diarrhea and jaundice develop days or weeks after the first milk ingestion, followed by dehydration, poor growth, parenchymal liver damage and, in one to two months, cataract formation. These problems, plus involvement of the central nervous system, progress unless a galactose-free (milk-free) diet is given. The earlier the diet is started the better the outcome.

Another enzymatic defect causes galactosemia without retardation. There are also transferase variants that retain some ability to metabolize galactose and may, as in the case of the Duarte variant, be entirely asymptomatic.

In the heterozygote carrier, Gal 1-P uridyl transferase activity in the blood is about

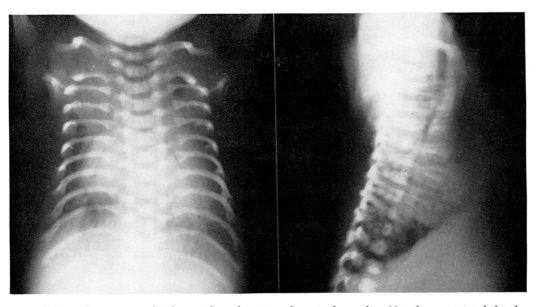

Figure 8-22. Chest x-rays of infant with asphyxiating thoracic dystrophy. Note how restricted the thoracic cavity is.

midway between that of the normal and the homozygote. The incidence of the disease is estimated to be of the order of 1:30,000 births, and the outlook for patients treated early appears to be good.

THE GLYCOGEN STORAGE DISEASES[42]

The glycogenoses are a group of diseases resulting from derangements in synthesis or degradation of glycogen. At least 15 enzyme defects of glycogen metabolism have been categorized, and there are still cases that do not fit readily into any of these categories. Some patients with combined defects have been observed. Von Gierke's disease has the distinction of being the first inborn error of metabolism in which the deficiency of a known tissue enzyme was demonstrated.

In general, the glycogenoses involve disorders of the liver or muscle, alone or in combination with heart, kidney and nervous system. The clinical manifestations of the disorders are, of course, related to the systems involved. For example, cardiomegaly may be present in any of the three entities (Pompe, limit dextrinosis, amylopectinosis) in which the heart is involved, although only in Pompe disease do the cardiac find-

ings consistently predominate. Hepatomegaly and hypoglycemia are prominent in the types that have liver involvement, and hypotonia is prominent in those with muscle and/or nervous system involvement.

The prognosis and severity vary both among and within the type of glycogenosis. In general, von Gierke disease (type Ia) is very severe, yet there are reports of survival to adulthood. In type VIa (Hers disease), the disease is generally milder, but severe involvement has been observed in some cases.

Table 8-4 lists some of the glycogenoses with the specific enzymes demonstrated to be absent or deficient in each disorder. As with the mucopolysaccharidoses, these categories (and those omitted) must be accepted with flexibility. Revisions will continue as the heterogeneity of these diseases becomes better appreciated.

HEMOPHILIA C (PTA OR FACTOR XI DEFICIENCY)[43]

Plasma thromboplastin antecedent deficiency is autosomal in inheritance in contrast to AHG and PTC deficiencies, which are sex-linked. Direct transmission has been reported in some pedigrees, but the ma-

TABLE 8-4.   Selected Glycogenoses

Disease	Organs Affected and Clinical Manifestations	Enzyme
Ia von Gierke	Liver, kidney, intestinal mucosa; hepatomegaly, hypoglycemia, growth retardation, bleeding, diathesis.	Glucose-6-phosphatase
IIa Pompe (cardiac)	Heart, muscle, liver, C.N.S.; cardiomegaly, hypotonia, death in infancy	Lysosomal alpha-1, 4-glycosidase (acid maltase)
IIIa Limit dextrinosis (Forbes, Cori)	Liver, muscle, heart; hepatomegaly, hypoglycemia, cardiomegaly.	Amylo-1, 6-glucosidase
IV Amylopectinosis	Liver, kidney, heart, muscle, C.N.S., R.E. system; hepatosplenomegaly, cirrhosis.	Amylo-1,4-1,6 transglucosidase
V McArdle	Muscle; appears in adult life as muscular fatigue and pain with exercise, myoglobinuria.	Muscle phosphorylase
VIa Hers	Liver; hepatomegaly, hypoglycemia, acidosis—mild to severe.	Liver phosphorylase
VII Tarui	See V—McArdle	Phosphofructokinase
VIII Thomson	Muscle weakness	Phosphoglucomutase

jority of cases appear to follow a recessive pattern. Clinically, this disorder is much milder than factor VIII or IX deficiencies. Bleeding is usually related to trauma, although spontaneous hemorrhage can occur. Hemarthroses are uncommon. Excessive bleeding may follow dental extraction, tonsillectomy or other surgical procedures. Diagnosis is confirmed by the thromboplastin generation test, which also differentiates this disorder from AHG or PTC deficiency. Treatment is with fresh plasma or blood.

HEPATOLENTICULAR DEGENERATION (WILSON DISEASE)[44]

The disease is usually characterized by a low ceruloplasmin, the copper-containing plasma protein, but there is a type with normal ceruloplasmin. The clinical effects, which become manifest in childhood or adult life, are liver disease, central nervous system symptoms and a pathognomonic Kayser-Fleischer ring, a golden discoloration around the cornea. Hepatomegaly, ascites, jaundice, cirrhosis and abnormal liver function tests call attention to the liver disease. Tremor (sometimes "wing-flapping"), indistinct speech, staring, drooling, hypertonicity, emotional lability and occasionally seizures are features of the central nervous system involvement. Laboratory confirmation comes from the demonstration of low plasma copper, low ceruloplasmin, high urinary copper and aminoaciduria. Defective radioactive copper uptake identifies cases with normal ceruloplasmin. Treatment with chelating agents may slow the progress of the disease, which usually is of several years' duration.

HYPOPHOSPHATASIA[45,46]

This disease, with skeletal abnormalities, low alkaline phosphatase, and hypercalcemia, described by Rathbun in 1948, is becoming recognized as having a spectrum of severity rather than necessarily being a disorder that terminates fatally in infancy. Over half of the patients die as infants, but others appear to survive to adult life with little or no detectable problem. The skeletal abnormalities include fragile bones with bowed legs, poorly mineralized skull with late closure of fontanelles and rachitic rosary (Fig. 8-23). Those who survive infancy have dental problems with defective dentin and premature loss of teeth. In the more severe cases there is respiratory insufficiency and hypotonia, failure to thrive and nephrocalcinosis. The homozygote has low serum alkaline phosphatase and high urinary excretion of phosphoethanolamine. The heterozygote may be observed to have low serum alkaline phosphatase. A "pseudohy-

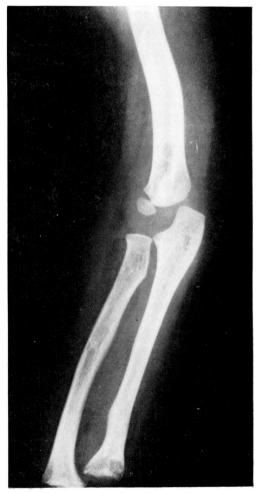

Figure 8-23. Metaphyseal rarefaction in hypophosphatasia.

pophosphatasia" has been described with the classic clinical picture but a normal phosphatase activity by the usual method of assay.

JAUNDICE, NONHEMOLYTIC (CRIGLER-NAJJAR SYNDROME)[47,48]

This rare disease is characterized by severe jaundice, high serum levels ($>$ 20 mg/100 ml) of indirect (unconjugated) bilirubin and kernicterus; it usually terminates fatally in infancy. The defect is a gross deficiency or absence of glucuronyl transferase necessary to conjugate bilirubin. The heterozygote may be detected by decreased glucuronide conjugation of menthol (despite normal excretion of injected bilirubin). Treatment by administration of barbiturates lowers serum bilirubin levels, perhaps through the induction of glucuronyl transferase. Two dominantly inherited conditions may be distinguished from the Crigler-Najjar syndrome: Gilbert syndrome and Dubin-Johnson syndrome (see Chapter 7).

LAURENCE-MOON-BIEDL SYNDROME[49]

This syndrome was recognized for its ophthalmologic abnormality and associated defects over 100 years ago. Retinitis pigmentosa is present in about two-thirds of the patients, and obesity, mental retardation, polydactyly (and syndactyly) are even more common (Fig. 8-24). Hypogonadism and genital hypoplasia are found in over half of these individuals. This syndrome should be distinguished on clinical grounds from the Prader-Willi syndrome, which has little risk of recurrence.

LEPRECHAUNISM (DONOHUE SYNDROME)[50]

This rare disorder deserves mention because it often appears in the differential diagnosis of infants with failure to thrive. It has been observed in siblings and with consanguinity. These small infants with their large eyes and ears, lack of adipose tissue and hirsutism look like the cartoon

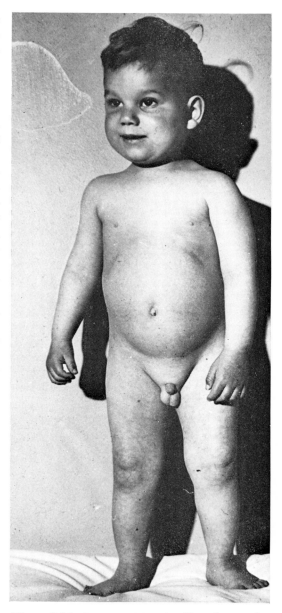

Figure 8-24. Laurence-Moon-Biedl syndrome. The only feature of the syndrome apparent in this photo is the obesity.

portrayals one has seen of leprechauns. They usually die in infancy and the basic metabolic defect remains obscure although they have endocrine derangement manifested by increased gonadotrophins, large phallus, breast hyperplasia, cystic ovaries

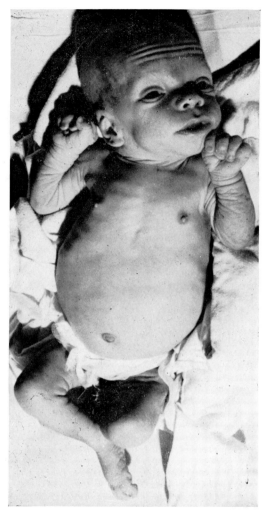

Figure 8-25. Severe failure to thrive and leprechaun face in infant diagnosed as Donohue syndrome, but in retrospect may represent cutis laxa.

and Leydig cell hyperplasia. Those patients who survive long enough for the observation to be made appear to be retarded.

THE LIPIDOSES[51,52]

As the title implies, this group of diseases is characterized by abnormalities of lipid metabolism with accumulation of lipids in viscera, brain and blood vessels, producing derangements of these systems. Table 8-5 presents a selection of lipidoses (including the classic disorders—Niemann-Pick, Gaucher and Tay-Sachs diseases) in which hepatosplenomegaly and neurologic deterioration predominate. The generalized gangliosidoses, GM (1), types I and II, and Farber disease, have features found in the mucopolysaccharidoses, as do the mucolipidoses, which are discussed in this connection and listed in Table 8-7. The three types of gangliosidosis GM(2) have clinical findings similar to the prototype of this group, Tay-Sachs disease. All of the lipidoses selected for presentation are autosomal recessive except for Fabry disease, which is X-linked recessive.

Table 8-5 also provides the salient clinical and laboratory features. It is recognized that Niemann-Pick, Gaucher and Tay-Sachs diseases may occur in individuals of various racial backgrounds, but that Jews are most often afflicted. Recently it has become clear that a catastrophic course and early death of patients with Niemann-Pick and Gaucher diseases is by no means invariable. Again the heterogeneity of types, presentations and clinical courses appears in this group of disorders as in so many others.

LIPODYSTROPHY (BERARDINELLI)[53]

This disorder (first reported by Berardinelli in 1954) consists of lipodystrophy, hepatomegaly, hyperlipemia and accelerated growth and maturation. The lipodystrophy involves a total loss of subcutaneous tissue of the face, trunk and limbs, with hypertrophy of skeletal muscle (Figs. 8-26, 8-27). Because of this, young patients appear much older than they are. Hyperglycemia, cataracts, cirrhosis of the liver and esophageal varices may develop. Mental retardation is found in some patients. This disorder, with its poor prognosis (death within the first two decades), is to be distinguished from partial lipodystrophy, which has a better outlook. In partial lipodystrophy the loss of fat may be mainly from the face or may include arms and trunk, but the legs are not involved.

TABLE 8-5. Selected Lipidoses

Disease	Laboratory Findings	Clinical Manifestations
Autosomal Recessive		
Niemann-Pick	Sphingomyelin accumulation; Niemann-Pick cells in bone marrow. Deficiency of sphingomyelin-splitting enzyme has been demonstrated in infantile type.	Four clinical types varying from degeneration and death by two years to survival to adult life with little or no handicap. Hepatosplenomegaly, mental retardation, neurologic deterioration.
Gaucher	Glucocerebroside accumulation; Gaucher cells in bone marrow. Deficiency of glucocerebroside-splitting enzyme.	Three clinical types; spectrum ranges from acute form in infancy with hepatosplenomegaly and neurologic deterioration with death in infancy or early childhood, to chronic form with onset in childhood or adulthood with hepatosplenomegaly, hypersplenism, bone and joint and neurologic involvement.
Farber	Ceramide and mucopolysaccharide accumulation.	Granulomatous lesions of skin, arthropathy, hoarse cry, irritability, failure to thrive.
Generalized gangliosidosis GM(1), Type I	Ganglioside GM(1) accumulation in brain and viscera, cytoplasmic vacuoles. Deficiency of A, B and C isozymes of beta-galactosidase.	Skeletal abnormalities suggestive of the Hurler syndrome, cherry-red macular spot, hepatosplenomegaly, death by age two years.
Generalized gangliosidosis GM(1), Type II	Ganglioside GM(1) accumulation in brain but not viscera. Deficiency of B and C isozymes of beta-galactosidase.	Similar to but later in onset than GM(1), Type I. Survival to ten years.
Gangliosidosis GM(2), Type I (Tay-Sachs disease; amaurotic family idiocy)	Tay-Sachs ganglioside GM(2) accumulation. Component A hexosaminidase deficient.	Onset in infancy of developmental retardation, blindness, paralysis, dementia and death by four years. Cherry-red macular spot.
Gangliosidosis GM(2), Type II (Sandhoff)	Ganglioside GM(2) accumulation in brain. Hexosaminidase A and B deficient.	Similar to Tay-Sachs. Not predominantly Jewish.
Gangliosidosis GM(2), Type III	Ganglioside GM(2) accumulation in brain. Hexosaminidase A partially deficient.	Later onset, non-Jewish origin. May survive to ten years.
X-linked Recessive		
Fabry	Cellular accumulation of ceramidetrihexoside. Deficiency of ceramidetrihexosidase.	Skin nodules, burning in hands and feet, progressive renal insufficiency, and death of affected males in thirties or forties.

METHEMOGLOBINEMIA[54]

Congenital methemoglobinemia is a recessive defect caused by congenital absence of DPNH-dependent methemoglobin reductase (diaphorase I). These patients equilibrate at about 40% methemoglobin. Generalized cyanosis is present. Occasional headaches may occur, but otherwise the patients are generally asymptomatic.

Differential diagnosis includes cyanotic congenital heart disease, hemoglobin M and acquired methemoglobinemia. Treatment consists of oral administration of methylene blue or ascorbic acid.

THE MUCOLIPIDOSES[55]

Mucolipidosis I (Lipomucopolysaccharidosis)

This disease has mild Hurler-like features without excess mucopolysacchariduria, but

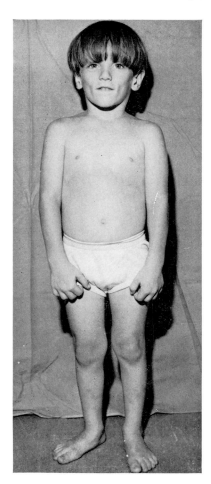

Figure 8-26. Berardinelli lipodystrophy. This four-year-old boy has an almost complete loss of subcutaneous fat over his entire body and has striking hypertrophy of skeletal muscle for his age. The loss of subcutaneous fat from his face makes him appear much older than he is.

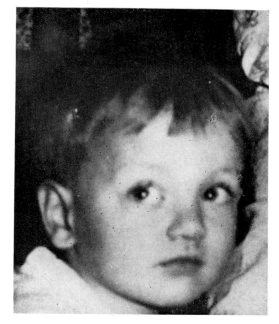

Figure 8-27. The patient in Figure 8-26 at two years of age before the lipodystrophy became evident.

Mucolipidosis II (Leroy Syndrome, I-Cell Disease)

This is another disease with clinical features of Hurler syndrome with no increase in mucopolysaccharides in the urine. It was first reported by Leroy and DeMars in 1967. Unusual cytoplasmic inclusions were noted by these authors in cultured fibroblasts, but metachromatic granules have not been observed in leucocytes. Growth and intellectual retardation, coarse Hurler-like facies, hyperplastic gums, stiff joints, congenital dislocation of the hip, kyphosis and x-ray findings compatible with MPS I are features of this syndrome. Hepatosplenomegaly is minimal and corneal clouding has not been noted. Prevalence and life expectancy are not known.

Mucolipidosis III (Pseudo-Hurler Polydystrophy)

This disorder was described by Maroteaux and Lamy in 1965. It is characterized by stiff joints, corneal clouding, coarse fa-

with peculiar fibroblast inclusions. Early psychomotor development is normal. Clinical features become apparent in the second and third year of life. Hepatosplenomegaly is inconstant. Joint mobility may be increased initially, but becomes restricted by four years of age. Patients may have cherry-red macular spots and, less frequently, corneal opacities. X-ray findings are similar to those of MPS III. Mental retardation is moderate.

cies, genu valgum, aortic valve disease and mild to moderate intellectual retardation. Metachromatic granules do not appear in the leucocytes but are visible in excess in the urine. Median nerve signs, which appear in these patients as in other disorders of this group, especially MPS V, are relieved by carpal tunnel release. Life expectancy and prevalence for this syndrome are not known.

THE MUCOPOLYSACCHARIDOSES[56]

This group of diseases has provided some of the most exciting advances in biochemical genetics in the past few years. Six types were distinguished on clinical and biochemical grounds: Hurler (I), Hunter (II—sex-linked recessive), Sanfilippo (III), Morquio (IV), Scheie (V) and Maroteaux-Lamy (VI). Recently it was shown that the accumulation of sulfated mucopolysaccharide in cultured fibroblasts of Hurler syndrome could be "cured" by culturing them with normal fibroblasts, or with cells from patients with Hunter or Sanfilippo disease. This showed that each was making a substance that the other lacked, and that the corrective factor (presumably an enzyme involved in the degradation of sulfated mucopolysaccharide) was present extracellularly. Furthermore, the Sanfilippo syndrome could be classified into two clinically indistinguishable types, with different enzymatic defects, each possessing the corrective factor lacking in the other. The second exciting advance is that the corrective factors appear to be therapeutically beneficial, at least in cases of the Hurler and Hunter syndromes. Surprisingly, cells from patients with Scheie disease and those with Hurler disease did not correct one another, indicating that they lacked the same substance, and that the mutant genes for these two diseases were allelic. This idea was confirmed by the discovery of patients with intermediate phenotypes, presumably compound heterozygotes. Finally a seventh type of disease has been described by Sly in which the enzyme beta-glucuronidase is missing. McKusick has therefore suggested reclassifying the mucopolysaccharidoses as shown in Table 8-6. Table 8-7 lists the mucopolysaccharidoses and mucolipidoses with their distinguishing features.

Patients with mucopolysaccharidoses have many common features but clinical as well as biochemical findings can be used to distinguish the various types. However, the clinical features may not be apparent in infants and even young children with MPS (except Leroy syndrome). Secondly, some patients with classic features of Morquio syndrome do not excrete keratosulfate in the urine. Patients with clinical signs of mucolipidoses also do not excrete mucopolysaccharides in the urine. Still other pa-

TABLE 8-6. Revised Classification of the Mucopolysaccharidoses

Type	Enzyme Defect	Inheritance	Classification Old	Classification New
Hurler	alpha-1-iduronidase	AR	I	IH
Scheie	" "	AR	V	IS
Hunter		SLR	II	II
Sanfilippo A	keratan sulfate sulfatase	AR	III	IIIA
Sanfilippo B	N-acetyl-alpha-D glucoaminidase	AR	III	IIIB
Morquio	?	AR	IV	IV
Sly	beta-glucuronidase		—	V
Maroteaux-Lamy			VI	VI

TABLE 8-7. Mucopolysaccharidoses, Mucolipidoses and Phenotypically Similar Diseases

Disease	Inheritance	Urine*	Meta-chromatic granules	Corneal Clouding	Mental Retardation	Other
MPS IH (Hurler)	AR	Ch.B. Hep. S.	++	++	++	Severe disease, heart, skeletal, dwarfing, hepatosplenomegaly.
MPS IS (Scheie)	AR	Ch.B.	+/−	++	0	Milder disease, skeletal, heart, psychosis.
MPS II (Hunter)	X-linked rec.	Ch.B. Hep.S.	+	0	+/−	Milder disease, heart, skeletal, dwarfing, deafness, hepatosplenomegaly.
MPS III (Sanfilippo)	AR	Hep.S.	+	0	++	Severe C.N.S., mild somatic, skeletal.
MPS IV (Morquio)	AR	Kerato-sulfate	+	+	0	Severe skeletal, heart, dwarfism.
MPS VI (Maroteaux-Lamy)	AR		+	+	0	Milder disease, skeletal, dwarfing, hepatosplenomegaly.
ML I (Lipomucopoly-saccharidosis)	AR	0	0	+/−	+	Skeletal and facial manifestations are mild.
ML II (Leroy syndrome; I-cell disease)	AR	0	0	0	++	Severe disease, skeletal, C.N.S.
ML III (Pseudo-Hurler polydystrophy)	AR	0	0	+	+	Milder disease, stiff joints, heart.
Generalized gangliosidosis GM(1) Type I	AR	0	0	0	++	Extremely severe C.N.S. involvement, death before 2 yrs.

*Ch. B. = chondroitin sulfate B. Hep. S. = heparitin sulfate.

tients with stigmata of MPS but no MPS excretion defy classification into the six major categories. It is clear that there is considerably greater heterogeneity within this group of disease than had been previously recognized. Cell culture techniques are helping to define more clearly the individual disorders within the mucopolysaccharidoses, mucolipidoses and gangliosidoses, and the categories presented at this time must be accepted with flexibility.

Mucopolysaccharidosis Type IH (Hurler Syndrome)[57,59]

History. Hurler published a description of this disorder in 1919. Dorfman and Lorincz discovered mucopolysacchariduria in

patients with the Hurler syndrome in 1957, establishing the nature of the disease.

Diagnostic Features. *General.* Progressive mental retardation. Equal sex distribution. Dwarfed, hirsute. Death usually in first decade.

Head. Large, bulging, scaphocephalic. Hydrocephalus, coarse facial features (gargoyle-like) (Figs. 8-28, 8-29).

Eyes. Cloudy corneas, retinal pigmentation, hypertelorism.

Ears. Occasional deafness.

Nose. Broad, wide nostrils, flat bridge, mucoid rhinitis.

Mouth. Full lips, enlarged tongue; teeth small, malformed; alveolar hypertrophy.

Neck. Short.

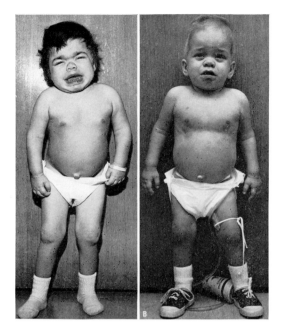

Figure 8-28. Two- and three-year-old siblings with Hurler syndrome. The "gargoyle" facies, claw hand and limitations in joint mobility may be appreciated.

Hands. Broad, "stiff" stubby fingers—flexion contractures (claw hand).

Skeletal. Generalized limitation in extensibility of joints, broad spatulate ribs, flaring rib cage, kyphosis and thoracolumbar gibbus secondary to anterior beaking of vertebral bodies.

Abdomen. Protuberant, hepatosplenomegaly, diastasis recti, umbilical hernia, inguinal hernia.

Cardiovascular. Deposition of mucopolysaccharides in cardiac valves and in coronary arteries, leading to congestive heart failure and coronary occlusion.

X-ray. "Shoe-shaped" sella, beaking of lumbar vertebrae, spatulate ribs, diaphyseal irregularities, short malformed phalangeal bones.

Laboratory. Chondroitin sulfate B and heparitin sulfate in urine; metachromatic granules in leucocytes.

Prevalence. 1:40,000.

Clinical Course. The patient appears normal at birth and during early growth and intellectual development. A gibbus may be observed during the first few months of life, but evidence of mental retardation is seldom recognized before six months to one year of age. Stiff joints, protuberant abdomen and persistent rhinitis are frequent reasons for initial medical consultation. Regression in mental and physical development becomes more apparent with increasing age. The joint stiffness becomes more generalized and involves wrists, knees, ankles and back.

At two to three years of age the clouding of the corneas and hepatosplenomegaly become increasingly obvious. Heart murmurs are heard and are probably related to the valvular depositions of mucopolysaccharides. The aortic and mitral valves are most often affected, but all four valves may be involved. The coronary arteries exhibit pronounced intimal thickening, which may produce coronary occlusion. The clinical course is one of progressive deterioration with a cardiac death in the first decade or early in the second decade.

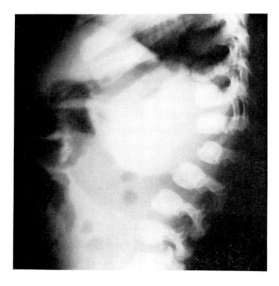

Figure 8-29. "Beaking" of lumbar vertebrae and gibbus in MPS IH (Hurler).

Treatment. Symptomatic. Recently there has been evidence that large infusions of human plasma produce clinical improvement, but this needs confirmation.

Differential Diagnosis. Although many diseases have various combinations of dwarfing, hepatosplenomegaly and mental retardation, the major differential is from other forms of mucopolysaccharidoses, mucolipidoses and gangliosidoses (Table 8-7).

Mucopolysaccharidosis II, or Hunter syndrome, is described in the chapter on sex-linked diseases.

Mucopolysaccharidosis Type IS (Scheie Syndrome)[58,59]

These patients, recognized by Scheie in 1962, have a normal to superior intellect and nearly normal height. They have stiff joints, claw hands and striking corneal clouding. Retinitis pigmentosa, hirsutism, a broad-mouthed face, and aortic valvular disease with aortic insufficiency are also found. Metachromatic granules are less easily detected than in the other mucopolysaccharidoses. The mucopolysaccharide excreted in excess in the urine is chondroitin sulfate B. The corneal clouding constitutes a significant problem. Efforts at corneal transplants have resulted in opacification of the grafts. Psychotic episodes have been reported. The life expectancy and prevalence of this disorder are as yet undetermined. The biochemical defect has been identified as involving the same enzyme as in Hurler syndrome.

Mucopolysaccharidosis Type IIIA and B (Sanfilippo A and B)[60]

In this disease, described by Sanfilippo and colleagues in 1963, the somatic manifestations are relatively mild but the mental retardation is severe. Heparitin sulfate, alone excreted in excess in the urine, differentiates this disease from MPS I and II. The intellectual deterioration, which is progressive throughout the school age period, is accompanied by reasonably good physical strength, making these patients manage-

ment problems requiring hospitalization. Dwarfing is not significant and stiffness of joints is less than in MPS I and II. Metachromatic granules are found in the lymphocytes. The corneas are clear. Patients with this syndrome generally survive several decades. Two distinct enzyme defects (Table 8-6) permit subdivision into type IIIA and type IIIB.

Mucopolysaccharidosis Type IV (Morquio Syndrome)[61,62]

Morquio and Brailsford described this syndrome independently in 1929, although Osler had reported siblings in 1897 as having achondroplasia who probably had MPS IV. In the literature one may see a distinction made between Morquio syndrome, Brailsford type, and Morquio syndrome Ullrich type, based on the presence of corneal clouding and keratosulfaturia in patients with the "Ullrich type" and the absence of these findings and a milder disease in the "Brailsford type."

We will follow the convention that patients with severe skeletal anomalies and keratosulfate in the urine have the Morquio syndrome—unqualified. The rare patients with the severe skeletal stigmata of the Morquio syndrome who do not secrete keratosulfate are called the nonkeratosulfate-excreting Morquio syndrome. There is reason to believe that patients previously classified as "Brailsford type" may well have had later onset of such extraskeletal manifestations as corneal clouding. The term "Brailsford type" has also been attached to patients with mild somatic findings suggestive of some form of mucopolysaccharidosis but without mucopolysacchariduria.

The Morquio syndrome may be difficult to distinguish from the Hurler syndrome during the first year of life on the basis of somatic features, but with increasing age the key differences become readily apparent. Patients with the Morquio syndrome are generally *not* retarded and the skeletal features are quite distinctive. They are severely dwarfed; the head seems to rest on a

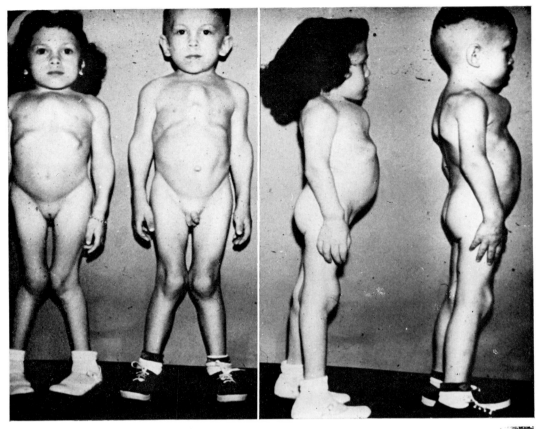

Figure 8-30.   Severe skeletal dysplasia of MPS IV (Morquio)—head resting on barrel chest, pigeon breast and knock-knees.

barrel chest. There is a pigeon breast. The joints are usually not stiff but the wrists and hands are deformed. Knock-knees and changes in the femoral heads may be noted as well as generalized osteoporosis and characteristically flat vertebrae. (See Figs. 8-30, 8-31.)

Corneal clouding may not be detectable until after ten years of age. Patients have a broad mouth with widely spaced teeth. Heart disease, specifically aortic insufficiency, has been observed. Metachromatic granules are found in cultured fibroblasts and the mucopolysacchariduria is specific for this syndrome—keratosulfate. The prevalence has been estimated at about 1: 40,000. Death commonly occurs between the second and fifth decades.

Mucopolysaccharidosis Type VI (Maroteaux-Lamy Syndrome)[63]

Maroteaux, Lamy and co-workers described this condition in 1963. Growth retardation, knock-knees, stiff joints and corneal clouding occur without mental retardation (Fig. 8-32). There are excessive chondroitin sulfate B in the urine and metachromatic granules in the leucocytes. The skeletal and growth abnormality is similar to MPS I, but the disease differs by virtue of the normal intelligence and lack of heparitin sulfate in the urine. The growth retardation of the trunk and limbs distinguishes this disease from MPS V, which also has only chondroitin sulfate B in the urine. Heart disease has not been described and

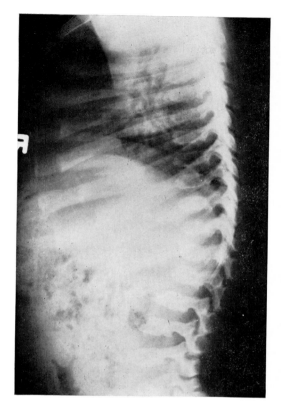

Figure 8-31. Flat thoracic vertebrae in patient with MPS IV.

prevalence and life expectancy have yet to be determined.

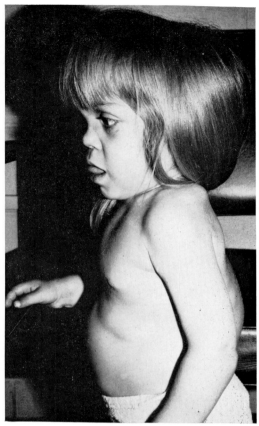

Figure 8-32. MPS VI (Maroteaux-Lamy) shares features of MPS IH and MPS IV. In contrast with MPS IH, there is normal intelligence.

MUSCULAR ATROPHY, PROGRESSIVE SPINAL (WERDNIG-HOFFMANN SYNDROME)[64]

This disease is one of the causes of extreme hypotonia of infancy. There is often a history of diminished or absent fetal movements. The hypotonia and areflexia are noted at birth or shortly after. The infant is limp, the muscles thin, and the only limb movements may be of the fingers. Progressive paralysis of respiratory muscles leads to death (often from respiratory infection) during the first year of life. Some patients have a later onset of the disease, with weakness becoming apparent at one or two years of age. These patients may survive adolescence. Muscle biopsy reveals fascicular atrophy. The basic abnormality is degeneration of the anterior horn cells with progressive loss of motor neurons.

MUSCULAR DYSTROPHY, RECESSIVE[65,66,67]

In this category, which comprises the largest group of muscle diseases of childhood, are disorders that are inherited by autosomal recessive, autosomal dominant and X-linked recessive modes. The three autosomal recessive forms are: muscular dystrophy I (limb-girdle, Leyden-Möbius) (Fig. 8-33); muscular dystrophy II, which resembles the X-linked Duchenne type; and a congenital muscular dystrophy that produces arthrogryposis. In all forms of this disease there is progressive weakness and

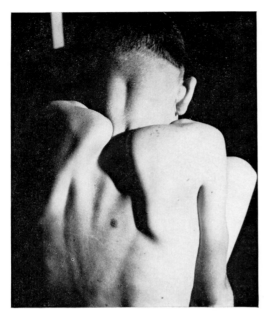

Figure 8-33. Muscular dystrophy I produces progressive atrophy and weakness of the limb girdle.

atrophy, with increasing disability and deformity. Early in the course of the Duchenne type and muscular dystrophy II there is pseudohypertrophy. A cardiomyopathy is present in many of the nosologic types, but less commonly in the autosomal forms.

OSTEOPETROSIS, RECESSIVE (ALBERS-SCHÖNBERG DISEASE; "MARBLE BONES")[68]

Two forms of this disorder exist, a mild autosomal dominant form and a severe recessive form that terminates fatally in infancy or early childhood, usually because of profound bone marrow depression. It is believed that there is defective resorption of immature bone. Other important clinical features are: progressive deafness, blindness and hydrocephalus due to compression of cranial foramina; hepatosplenomegaly; and characteristic x-ray appearance of "marble bones," "bone within bone," broad metaphyses and vertical striations at the metaphyseal-diaphyseal juncture (Fig. 8-34). The abnormal bone x-ray appearance has been detected before the birth of the affected fetus.

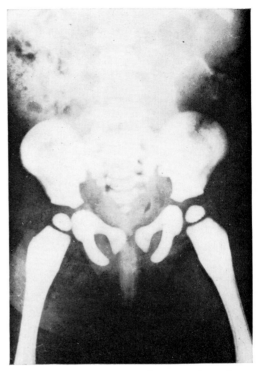

Figure 8-34. Dense mineralization gives characteristic x-ray appearance of "marble bones" in osteopetrosis.

PANCREATIC EXOCRINE DEFICIENCY (SCHWACHMAN SYNDROME)[69]

Leukopenia and lack of exocrine pancreas are the features of this syndrome. The exocrine pancreas is replaced by adipose tissue. The patients, therefore, lack trypsin, lipase and amylase. Steatorrhea is not a feature. Duodenal secretions have normal viscosity in contrast to cystic fibrosis and the sweat test is normal. Some patients respond dramatically to enzyme replacement while others do not. Leukopenia is variable and may lead to frequent bacterial infections. Leukemia is being recognized more frequently as an eventual complication.

POLYCYSTIC DISEASE OF KIDNEYS AND LIVER WITH CHILDHOOD ONSET[70]

There are several genetically distinct forms of childhood polycystic kidney disease with liver involvement, as well as the dominantly inherited adult form. According to a recent classification these childhood types can be classified as follows:

The Perinatal Type. These children present at birth with very marked abdominal distension due to huge symmetric renal masses; they die within six weeks. There is cystic formation, appearing as longitudinal dilatation, of 90% of the renal tubules, and ectasia of the bile ducts with minimal periportal fibrosis. A "Potter's facies," with lowset floppy ears, micrognathia and snub nose, is often present.

The Neonatal Type. In this group the kidney enlargement becomes manifest within the first month of life and death occurs within one year. The kidneys are entirely cystic, with over 60% of the tubules involved. In the liver there are several diffusely scattered cystic portal areas, and dilatation of all the intrahepatic bile ducts.

The Infantile Type. These children usually present in the first six months with enlargement of the liver, with or without palpable enlargement of kidneys and/or spleen. They may present with signs of renal failure or portal hypertension. The kidneys are cystic with involvement of about 25% of the tubules, and the liver shows dilatation and infolding of the intrahepatic bile ducts and ductules with moderate periportal fibrosis.

The Juvenile Group. In this group the child usually presents between one and five years with enlargement of the liver, splenic enlargement and variable kidney enlargement. The clinical picture is that of portal obstruction. The liver is hard and finely mottled with biliary dilatation and infolding, and marked biliary fibrosis. The kidneys show dilation of about 10% of tubules or less.

POLYCYSTIC KIDNEYS, POLYDACTYLY AND ENCEPHALOCELE (MECKEL SYNDROME)[71]

In this rare syndrome, occipital encephalocele, polycystic kidneys and postaxial polydactyly are often associated with microcephaly, microphthalmia, cleft palate, congenital heart defects and club feet.

PORPHYRIA, ERYTHROPOIETIC, CONGENITAL[72]

The hepatic porphyrias are inherited as dominant traits; the rare congenital erythropoietic porphyria is autosomal recessive. Burgundy red urine is a constant finding. Splenomegaly and cutaneous mutilation are features. Onset is in infancy. The acute visceral and neurologic attacks that characterize the hepatic forms are absent in this disorder. Another point of differentiation is that porphyrins are present in the erythrocytes of erythropoietic porphyria but not in hepatic porphyria. The defect appears to be in the conversion of porphobilinogen to uroporphyrinogen in the developing erythrocyte.

THE PREMATURE SENILITIES

Cockayne Syndrome[73]

Cockayne described this syndrome of senile appearance in sibs in 1946. Growth failure and loss of adipose tissue becomes apparent during late infancy. Cataracts, mental retardation, hearing loss, unsteady gait, retinal degeneration, marble epiphyses and dermal photosensitivity are observed in a child who fails to grow and has the appearance of a "little, old man" (Fig. 8-35). There is no specific treatment other than supportive and symptomatic care for the syndromes of senile appearance of Cockayne, Werner, Rothmund and Hutchinson-Gilford (progeria).

Poikiloderma Congenitale of Rothmund[74]

Patients with this disorder of the skin and eyes may initially appear to have an ectodermal dysplasia or a disorder of senile appearance. Between three to 12 months of age the skin begins to show a marbled surface pattern produced by an erythema that progresses to telangiectasia, scarring and atrophy (Fig. 8-36). Juvenile cataracts develop between 18 months and ten years of age. The typical patient will be short, and has cataracts, sparse, prematurely gray hair, deficiencies of teeth and dystrophy of

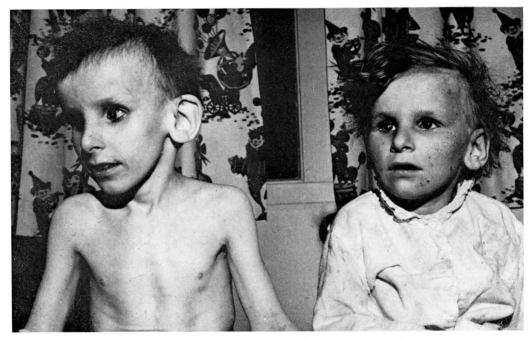

Figure 8-35.   Senile appearance in ten- and seven-year-old siblings with Cockayne syndrome.

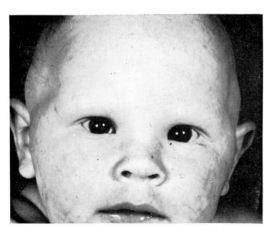

Figure 8-36.   Alopecia and "marbled-skin" pattern in patient with Rothmund syndrome (age six years).

the nails. The skin shows punctate areas of atrophy, telangiectasia and hyperpigmentation.

Progeria (Hutchinson-Gilford Syndrome)[75]

The autosomal recessive mode of inheritance of this very rare syndrome is sus-

pected from its occurrence in sibs, though family data are scarce. However, the presentation of this disorder in the context of other diseases of senile appearance seems reasonable. Hutchinson, in 1886, and Gilford, in 1904, made the early observation of this syndrome. As in Cockayne syndrome the infant appears normal at birth, and it is not for several months to as long as two years that the suspicion of abnormal development occurs. Unlike Cockayne syndrome, intelligence does not appear to be impaired. Baldness is early in onset. Growth reaches a plateau at about 18 months and the eventual height attainment may be that of a five-year-old. There are loss of fat, periarticular fibrosis with joint-stiffening, and skeletal abnormalities, such as hypoplasia, dysplasia and a characteristic degeneration of the clavicle and distal phalanges (Fig. 8-37). Generalized atherosclerosis progresses from as early as five years to the time of death in the second decade, often of coronary artery disease.

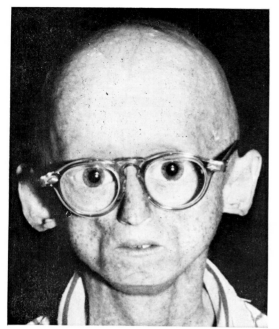

Figure 8-37.   Appearance of advanced age in 15-year-old child with progeria.

Werner Syndrome[76]

In this syndrome the appearance of premature senility begins in young adult life, although the effects of the disease have had an earlier onset as manifested by moderate growth retardation with decreased height attainment. There is thin skin with loss of subcutaneous fat and replacement by fibrous, thick subcutaneous tissue. Other findings include premature graying and balding, cataracts, atherosclerosis, osteoporosis, muscle hypoplasia, thin extremities, pinched face, reduced fertility, diabetes and liver atrophy.

PSEUDOXANTHOMA ELASTICUM[77,78]

Various aspects of this disease have been reported by a number of authors since the 1880's. The three major areas of involvement are the skin, the eyes and the cardiovascular system. The skin becomes thickened, yellowed, grooved and redundant, usually beginning in the second decade. In the eye angioid streaks, which are cracks in

the membrane beneath the retina, develop in the fundus. Hemorrhage and chorioretinal scarring and severe visual impairment occur. Cardiovascular involvement is manifested by weak pulses, arterial insufficiency, intermittent claudication, calcification of peripheral arteries, coronary occlusion, hypertension and bouts of gastrointestinal hemorrhage. Psychiatric disorders and early neurologic deterioration may be attributed to cerebral vascular changes.

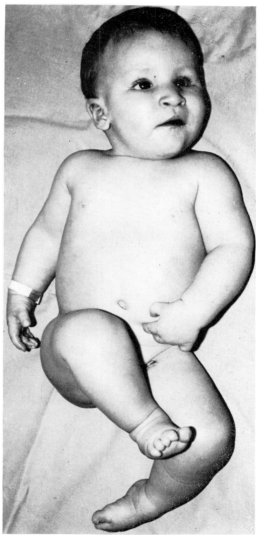

Figure 8-38.   Full body view of patient with Smith-Lemli-Opitz syndrome.

SMITH-LEMLI-OPITZ SYNDROME[79,80]

The clinical features of this syndrome are failure to thrive, mental retardation, microcephaly, low-set ears, ptosis, broad nose with upturned nares, micrognathia, high palate, broad alveolar ridge, short neck, simian crease, flexed fingers, syndactyly between second and third toes, clubbed feet and cryptorchism and/or hypospadias (Figs. 8-38 to 8-41). Other features sometimes found include breech birth, low birth weight, epicanthic folds, strabismus, cleft palate, heart defect and pyloric stenosis. Probably no one feature is always present.

Because of the poor prognostic outlook, one must be cautious neither to overdiagnose this syndrome in patients with syndactyly of the second and third toes and few other defects, nor to fail to recognize the associated anomalies leading to a diagnosis of Smith-Lemli-Opitz syndrome, with all that this implies.

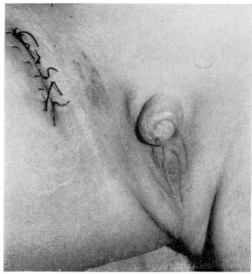

Figure 8-40. Hypospadias and cryptorchism are features of Smith-Lemli-Opitz and congenital heart disease is common (note stitches and incision of recent cardiac catheterization).

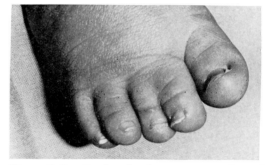

Figure 8-41. Syndactyly between second and third toes is an important feature of Smith-Lemli-Opitz, but it is also found in otherwise normal individuals.

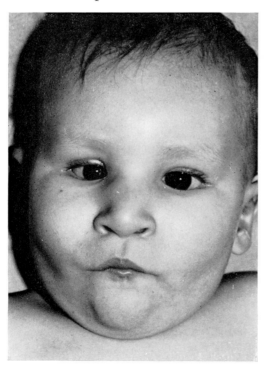

Figure 8-39. Anteverted nares, epicanthic folds and strabismus contribute to characteristic facies of Smith-Lemli-Opitz.

SPHEROPHAKIA WITH BRACHYMORPHY (WEILL-MARCHESANI SYNDROME)[81]

The mode of inheritance of this syndrome is not well established, but is probably autosomal recessive in most families, with brachymorphism sometimes occurring in the heterozygote. The lens is small and round, and may be subluxated with secondary glaucoma. There is short stature with short neck and stocky build, and short, stiff hands and feet.

REFERENCES

Adrenal Cortical Hyperfunction, Inherited

1. Bongiovanni, A. M.: Disorders of adrenocortical steroid biogenesis. *In* Stanbury, J. B., et al. (ed.): Metabolic Basis of Inherited Disease. 3rd ed. New York, McGraw-Hill, 1972, p. 857.

Agammaglobulinemia, Swiss Type

2. Haworth, J. C., Hoogstraten, J., and Taylor, H.: Thymic alymphoplasia. Arch. Dis. Child., 42:42, 1967.

Albinism

3. Witkop, C. J.: Albinism. *In* Hirschhorn, K., and Harris, H. (eds.): Advances in Human Genetics. vol. 2. New York, Plenum Press, 1971, p. 61.

Alpha-l-Antitrypsin Deficiency

4. Gans, H., Sharp, H. L., and Tans, B. H.: Antiprotease deficiency and familial infantile liver cirrhosis. Surg. Gynec. Obstet., 129:289, 1969.
5. Talamo, R. C., Levinson, H., and Lynch, M. J.: Symptomatic pulmonary emphysema in childhood associated with alpha-1-antitrypsin and elastase inhibitor deficiency. J. Pediat., 79:20, 1971.

Amino Acid Metabolism, Inborn Errors

6. Stanbury, J. B., Wyngaarden, J. B., and Fredrickson, D. S. (eds.): The Metabolic Basis of Inherited Disease. 3rd ed. New York, McGraw-Hill, 1972.
7. Clow, C. L., Reade, T. M., and Scriver, C. R.: Management of hereditary metabolic disease. New Eng. J. Med., 284:1292, 1971.

ALKAPTONURIA

8. La Du, B. N., et al.: The nature of the defect in tyrosine metabolism in alcaptonuria. J. Biol. Chem., 230:251, 1958.

CYSTINURIA

9. Rosenberg, L. E., et al.: Cystinuria: biochemical evidence for three genetically distinct diseases. J. Clin. Invest., 45:365, 1966.

HISTIDINEMIA

10. La Du, B. N.: Histidinemia: Current status. Amer. J. Dis. Child., 113:88, 1967.

HOMOCYSTINURIA

11. Mudd, S. H., et al.: Homocystinuria due to cystathionine synthase deficiency: The effect of pyridoxine. J. Clin. Invest., 49:1762, 1970.

MAPLE SYRUP URINE DISEASE

12. Westall, R. G., Dancis, J., and Miller, S.: Maple sugar urine disease. A.M.A. J. Dis. Child., 94:571, 1957.
13. Westall, R. G.: Dietary treatment of maple syrup urine disease. Amer. J. Dis. Child., 113: 58, 1967.

PHENYLKETONURIA

14. Hsia, D. Y.-Y.: Phenylketonuria and its variants. Prog. Med. Genet., 7:29, 1970.

TYROSINEMIA

15. Scriver, C. R., La Rochelle, J., and Silverberg, M.: Hereditary tyrosinemia and tyrosyluria in a French Canadian geographic isolate. Amer. J. Dis. Child., 113:41, 1967.

Anemias

CONSTITUTIONAL APLASTIC ANEMIA (FANCONI PANCYTOPENIA)

16. Fanconi, G.: Die familiare Panmyelopathie. Schweiz. Med. Wschr., 94:1309, 1964.

HEMOGLOBINOPATHIES (C AND S)

17. Lehmann, H., and Huntsman, R. G.: The hemoglobinopathies. *In* Stanbury, J. B., et al. (eds.): Metabolic Basis of Inherited Disease. New York, McGraw-Hill, 1972, p. 1398.

PYRUVATE KINASE DEFICIENCY

18. Zuelzer, W. W., Robinson, A. R., and Hus, T. H. J.: Erythrocyte pyruvate kinase deficiency in nonspherocytic hemolytic anemia: A system of multiple genetic markers. Blood, 32:33, 1968.

THALASSEMIAS

19. Weatherall, D. J.: The genetics of the thalassemias. Brit. Med. Bull., 25:24, 1969.

Ataxia, Friedreich

20. Hartman, J. M., and Booth, R. W.: Friedreich's ataxia: a neurocardiac disease. Amer. Heart J., 60:716, 1960.

Ataxia Telangiectasia (Louis-Bar Syndrome)

21. Tadjoedin, M. K., and Fraser, F. C.: Heredity of ataxia-telangiectasia (Louis-Bar syndrome). Amer. J. Dis. Child., 110:64, 1965.

Color Blindness, Total

22. Harrison, R., Hofnagel, D., and Hayward, J. N.: Congenital total color blindness. Arch. Ophthal., 64:685, 1960.

Cretinism

23. Stanbury, J. B.: Familial goiter. *In* Stanbury, J. B., et al. (eds.): The Metabolic Basis of Inherited Disease. 3rd ed. New York, McGraw-Hill, 1972, p. 223.

Cutis Laxa Syndrome

24. Hajjar, B. A., and Joyner, E. N.: Congenital cutis laxa with advanced cardiopulmonary disease. J. Pediat., 73:116, 1968.

Cystic Fibrosis (Mucoviscidosis)

25. Mangos, J. A., and McSherry, N. R.: Sodium transport: inhibitory factor in sweat of patients with cystic fibrosis. Science, 158:135, 1967.
26. Rao, C. J. S., and Nadler, H. L.: Deficiency of trypsin-like activity in saliva of patients with cystic fibrosis. J. Pediat., 80:573, 1972.

Deafness

27. Konigsmark, B. W.: Hereditary deafness in man. New Eng. J. Med., 281:713, 774, 827, 1969.
28. Stevenson, A. C., and Davison, B. C. C.: Genetic Counselling. London, Heinemann, 1970.

Diplegia, Ichthyosis, Mental Retardation
(*Sjögren-Larsson Syndrome*)

29. Selmanowitz, V. J., and Porter, M. J.: The Sjögren-Larsson syndrome. Amer. J. Med., 42:412, 1967.

Dysautonomia (Riley-Day Syndrome)

30. Goldstein-Nieviazhski, C., and Wallis, K.: Riley-Day syndrome (familial dysautonomia). Survey of 27 cases. Ann. Paediat., 206:188, 1966.

Dwarfism
BIRD-HEADED DWARFS (SECKEL SYNDROME)

31. Seckel, H. P. G.: Bird-Headed Dwarfs. Springfield, Ill., Charles C Thomas, 1960, p. 241.

BLOOM SYNDROME

32. Sawitsky, A., Bloom, D., and German, J.: Chromosomal breakage and acute leukemia in congenital telangiectatic erythema and stunted growth. Ann. Intern. Med., 65:487, 1966.

CARTILAGE-HAIR HYPOPLASIA

33. McKusick, V. A., et al.: Dwarfism in the Amish. II Cartilage-hair hypoplasia. Bull. Hopkins Hosp., 116:285, 1965.
34. Lux, S. E. et al.: Chronic neutropenia and abnormal cellular immunity in cartilage-hair hypoplasia. New Eng. J. Med., 282:231, 1970.

CHONDRODYSTROPHIA CALCIFICANS CONGENITA (CONRADI DISEASE)

35. Spranger, J. W., Opitz, J. M., and Bidder, V.: Heterogeneity of chondrodysplasia punctata. Humangenetik, 11:190, 1971.

CHONDROECTODERMAL DYSPLASIA (ELLIS-VAN CREVELD SYNDROME)

36. McKusick, V. A., et al.: Dwarfism in the Amish. The Ellis-van Creveld syndrome. Bull. Hopkins Hosp., 115:306, 1964.
37. Metrakos, J. D., and Fraser, F. C.: Evidence for a hereditary factor in chondroectodermal dysplasia (Ellis-van Creveld syndrome). Amer. J. Hum. Genet., 6:260, 1954.

DIASTROPHIC DWARFISM

38. Langer, L. O., Jr.: Diastrophic dwarfism in early infancy. Amer. J. Roentgen., 93:399, 1965.

THORACIC DYSTROPHY, ASPHYXIATING (JEUNE SYNDROME)

39. Jeune, M., Beraud, C., and Carron, R.: Dystrophie thoracique asphyxiante de caractère familial. Arch. Franç. Pédiat., 12:886, 1955.

40. Pirnar, T., and Neuhauser, E. B. D.: Asphyxiating thoracic dystrophy of the newborn. Amer. J. Roentgen., 98:358, 1966.

Galactosemia

41. Hsia, D. Y.-Y.: Galactosemia. Springfield, Ill., Charles C Thomas, 1969.

Glycogen Storage Diseases

42. Sidbury, J. B., Jr.: The genetics of the glycogen storage disease. In Steinberg, A. G., and Bearn, A. G.: Progress in Medical Genetics. vol. 4. Grune & Stratton, 1965.

Hemophilia C (PTA or Factor XI Deficiency)

43. Rapaport, S. I., et al.: The mode of inheritance of PTA deficiency; evidence for the existence of major PTA deficiency and minor PTA deficiency. Blood, 18:149, 1961.

Hepatolenticular Degeneration (Wilson Disease)

44. Bearn, A. G.: Wilson's disease. In Stanbury, J. B., et al. (eds.): The Metabolic Basis of Inherited Diseases. 3rd ed. New York, McGraw-Hill, 1972, p. 1033.

Hypophosphatasia

45. Rathbun, J. C., et al.: Hypophosphatasia: a genetic study. Arch. Dis. Child., 36:540, 1961.
46. Teree, T. M., and Klein, L.: Hypophosphatasia: Clinical and metabolic studies. J. Pediat., 72:41, 1968.

Jaundice, Nonhemolytic
(*Crigler-Najjar Syndrome*)

47. Gardner, W. A., Jr., and Konigsmark, B. W.: Familial nonhemolytic jaundice. Pediatrics, 43:365, 1969.
48. Karon, M., Imach, D., and Schwartz, A.: Effective phototherapy in congenital nonobstructive, nonhemolytic jaundice. New Eng. J. Med., 282:377, 1970.

Laurence-Moon-Biedl Syndrome

49. Bell, J.: The Laurence-Moon syndrome. In Penrose, L. S. (ed.): The Treasury of Human Inheritance. vol. 5, part 3. London, Cambridge University Press, 1958.

Leprechaunism (Donohue Syndrome)

50. Donohue, W. L., and Uchida, I.: Leprechaunism: An euphuism for a rare familial disorder. J. Pediat., 45:505, 1954.

Lipidoses

51. Knudson, A. G., Jr., and Kaplan, W. D.: Genetics of the sphingolipidoses. In Aaronson, S. M., and Volk, B. W. (eds.): A Symposium on Tay-Sachs Disease. New York, Academic Press, 1962, p. 395.
52. O'Brien, J. S.: Ganglioside storage diseases. In Harris, H., and Hirschhorn, K. (eds.): Advances in Human Genetics. vol. 3. New York, Plenum Press, 1972, p. 39.

Lipodystrophy (Berardinelli)

53. Senior, B., and Gellis, S. S.: The syndromes of total lipodystrophy and of partial lipodystrophy. Pediatrics, 33:593, 1964.

Methemoglobinemia

54. Cawein, M., *et al.*: Hereditary diaphorase deficiency and methemoglobinemia. Arch. Intern. Med., 113:578, 1964.

Mucolipidoses

55. Spranger, J. W., and Wiedemann, H.-R.: The genetic mucolipidoses. Humangenetik, 9:113, 1970.

Mucopolysaccharidoses

56. McKusick, V. A., *et al.*: Allelism, non-allelism and genetic compounds among the mucopolysaccharidoses. Lancet, 1:993, 1972.

MUCOPOLYSACCHARIDOSIS TYPE IH
(HURLER SYNDROME)

57. Leroy, J. G., and Crocker, A. C.: Clinical definition of the Hurler-Hunter phenotypes. A review of 50 patients. Amer. J. Dis. Child., 112:518, 1966.

MUCOPOLYSACCHARIDOSIS TYPE IS
(SCHEIE SYNDROME)

58. Scheie, H. G., Hambrick, G. W., Jr., and Barness, L. A.: A newly recognized forme fruste of Hurler's disease (gargoylism). Amer. J. Ophthal., 53:753, 1962.
59. Weismann, V., and Neufeld, E. F.: Scheie and Hurler syndromes: apparent identity of the biochemical defect. Science, 169:72, 1970.

MUCOPOLYSACCHARIDOSIS TYPE IIIA AND IIIB
(SANFILIPPO A AND B)

60. Sanfilippo, S. J., Podosin, R., Langer, L., and Good, R. A.: Mental retardation associated with acid mucopolysacchariduria (heparitin sulfate type). J. Pediat., 63:837, 1963.

MUCOPOLYSACCHARIDOSIS TYPE IV
(MORQUIO SYNDROME)

61. Langer, L. O., and Carey, L. S.: The roentgenographic features of the KS mucopolysaccharidosis of Morquio (Morquio-Brailsford's disease). Amer. J. Roentgen., 97:1, 1966.
62. Linker, A., Evans, L. R., and Langer, L. O.: Morquio's disease and mucopolysaccharide excretion. J. Pediat., 77:1039, 1970.

MUCOPOLYSACCHARIDOSIS TYPE VI
(MAROTEAUX-LAMY SYNDROME)

63. Maroteaux, P., and Lamy, M.: Hurler's disease, Morquio's disease, and related mucopolysaccharidoses. J. Pediat,, 67: 312, 1965.

*Muscular Atrophy, Progressive Spinal
(Werdnig-Hoffmann Syndrome)*

64. Gamstorp, I.: Progressive spinal muscular atrophy with onset in infancy or early childhood. Acta Paediat. Scand., 56:408, 1967.

Muscular Dystrophy, Recessive

65. Jackson, C. E., and Carey, J. H.: Progressive muscular dystrophy: autosomal recessive type. Pediatrics, 28:77, 1961.
66. Kloepfer, H. W., and Talley, C.: Autosomal recessive inheritance of Duchenne-type muscular dystrophy. Ann. Hum. Genet., 22:138, 1958.
67. Banker, B. Q., Victor, M., and Adams, R. D.: Arthrogryposis multiplex due to congenital muscular dystrophy. Brain, 80:319, 1957.

*Osteopetrosis, Recessive
(Albers-Schonberg Disease)*

68. Enell, H., and Pehrson, M.: Studies on osteopetrosis. I. Clinical report of three cases with genetic considerations. Acta Paediat. Scand., 47:279, 1958.

*Pancreatic Exocrine Deficiency
(Schwachman Syndrome)*

69. Schwachman, H., *et al.*: Pancreatic insufficiency and bone marrow dysfunction. A new clinical entity. J. Pediat., 63:835, 1963.

Polycystic Disease of Kidneys and Liver

70. Blyth, H., and Ockenden, B. G.: Polycystic disease of kidneys and liver presenting in childhood. J. Med. Genet., 8:257, 1971.

*Polycystic Kidneys, Polydactyly and
Encephalocele (Meckel Syndrome)*

71. Meckel, S., and Passarge, E.: Encephalocele, polycystic kidneys and polydactyly. Ann. Genet., 14:97, 1971.

Porphyria, Erythropoietic, Congenital

72. Marver, H. S., and Schmid, R.: *In* Stanbury, J. B., *et al.* (eds.): The Metabolic Basis of Inherited Diseases. 3rd ed. New York, McGraw-Hill, 1972, p. 1104.

Cockayne Syndrome

73. Cockayne, E. A.: Dwarfism with retinal atrophy and deafness. Arch. Dis. Child., 21:52, 1946.

Poikiloderma Congenitale of Rothmund

74. Taylor, W. B.: Rothmund's syndrome—Thomson's syndrome. Arch. Derm., 75:236, 1957.

Progeria (Hutchinson-Gilford Syndrome)

75. DeBusk, F. L.: The Hutchinson-Gilford progeria syndrome. J. Pediat., 80:697, 1972.

Werner Syndrome

76. Epstein, C. J., *et al.*: Werner's syndrome. Medicine, 45:177, 1966.

Pseudoxanthoma Elasticum

77. Berlyne, G. M., Bulmer, M. G., and Platt, R.: The genetics of pseudoxanthoma elasticum. Quart. J. Med., 30:201, 1961.

7

78. Coffman, J. D., and Sommers, S. C.: Familial pseudoxanthoma elasticum and valvular heart disease. Circulation, 19:242, 1959.

Smith-Lemli-Opitz Syndrome

79. Smith, D. W., Lemli, L., and Opitz, J. M.: A newly recognized syndrome of multiple congenital anomalies. J. Pediat., 64:210, 1964.
80. Dallaire, L., and Fraser, F. C.: The syndrome of retardation with urogenital and skeletal anomalies in siblings. J. Pediat., 69:459, 1966.

Spherophakia With Brachymorphia (Weill-Marchesani Syndrome)

81. Feinberg, S. B.: Congenital mesodermal dysmorphodystrophy (brachymorphic type). Radiology, 74:218, 1960.

Chapter 9

SEX-LINKED (X-LINKED) DISEASES

As the chapter title implies, sex-linked diseases (with one exception) are X-linked diseases and the great majority are X-linked recessive. Only a few decades ago, there was a sizable catalogue of supposedly Y-linked (holandric) disorders. Critical review has progressively reduced this list to one abnormality: hairy ears. We prefer not to explore the question of Y-linked conditions, except to note that the progressive number of behavioral and physical abnormalities observed in patients with the XYY chromosomal constitution leads one to suspect that the Y chromosome may contain more genetic information than that required to determine the male sex and produce hairy ears. The possibility of homologous loci on the X and Y chromosomes remains a subject for investigation.

X-LINKED DISEASES

From the discussion of the Lyon hypothesis in Chapter 4, it would be expected that the heterozygote (female carrier) of a recessive X-linked single mutant gene would show variable manifestations of the disease, depending on what proportion of her cells show the normal vs. the mutant phenotype. In autosomal recessive diseases the heterozygote has approximately 50% of the normal gene product, which under normal circumstances is sufficient to prevent unfavorable manifestations of the mutant gene. This is quite a different matter than having about 50% mutant and 50% normal cells. Furthermore, the random inactivation of the X chromosome, as visualized in the Lyon hypothesis, does not necessarily lead to 50% of the cells carrying the mutant gene being inactivated. Randomly a 60-40, 75-25 or even 90-10 partition could occur. Under these circumstances the "protective influence" of the normal gene product may be so diminished as to permit manifestations of the disease in the heterozygote. For instance, hemophilia A is a disease of males, but minor or occasionally major expression due to Lyonizing may be found in some female carriers—presumably those in which, by chance, a high proportion of the X's carrying the normal allele were inactivated. Fundamental and clinical aspects of the Lyon hypothesis have been extensively investigated in G6PD deficiency, which will be discussed later in this chapter.

The term "hemizygote" is used in the male to emphasize that the X and Y chromosomes do not represent homologous pairs as do the autosomes. An X-linked mutant gene that is transmitted as a recessive becomes manifest in the male because there is no "protection" from a homologous locus on the Y chromosome as there would be in an autosomal recessive.

An X-linked recessive disease, in the usual random-mating situation, is transmitted by the usually unaffected heterozygous carrier female to half of her sons. (The carrier state is transmitted to half of her daughters.) The affected male does not transmit the disease. All of his sons will be free of the disease, but *all* of his daughters will be carriers.

The transmission of the X-linked dominant diseases is from the affected male to all of his daughters and none of his sons. The heterozygous female is, by definition, always affected in X-linked dominant diseases, but the disease is generally milder than in the affected male. In her offspring half would be affected irrespective of sex.

SEX-LIMITED AND SEX-CONTROLLED TRAITS

Certain genes that are present in both sexes act only in one sex. An example is milk-yield genes in cows. Beard growth, hair distribution, and possibly male-pattern baldness may represent examples of **sex-limited traits** in humans.

The term **sex-controlled trait** is usually used in the context of multifactorial inheritance. Certain diseases affect one sex more than another, and it is presumed that the slight "environmental" difference provided by a difference in sex is sufficient to influence the threshold of a polygenic predisposition. Examples are the predominance of females with congenital dislocation of the hip, patent ductus arteriosus and atrial septal defect, and the predominance of males with pyloric stenosis, coarctation of the aorta and transposition of the great vessels.

CLINICAL EXAMPLE

Perhaps the most widely-known example of a genetically determined disease is classic hemophilia (hemophilia A), which has afflicted the royal families of Europe and which probably arose as a fresh mutation in Queen Victoria. An abbreviated pedigree of this family is presented in Figure 9-1. The counseling situation in a less conspicuous family that also has hemophilia A follows (see Fig. 9-2).

Case History. This 24-year-old mother of one apparently normal three-year-old son, who has a brother and an uncle with es-

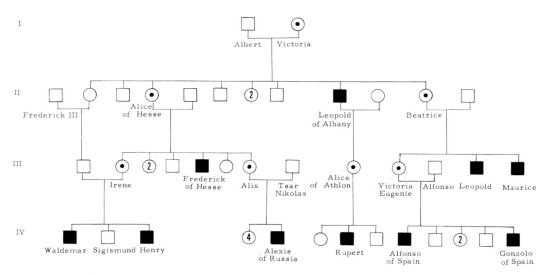

Figure 9-1. Pedigree of hemophilia A in royal families of Europe.

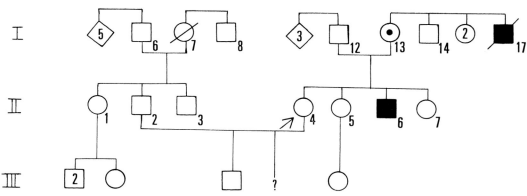

Figure 9-2. Pedigree of hemophilia A in a North American family.

tablished diagnosis of hemophilia A, was referred to our service. Her physician prior to her marriage and first pregnancy had not acquainted her with the possibility of genetic counseling, but her present physician, when consulted about the advisability of another pregnancy, suggested that a pregnancy not be entertained until the genetic risks were defined.

The family history is shown in Figure 9-2. Only two recognized patients in this family have had hemophilia A. The affected uncle (I-17) died of a gastrointestinal hemorrhage at 28 years of age, having been bedridden for three years with hemarthroses. The mother (I-13) of our patient is an established carrier, having both a brother and a son (II-6) with the disease.

The questions were: was our patient a carrier and was her apparently normal son truly free of the disease? Previous clotting studies had suggested that her son did not have hemophilia A, and our studies including assay of antihemophilic globulin (AHG) confirmed the earlier results. However, our hematology service felt that they could not distinguish the carrier state in the mother by her AHG level. So we were still left with a strong probability that the mother was a carrier. The method of calculating this probability is developed in Chapter 5. The probability that this patient did not inherit the gene is 1/2. The probability that she did inherit the gene and has one normal son is

$1/2 \times 1/2 = 1/4$. The probability that she is a carrier is $\dfrac{1/4}{1/4 + 1/2} = 1/3$

If this mother were known to be a carrier (as her mother was), the probability of her having an affected son would be 1/4 (probability of 1/2 of having a son × 1/2, the probability of receiving the X chromosome with the mutant gene). If she had not had a normal son, the chances of her having an affected son would be 1/2 (the probability that she is a carrier) × 1/4 (the probability of having an affected son) = 1/8. Having had a normal son reduces the probability of her being a carrier from 1/2 to 1/3, and the probability of her having an affected son from 1/8 to 1/12 (1/3 × 1/4).

This is still a high risk and the mother was so informed. The available options, as of the time of this counseling, were discussed with her. The possibility was mentioned that AHG assays (or some other laboratory test) should eventually be refined to the point that a confident diagnosis of the carrier state could be advanced. For the present, the most that could be offered was amniocentesis should pregnancy occur. The only usable information to be gained from an amniotic fluid specimen, at about 16 weeks gestation, would be the sex of the fetus. If a recommendation were made, it would be to terminate the pregnancy if the fetus were male.

X-LINKED RECESSIVE DISORDERS

Agammaglobulinemia (Bruton Disease, Hypogammaglobulinemia)[1]

This is the commonest of the immune deficiency diseases. The pattern of inheritance is X-linked recessive; therefore, the affected patients are males.

Diagnostic Features and Clinical Course. A history of frequently recurring severe bacterial infections, such as pneumonia and sepsis in a male child, is the initial basis for entertaining the diagnosis. A family history of other males dying of overwhelming infection might also be obtained. Immunoelectrophoresis and quantitative immunoglobulin determinations reveal absence or virtual absence of IgG, IgM and absence of IgA. Plasma cells are rarely found, but lymphocytes are present. Isohemagglutinins are either absent or present in low titer. The tonsils are unusually small and adenoids are not visible by lateral pharyngeal x-rays. These patients have adequate cellular immunity and ability to reject allografts. There is no excessive vulnerability to viral and fungal infections. Patients recognized early and treated promptly with gamma globulin and chemotherapy may do quite well during childhood. Complications of adolescence and early life include a dermatomyositis-like syndrome of arthritis, contractures and brawny edema that ends fatally.

Treatment. Gamma globulin is administered regularly in monthly maintenance therapy after the initial loading dose to raise the IgG level about 200 mg/ml. Vigorous specific antimicrobial therapy is given for individual bacterial infections.

Angiokeratoma, Diffuse (Fabry Disease)[2]

Small dark nodular lesions clustered in the umbilical area, around the buttocks, genitalia, knees and mucous membranes may first be noted in early childhood. Burning pain of the hands and feet associated with fever heat, cold or exercise is often the first symptom. Progressive renal insufficiency is the critical feature and is usually responsible for the death of affected males in their thirties or forties. As in other X-linked recessive disorders, heterozygous females may be mildly affected. The biochemical defect is a deficiency of the enzyme ceramidetrihexosidase, which leads to a cellular accumulation of ceramidetrihexoside. The carrier female has enzyme levels that fall between those of the affected male and the normal. Other findings in affected individuals may include seizures, diarrhea, hemoptysis and nosebleeds.

Color Blindness[3]

Several types of X-linked color blindness have been described. Eight per cent of western European males and between 5 and 9% of men in different white populations are estimated to be color-blind. This topic is developed in Chapter 10.

Diabetes Insipidus[4,5]

Two types of X-linked diabetes insipidus are known: nephrogenic and neurohypophyseal. An autosomal dominant neurohypophyseal type has also been recognized. In the nephrogenic form there is failure of renal tubular response to antidiuretic hormone (pitressin-resistant) in the male and partial defect in the female. The neurohypophyseal type responds to pitressin and may follow an X-linked or occasionally an autosomal dominant pattern. Deficiency in hypothalamic nuclei has been demonstrated in some of these patients.

Ectodermal Dysplasia, Anhidrotic[6]

This X-linked recessive disorder is seen in the full-blown clinical picture in males; however, some features have been found in heterozygous carrier females. The major findings are absence of teeth, hair and sweat and mucous glands. Darwin described the "toothless men of Sind" in 1875, noting that there was a total of only 12 teeth distributed among the ten affected men in the Hindu family he observed.

Male patients with this disease suffer during hot weather because of their inability to sweat. Scalp and body hair is sparse and complete baldness occurs early in life. Some observers believe that they have recognized a mosaic patchy distribution of skin abnormalities in some mildly affected female carriers of this disorder, reminiscent of the distribution of hair color in the heterozygote tabby mouse.

Problems early in life from this disease are the not insignificant threat to life from hyperthermia and difficult respiratory infections, complicated by the absence of mucous glands. In later life the alimentary and cosmetic problems are managed by false teeth and wigs.

The inability to sweat distinguishes this disorder clinically from the hidrotic ectodermal dysplasias that are mainly autosomal dominant.

Glucose 6-Phosphate Dehydrogenase (G6PD) Deficiency[7,8]

This disorder is one of the more informative genetic diseases and one that continues to stimulate intensive investigative efforts. The G6PD variants are increasing at such a rapid rate that it is not too meaningful to report the number (approximately 80 at the time of this writing). Whether or not each newly discovered variant represents a distinct entity awaits the comparison of physicochemical test results with the findings in established variants.

The categorization of variants has also been subject to a change. Presently there is division into five classes.

Class 1. Severe enzyme deficiency with chronic nonspherocytic hemolytic anemia.

Class 2. Severe enzyme deficiency (10% of normal)

Class 3. Moderate enzyme deficiency (10 to 60% of normal)

Class 4. Mild to no enzyme deficiency (60 to 100% of normal)

Class 5. Increased enzyme activity (2× normal)

Within each class the variants may be categorized into four subgroups:

Group I. Well characterized and distinctive.

Group II. Insufficient information to establish that the variant is distinct. (Such variants are shown in quotation marks.)

Group III. Insufficient data to justify tabulation.

Group IV. Seem to be identical with previously described variants.

G6PD deficiency is widely distributed throughout the world; however, certain populations, such as African and Mediterranean, have a high frequency of involvement. Sephardic Jews and Iranians are also frequently affected. The deficiency is present in approximately 10% of males and 2% of females in the black North American population and is as high as 25 to 30% in males in parts of Africa and Sardinia.

In patients with severe enzyme deficiency, episodic hemolysis of older red blood cells may follow exposure to environmental triggers such as drugs, infections, fava beans and moth balls. Primaquine, salicylates and sulfa preparations are frequently implicated drugs. Chronic hemolytic anemia, apparently unassociated with distinct episodes, is the alternative presentation in patients with severe enzyme deficiency.

Diagnostic tests include glutathione stability and methemoglobin reduction screening. More sophisticated physicochemical tests are required to distinguish the variants; these include assay of red blood cell enzymatic activity, electrophoretic mobility, 2-d G6P and deamino NADP utilization, K_mG6P and K_mNADP.

One of the earliest and most convincing studies in the human supporting the single-active-X hypothesis was that of Beutler and co-workers using G6PD deficiency as a marker to demonstrate that the human female is a mosaic of X chromosome activity. Two populations of cells, one normal and one deficient in G6PD, were found in heterozygous females when studied by gluta-

in the first months of life. The X-linked form is also seen at birth, but is not as extensive, having a predilection for head, abdomen and flexures. The dominant form (ichthyosis vulgaris), which is characterized histologically by epidermal atrophy, is not usually recognized for several months after birth and is most noticeable on palms and soles; throughout life it may be appreciated only as excessive dryness and shininess of the skin of the extremities. The X-linked form has histologic findings of hypertrophy of the epidermis and a more striking "fish-skin" appearance.

Kinky Hair Syndrome (Menkes Syndrome)[13]

This progressive brain disease, first recognized by Menkes in 1962, is characterized by pili torti, scorbutic changes in the metaphyses of the long bones, tortuosity of the cerebral and other arteries, which may lead to vascular occlusion, hypothermia, and death within three years, with progressive brain degeneration. The kinky hair, fragmentation of the internal elastic lamina in the arteries, and bone changes have recently been traced to a defect in the intestinal absorption of copper. The pili torti only develops after several weeks, and the disease may be more common than presently realized.

Lowe Oculo-cerebro-renal Syndrome[14]

This syndrome of cataracts, hydrophthalmos, mental retardation and renal tubular dysfunction was reported by Lowe and colleagues in 1952. Growth and mental development are poor. The patients are both hyperactive and hypotonic. Deep tendon reflexes are diminished. Congenital cataracts and frequently glaucoma are present (Fig. 9-3). The renal tubular dysfunction is characterized by poor ammonium production, hyperchloremic acidosis, phosphaturia with hypophosphatemia, aminoaciduria and albuminuria. Osteoporosis and vitamin D-resistant rickets develop. Cryptorchism is common. These severe manifestations are confined to the male. The heterozygous car-

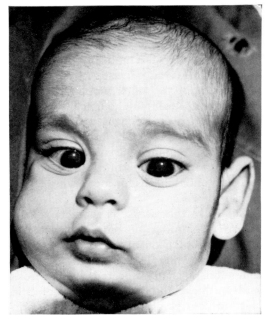

Figure 9-3.   Facies in Lowe oculo-cerebro-renal syndrome. The hydrophthalmos and cataracts may be seen in this photograph.

rier female may show some fine opacities of the lens, presumably reflecting the Lyon hypothesis and the results of random inactivation of X chromosomes. Renal insufficiency and dehydration are commonly responsible for death. Treatment with vitamin D and alkali and surgical attention to the ocular problems have been recommended.

Mucopolysaccharidosis II (Hunter Syndrome)[15]

The other mucopolysaccharidoses and mucolipidoses are autosomal recessive disorders and are discussed in Chapter 7. It is curious that Hunter's detailed report in 1917 of a mucopolysaccharidosis, although published two years earlier than Hurler's report, received little attention. Follow-up evidence has suggested that Hunter's patients probably suffered from the X-linked form of the disease.

Patients with the Hunter syndrome have milder disease than those with Hurler syndrome. Mental retardation may be minimal or absent; we have investigated a pedigree in which one affected individual was an engineer. The skeletal abnormality may not be as debilitating as in MPS I, but the features are similar—claw hand, stiff joints (Figs. 9-4, 9-5). There is, however, no gibbus. The facies is coarse (gargoylism) and there is hepatosplenomegaly. Deafness is a more frequent and severe problem in MPS II than in the other diseases in this group, in all of which it may also occur. Metachromatic granules are found more readily in lymphocytes than in polymorphs and less readily in these patients than in patients with the Hurler syndrome. Urine mucopolysaccharide excretion is similar to MPS I: chondroitin sulfate B and heparitin sulfate.

A clinical differentiating point between MPS I and MPS II is the absence of corneal clouding in patients with the Hunter syndrome. However, retinal changes may occur and diminish or terminate vision. Heart disease is prominent in these patients and is similar to the cardiac pathology in MPS I (coronary artery disease). A cardiac death is likely between the second and fifth decades. The prevalence is estimated at 1:200,000.

Muscular Dystrophy[16]

At least three X-linked forms of muscular dystrophy have been described, including the most common form, pseudohypertrophic

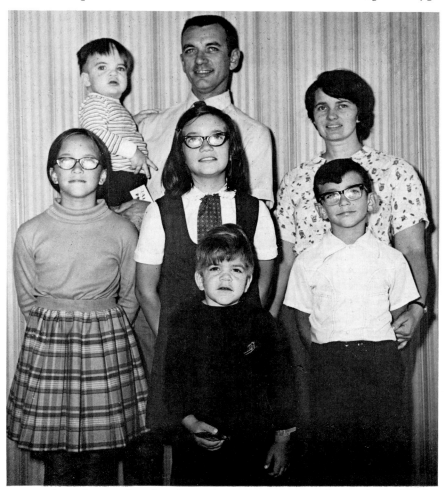

Figure 9-4. Family with two affected males with Hunter syndrome, who may be readily distinguished from their siblings.

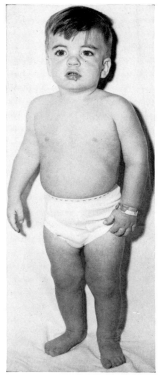

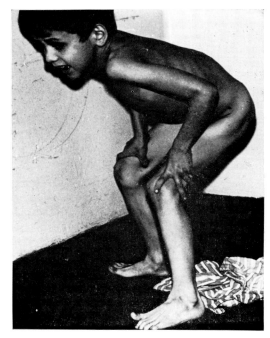

Figure 9-6. Patient with Duchenne muscular dystrophy "climbing up himself."

Figure 9-5. Hunter syndrome. Note the facies and the "claw hand."

muscular dystrophy (Duchenne type), and the less common tardive type of Becker and tardive type of Dreifuss. Autosomal recessive and dominant forms also exist.

The patient with the Duchenne type of pseudohypertrophic disease becomes symptomatic by the time he is five years old. The muscles, especially of his lower limbs, appear to be unusually well-developed, yet he is weak and unable to walk well, pedal a tricycle or climb stairs. From a sitting position on the floor he characteristically "climbs up himself" (Fig. 9-6). By the time the patient is ten years old he is usually confined to a chair and death usually occurs before 20 years of age. The muscle of the heart, as well as skeletal muscle, is affected. Myocardial disease and congestive heart failure are observed. Mental retardation is present in about one-third of the patients. Creatinuria accompanies the disease and creatine

phosphokinase (CPK) has been reported as being elevated in about 70% of female carriers.

The tardive type of Becker is later in onset (twenties and thirties) and milder in course, permitting survival to more advanced ages.

In the tardive type of Dreifuss the onset may be as early as in the Duchenne type, but the progress is considerably slower, so that these patients may be gainfully employed. The shoulder-girdle musculature and the heart become involved, but there is no pseudohypertrophy. Flexion deformities of the elbows are characteristic.

Testicular Feminization Syndrome[17]

This syndrome offers an exception to the rule regarding chromosomal determination of phenotypic sex. In the human being, the presence of a Y chromosome produces the male phenotype and the absence of a Y chromosome allows the more passive line of development of the female, no matter what the number of X chromosomes. It is probably more precise to say that the Y chromosome leads to the development of testes and that the testes usually produce male sexual characteristics. Castrated male rat or rabbit embryos develop female genitalia. However, in the case of testicular feminization, testes are present and their androgen production is normal, but an abnormality at some point in the metabolic pathway leads to the development of female rather than male external genitalia, sparse growth of pubic and axillary hair and the adult attainment of a frequently voluptuous feminine habitus. In some cases the metabolic defect probably involves the conversion of testosterone to dihydrotestosterone, which in normal females proceeds more rapidly in the sexual skin (e.g., of the labia) than in ordinary skin. In individuals with the syndrome, the conversion in the sexual skin resembles that of ordinary skin. However, there seems to be some genetic heterogeneity.

Patients with this syndrome are usually brought to medical attention as teenagers because of delay in menstruation, or they are discovered in early childhood because of "inguinal hernias" that are not hernias but testes in the inguinal canal. Further examination reveals a shortened vagina and the absence of uterus and adnexa. The buccal smear is negative and the karyotype is that of a normal male: 46,XY. Hormonal assays are normal.

The familial transmission of the disorder fits the expectation for X-linked recessive inheritance, although the alternative of an autosomal gene dominant in males and recessive in females has not yet been excluded, since affected individuals do not have children.

Wiskott-Aldrich Syndrome[18]

This syndrome of eczema, thrombocytopenia and frequent infections was described in three brothers by Wiskott in 1937. Aldrich defined the X-linked recessive mode of inheritance in 1954. Eczema and bloody diarrhea (with thrombocytopenia) are the usual manifestations early in infancy. Later in infancy infections, particularly of the skin, middle ears and lungs, become a more prominent problem. The immunologic deficiency is somewhat variable and may involve both cellular and humoral immunity. IgM and isohemagglutinins are usually diminished. There is often lymphopenia and thymic hypoplasia. Malignancies such as leukemia and lymphoma occur. Death is usual in infancy or early childhood.

X-LINKED DOMINANT DISORDERS

Brown Teeth

This disorder is presented not because of its clinical importance, but because it has provided some interesting pedigrees of X-linked dominant inheritance. There has been direct transmission from males to all their daughters and none of their sons and from females to half their daughters and half their sons. (There have also been pedigrees of brown teeth transmitted by an autosomal dominant mode.)

Hypophosphatemic Rickets (Vitamin D-resistant Rickets)[19,20]

This X-linked dominant disorder is transmitted directly from an affected female to half of her sons and half of her daughters, and from an affected male to all of his daughters and to none of his sons. Affected females appear to have a somewhat milder form of the disease than males. The hypophosphatemia is secondary to diminished tubular resorption of the phosphorus and possibly decreased gastrointestinal resorption of phosphorus and calcium. Growth in early infancy is normal until the serum phosphorus drops to a low level around six months of age. Clinical and roentgen evidence of rickets becomes gradually apparent (Fig. 9-7). The lower limbs bow with weight bearing. Growth is slow and ultimate height attainment is decreased. The gait may become waddling. Dolichocephaly, pseudofractures and enamel hypoplasia are sometimes observed. Careful control of

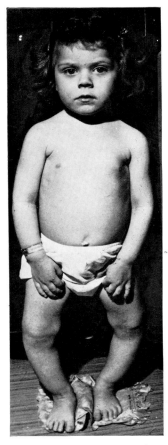

Figure 9-7. Skeletal deformity in hypophosphatemic rickets.

serum phosphorus levels may permit normal growth.

Incontinentia Pigmenti[21]

This disorder, like OFD I, is thought to be X-linked dominant with lethality in the male. All patients are female and there is a 2:1 ratio of liveborn females to males in affected families. The consistent feature is lesions of the skin, which may be vesicular, inflammatory, atrophic or verrucous, but most characteristically is a "chocolate swirl ice cream" effect on the trunk and extremities. Patchy alopecia, incomplete dentition with malformed teeth, strabismus, keratitis, cataracts, blue sclerae, syndactyly, hemivertebrae, microcephaly and cardiac dis-

ease are frequent findings. The skin lesions, which begin as inflammatory in appearance, progress through the "chocolate swirl" appearance and are usually gone by 20 years of age. The most serious problem for the affected individual is central nervous system involvement. About one-third of the patients have varying degree of mental retardation and spasticity; some have sei-

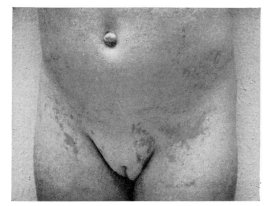

Figure 9-8. Skin lesions of incontinentia pigmenti.

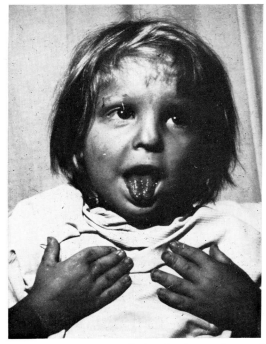

Figure 9-9. Hand and facial abnormalities of oral-facial-digital syndrome (OFD I).

zures. The counseling revolves around the specific clinical problems for the patient and what risks may be anticipated for her future offspring: one-third affected females, one-third normal females, and one-third normal males.

Oral-facial-digital Syndrome (OFD I)[22]

This syndrome is found only in females and pedigree analysis of their families has

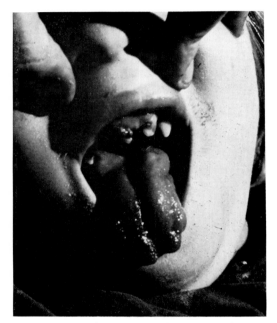

Figure 9-10. Close-up of cleft tongue and irregular dentition of OFD I.

revealed an approximate 2:1 female ratio, suggesting that this disease is lethal in the male. The most reasonable explanation of the cause of this mode of inheritance is an X-linked dominant mutant gene. Because of lethality in the male, the genetic counseling risk is: two-thirds of the offspring of an affected mother would be female and one-half of these females would be affected; the one-third of the offspring who would be live-born males would be normal. Thus, the risks would be: one-third affected females; one-third normal females; and one-third normal males.

Diagnostic Features (Figs. 9-9 to 9-11). *Oral.* Partial clefts in tongue, upper lip, alveolar ridge, palate. Irregularities of dentition (absence of teeth, supernumerary teeth). Webs between buccal mucosa and alveolar ridge. Hamartoma of tongue.

Facial. Laterally placed inner canthi, hypoplasia of alar cartilages, short philtrum, malar hypoplasia.

Digital. Asymmetric shortening of digits, some partial syndactyly, clinodactyly and *unilateral* polydactyly.

Other. Moderate retardation, alopecia and trembling.

Differential Diagnosis. *OFD II (Mohr syndrome).* This syndrome has many of the features of OFD I, but also has conductive hearing loss and bilateral polydactyly. OFD II is inherited as an autosomal recessive.

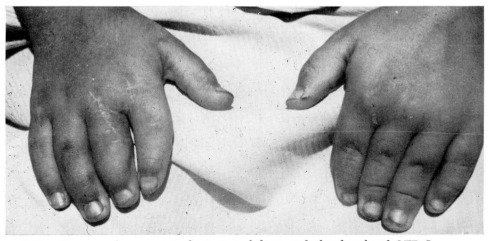

Figure 9-11. Close-up of asymmetric shortening of digits and clinodactyly of OFD I.

REFERENCES

Agammaglobulinemia (Bruton Disease)

1. Seligman, M., Fudenberg, H. H., and Good, R. A.: A proposed classification of primary immunologic deficiencies. Amer. J. Med., 45: 817, 1968.

Angiokeratoma, Diffuse (Fabry Disease)

2. Opitz, J. M. *et al.*: The genetics of angiokeratoma corporis diffusum (Fabry's disease) and its linkage relations with the Xg locus. Amer. J. Hum. Genet., 17:325, 1965.

Color Blindness

3. Kalmus, H.: Diagnosis and Genetics of Defective Color Vision. Oxford, Pergamon Press, 1965.

Diabetes Insipidus

4. Forssman, H.: Two different mutations of the X-chromosome causing diabetes insipidus. Amer. J. Hum. Genet., 7:21, 1955.
5. Abelson, H.: Nephrogenic diabetes insipidus. Pediat. Res., 2:271, 1968.

Ectodermal Dysplasia, Anhidrotic

6. Lowry, R. B., Robinson, G. C., and Miller, J. R.: Hereditary ectodermal dysplasia. Symptoms, inheritance patterns, differential diagnosis, management. Clin. Pediat., 5:395, 1966.

Glucose 6-Phosphate Dehydrogenase (G6PD) Deficiency

7. Beutler, E., Yeh, M., and Fairbanks, V. F.: The normal human female as a mosaic of X-chromosome activity: studies using the gene for G-6-PD deficiency as a marker. Proc. Nat. Acad. Sci., 48:9, 1962.
8. World Health Organization: Nomenclature of glucose-6-phosphate dehydrogenase in man. Bull. WHO, 36:319, 1967.

Hemophilia A (Classic Hemophilia)

9. Bennett, E., and Huehns, E. R.: Immunological differentiation of three types of hemophilia and identification of some female carriers. Lancet, 2:956, 1970.

Hemophilia B (Christmas Disease)

10. Brown, P. E., Hougie, C., and Roberts, H. R.: The genetic heterogeneity of hemophilia B. New Eng. J. Med., 283:61, 1970.

Hyperuricemia (Lesch-Nyhan Syndrome)

11. Demars, R., *et al.*: Lesch-Nyhan mutation: prenatal detection with amniotic fluid cells. Science, 164:1303, 1969.

Ichthyosis

12. Schnyder, U. W.: Inherited ichthyoses. Arch. Derm., 102: 240, 1970.

Kinky Hair Syndrome (Menkes Syndrome)

13. Danks, D. M., *et al.*: Kinky hair disease. Pediatrics, 50:181, 1972.

Lowe Oculo-cerebro-renal Syndrome

14. Richards, W., *et al.*: The oculo-cerebro-renal syndrome of Lowe. Amer. J. Dis. Child., 109: 185, 1965.

Mucopolysaccharidosis II (Hunter Syndrome)

15. Leroy, J. G., and Crocker, A. C.: Clinical definition of the Hurler-Hunter phenotypes. A review of 50 patients. Amer. J. Dis. Child., 112:518, 1966.

Muscular Dystrophy

16. Morton, N. E., and Chung, C. S.: Formal genetics of muscular dystrophy. Amer. J. Hum. Genet., 11:360, 1959.

Testicular Feminization Syndrome

17. Mouvais-Jarvis, P., *et al.*: Studies on testosterone metabolism in subjects with testicular feminizing syndrome. J. Clin. Invest., 49: 31, 1970.

Wiskott-Aldrich Syndrome

18. Wolff, J. A.: Wiskott-Aldrich syndrome: clinical, immunologic, and pathologic observations. J. Pediat., 70:221, 1967.

Hypophosphatemia (Vitamin D-resistant Rickets)

19. Winters, R. W., *et al.*: A genetic study of familial hypophosphatemia and vitamin D resistant rickets with a review of the literature. Medicine, 37:97, 1958.
20. Glorieux, F. H., *et al.*: Prevention of dwarfism and rickets in X-linked hypophosphatemia. New Eng. J. Med., 287:481, 1972.

Incontinentia Pigmenti

21. Carney, R. G., and Carney, R. G., Jr.: Incontinentia pigmenti. Arch. Derm., 102:157, 1970.

Oral-facial-digital Syndrome (OFD I)

22. Gorlin, R. J., and Psaume, J.: Orodigitofacial dysostosis—a new syndrome. J. Pediat., 61: 520, 1962.

Chapter 10

NORMAL VARIATION

I am the family face;
Flesh perishes, I live on,
Projecting trait and trace
Through time to finis anon,
And leaping from place to place
Over oblivion.

Thomas Hardy

NORMAL PHYSICAL FEATURES

Interest is taken by nearly everyone in the inheritance of physical features and it is rather disappointing that so few of them show clear-cut mendelian pedigree patterns. One difficulty is that normal physical differences often do not fall into sharply different classes, so that it is difficult to know how to classify individuals in the overlap range. Nevertheless, there is a great deal of data about the inheritance of normal features, as well as a good many misconceptions. The reader is referred to Amram Scheinfeld's book *Your Heredity and Environment* for an interesting and detailed coverage of inherited normal variations.[2] We will touch only lightly on the subject.

Eye Color. Probably the example of simple mendelian inheritance in man most frequently cited in elementary texts and popular articles is eye color. This has the advantage of being a trait with which almost everyone is familiar, but it also has a disadvantage. It is not an example of *simple* mendelian inheritance, as a modicum of observation and a little thought will tell you. Eye color is clearly a graded character, with many possible shades of color as well as innumerable patterns. That it is genetically determined is clear from the striking resemblances in color and pattern between monozygous twins. The color is determined in part by the amount and distribution of melanin in the iris. Albinos have none at all so the iris appears red because it transmits light reflected from the fundus. "True blue" eyes have virtually no pigment in the anterior part of the iris, but some in the posterior layers, and darker colors have progressively more melanin (yellow or brown) present. The structure of the iris will also modify the shade. In general the genes for the darker colors tend to be dominant to those for the lighter, but the situation is complex: a child with eyes darker than those of both parents is not necessarily cause for divorce!

Remember that the iris may darken considerably for some months or even years after birth.

Hair Color. The innumerable shades of hair color also attest to complex inheritance, as well as a considerable amount of environmental modification, at least in some populations. Again, the various shades of blond through black are determined by the concentration and type of melanin, and the genes causing the darker colors tend to dominate those for the lighter ones.

Red hair results from another pigment that appears to be under the control of a separate gene locus. Presence of the red pigment is recessive to its absence, but of course the difference between red and not-red is only visible if the hair is fair. That is, the dark-hair genes are epistatic to the red hair locus.

Hair Form. The form or texture of the hair depends on its cross-sectional shape, which is round in straight hair and elliptic in curly hair. A case has been made for a single locus, with curly hair resulting from homozygosity for one allele, straight hair from homozygosity for the other allele, and wavy hair from heterozygosity, but the situation is hardly as simple as that, as there are many degrees of waviness. Kinky hair in Caucasians shows dominant inheritance, and the straight hair of Orientals is also said to be dominant, but there is a lack of critical data.

Baldness. Hair loss in older age is presumably determined multifactorially. Pattern baldness, with onset before 30 years of age, is one of the few common traits that seems to fit mendelian expectations. It is caused by an autosomal gene that expresses itself in the heterozygote in males but not in females. Presumably androgen makes the difference, and its lack may also prevent expression of the gene in homozygous fe-males; otherwise, there should be more pattern-bald women than there appear to be.

Skin Color. Once again, it should be evident that skin color is multifactorially determined, since there is a continuous range of shades from "black" to "white." Davenport's original proposal that the Negro-Caucasian skin color difference is due to two independent loci, each showing intermediate dominance, is an oversimplification. Gate's scheme involving three loci contributing different amounts of melanin (dark, beige, and dark brown) allows for 18 possible shades and fits observed family patterns reasonably well. Either scheme implies that a "dark" person and a "white" mate cannot have a baby much darker than the dark parent, thus disposing of the myth that Negro ancestry on one side of the family can result in a "black" baby even though both parents are light-skinned.

Attached Ear Lobes. Most ear lobes extend below the point of attachment of the ear, but some merge with the facial skin along the anterior border, making it difficult to wear earrings. The attached lobe is said to be recessively inherited, but in some people it is difficult to decide whether the lobe is attached or not.

Ear Pits. Small pits in the skin, in the ear lobe as if it had not quite been pierced for earrings, or in the skin just anterior to the attachment of the ear are said to show recessive inheritance.

Tongue Rolling. The ability to roll the tongue into a trough or even tube is said to be dominant to the inability, but there are exceptions.

Handedness. Left-handedness is certainly familial, but how much of the tendency to resemble parents is cultural is not at all clear. In one study the frequency of left-handedness was about 6% when both parents were right-handed, 17% when one parent was left-handed, and 50% when both parents were left handed. This can be made to fit a single locus scheme if the heterozygotes are postulated as being either right-

or left-handed, depending on subtle environmental variations.

Hand Clasping. When you fold your hands, which thumb is on top? This is a sharply determined characteristic, with about 50% of Caucasians preferring one hand to be uppermost and 50% preferring the other hand. It does not seem to be related to handedness and has only a slight tendency to be familial.

"Hitch-hiker's Thumb." The ability to extend the terminal phalanx of the thumb more than 30° from the axis of the second phalanx is said to be recessive, but a number of people fall in the intermediate range.

Dental Anomalies. Inherited variations in tooth morphology are numerous and cannot be reviewed adequately here. One of the most striking is the dominant gene that causes peg-shaped or missing lateral incisors.

Webbed Toes. Partial webbing of varying degrees is an anomaly so frequent that it may be included among the normal variations. Autosomal dominant inheritance is the usual pattern, though in some families it only appears in females.

NORMAL PHYSIOLOGIC VARIATIONS

In addition to "normal" morphologic variants, a number of interesting physiologic variants have been identified. We will exclude the biochemical polymorphisms here.

PTC Taste Threshold. The ability to taste phenylthiocarbamide or related goitrogenic chemicals with the N—C=S group shows marked variation among individuals. The majority of people can taste very weak concentrations of the compound (tasters), but (in Caucasians) about one out of three people can only taste much higher concentraitons (nontasters). This striking physiologic difference is determined by a single locus, the nontaster allele being recessive. It is not related to taste acuity in general. If taste thresholds are carefully measured, a few individuals fall into the intermediate range, but if due allowance is made for general taste sensitivity, quite good discrimination can be achieved and the heterozygotes can be shown to have somewhat higher taste thresholds for PTC than the homozygous tasters.[1] As with other polymorphisms, there are wide variations in gene frequency in different populations, and there is some evidence to suggest that the nontaster genotype predisposes to the development of nodular goiter.

Ear Wax. Almost all Caucasians and Negros have brown, wet, sticky ear wax, but in the Japanese the common type is grey, dry and flaky. The dry type is also frequent in American Indians and Eskimos and appears to be dominantly inherited.

Color Blindness. Lack of the chlorolobe pigment in the retinal cone cells results in inability to discriminate green colors, or **deuteranopia.** The responsible mutant gene is on the X chromosome and is carried by about 5% of Caucasian males. A second allele, with a frequency of about 1.5%, causes a partial defect in green discrimination or **deuteranomaly.** Similarly, a lack of the erythrolobe pigment, necessary for discrimination in the red end of the spectrum, results in **protanopia** (1% of males), and a partial defect results in **protanomaly** (1%). This gene is also X-linked and appears to be quite close to the deuteranopia locus.

Beetroot Urine. An autosomal recessive gene results in the appearance of red pigment in the urine after eating beets.

CONCLUSION

Much of the data on normal variations cited in this chapter is uncritical, and should not be taken too seriously. Part of the difficulty lies in the quantitative nature of many of these traits, and the situation may improve as specific components of the total variation are identified.

REFERENCES

1. Kalmus, H.: Improvements in the classification of taster genotypes. Ann. Hum. Genet., 22:200-212, 1958
2. Scheinfeld, A.: Your Heredity and Environment. Philadelphia, J. B. Lippincott, 1964.

Chapter 11

THE FREQUENCIES OF GENES IN POPULATIONS

Man is graced by numerous advantageous genes and plagued by deleterious ones. What determines their proportions? The question is important for several reasons. Gene frequencies are being changed by the effects of radiation and other environmental mutagens. Are these changes large enough to worry about? Gene frequencies are also changing because of marked changes in population structure resulting from the widespread use of contraceptives and many other factors influencing the birth and death rates of various social and ethnic groups. Are our tax structures dysgenic? Medical advances have improved the fertility of patients with many hereditary diseases. Will we thereby become a species of malformed morons? Finally, the ability to estimate the frequencies of heterozygotes for genes causing recessively inherited diseases may be useful to the genetic counselor.

In this context we must stop thinking of genes segregating in families and consider the population as a pool of genes, from which any individual draws two for each locus.

THE HARDY-WEINBERG EQUILIBRIUM

Consider a particular gene locus "D" with two alleles D and d in a population in which, for simplicity's sake, we will assume there is no mutation and no selection. Suppose that the dd genotype causes a recessively inherited disease. Assume also that the frequency of the d allele is 1%, and that of the D allele is 99%. If mating is at random (except with respect to sex, of course), each individual can be considered as drawing two of the "D"-locus genes (either D or d), one from the father and one from the mother, and will have one of three possible genotypes—DD, Dd, or dd.

What is the probability that the individual will draw two d alleles and have the disease? There is a 1% chance that he will draw a d allele from his mother, and also a 1% chance that he will draw one from his father, so the probability that he will do both and be homozygous dd is $1/100 \times 1/100 = 1/10,000$. Note that this is the frequency of the disease, which can be measured. Thus we have developed an important rule: **In a population in equilibrium the frequency of a disease caused by an autosomal recessive gene is the square of the frequency of the recessive gene.**

In practice, we usually proceed in the other direction; that is, we measure the frequency of the disease and take the square root of this to estimate the gene frequency. Thus we may state the rule conversely: **The frequency of a gene is the square root of the frequency of the homozygote for that gene.**

Similarly we may deduce the frequency of heterozygotes—a question that sometimes comes up in genetic counseling. An individual may draw a *d* allele from the mother (1/100) and a *D* allele from the father (99/100), so the probability that he will do both is 1/100 × 99/100 or 99/10,000. But it can also happen that he draws a *d* allele from his father and a *D* allele from his mother, and the probability that he does both is again 1/100 × 99/100. Since these are alternative possibilities, the total probability of the individual being heterozygous (*Dd*) is found by adding the two alternative probabilities, and is thus 2 × 1/100 × 99/100, or 198/10,000. (For convenience this may be rounded off to 200/10,000 or 1/50.) Our second rule will therefore be: **The frequency of the heterozygote for two alleles is the frequency of one allele multiplied by the frequency of the other allele, times two.**

These principles were first developed independently by an English mathematician, Hardy, and a German ophthalmologist, Weinberg, shortly after the rediscovery of mendelism, and they are known collectively as the **Hardy-Weinberg law.** In algebraic terms it states that, in a population in equilibrium, if a genetic locus has alleles *D* and *d*, with frequencies p and q, **the frequencies of the genotypes DD, Dd and dd will be p^2, 2 pq and q^2.**

The significance of this relationship in genetic counseling was illustrated in Chapter 5, p. 80.

FACTORS ALTERING THE FREQUENCIES OF GENES[1,2]

Mutation. A mutation may be defined as a change in the genetic constitution from one stable state to another. Strictly speaking, a mutation can be either a chromosomal alteration or a point mutation—that is, a change in the DNA from one nucleotide to another, resulting in a change in the messenger RNA from the locus involved, and a corresponding amino acid substitution in the polypeptide change for which the gene codes. It is the latter sense that is commonly used in population genetics.

Mutations are beneficial in the sense that they provide genetic variation, without which evolution could not take place. On the other hand, most mutations with overt effects are harmful, since they are random changes in a system that has already incorporated most of the possible improvements. Throwing a spanner into a running motor would hardly ever improve its function.

Selection. A mutation that is harmful, through causing a deformity or disease or otherwise impairing function and thus reducing fertility, will have less chance of being passed on to the next generation than its normal allele. In other words, it will be selected against, and will have a lower frequency than the normal allele.

Selection can be expressed mathematically as the probability of the mutant gene being passed on to the next generation, relative to that of the normal allele. If this probability is low, there is strong negative selection. The converse of this is "fitness." The stronger the selection against a gene, the less "fit" it is.

The Balance Between Mutation and Selection. The more harmful a mutation is, the stronger the selection against it and the less frequent the gene will be. On the other hand, the higher the mutation rate, the more frequent it will be. Thus **the frequency of any given allele reflects a balance between the rate at which alleles of this kind are being removed from the population by selection and the rate at which new ones are being created by mutation.**

Consider a locus *A* at which a mutation to an allele A^L occurs in one of every 100,000 gametes that contribute to the next generation. Suppose that A^L is dominant and causes a disease that causes death before puberty or produces sterility. Thus the gene would not be passed on to the next generation, a fitness of 0. What will be the frequency of the disease? Since 100,000 gametes give rise to 50,000 people, if 1/100,000 gametes carries the mutant gene, 1/50,00 people will have the disease. Thus, **for a dominant lethal gene the disease frequency will be twice the mutation rate,** or in algebraic terms,

$$X = 2m$$

where X is the frequency of the disease and m is the mutation rate.

Suppose circumstances now changed so that the allele had a fitness of 0.5; that is, the mutant allele had half as much chance of contributing to the next generation as the normal allele. Since selection would remove fewer genes than before, but mutation would still be providing new ones, the frequency of the allele would increase and the disease frequency would increase (Fig. 11-1). When the frequency of A^L reached two per 100,000 genes, there would be four per 100,000 diseased individuals. Since only half the mutant genes would be transmitted to the next generation, the other half, or one per 100,000 would be lost. Thus selection would remove one per 100,000 A^L mutant genes per generation, and mutation would create one per 100,000 new mutant

alleles. A new equilibrium would have been reached at a higher frequency of the mutant gene, where the loss of A^L alleles by selection was balanced by the input of new A^L alleles through mutation. Algebraically the relationship is

$$X = 2m/(1-f)$$

where f is the fitness of the mutant allele, measured as the proportion of mutant to normal alleles that are transmitted to the next generation.

For recessive genes in which selection only acts on the homozygote, each death due to the mutant gene removes two mutant alleles rather than one, and the equation is:

$$X = m/(1-f)$$

Heterozygote Advantage. The foregoing discussion has assumed that in the case of a dominant mutation the mutant allele is so rare that the homozygotes can be ignored, and that in the case of recessive mutations the mutant gene does not affect the fitness of the heterozygote. It sometimes happens, however, that the heterozygote is fitter than either homozygote. The best known example is sickle cell anemia.

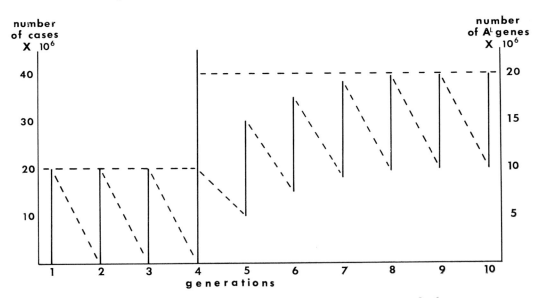

Figure 11-1.   Diagram illustrating the relation of gene frequency to mutation and selection.

In nontropical countries the gene for sickle cell disease, β^S, produces a serious and often lethal disease in the homozygote and only mild symptoms, if any, in the heterozygote. However, the heterozygous individual is more resistant to falciparum malaria than the normal homozygote, so that in countries where falciparum malaria is endemic, the β^S gene in heterozygous individuals has a better chance of being transmitted to the next generation than the normal β^A gene. This provides a mechanism for increasing the frequency of the mutant allele, and explains why the sickle cell gene is so frequent in certain races of African origin.

Heterozygote advantage is therefore a means of increasing the frequency of a given gene other than by mutation. It may explain why certain diseases such as cystic fibrosis of the pancreas or infantile amaurotic idiocy (in Ashkenazi Jews) are so frequent. Cystic fibrosis of the pancreas may involve one in 3,600 births or more in some populations, and since fitness is close to 0 it would require a mutation rate of about one in 3,600 to maintain the gene frequency if selection occurred only in the homozygote. This is higher than any known mutation rate. However, a fairly small heterozygote advantage—too small to detect by the usual family studies—would be enough to maintain this high a frequency without involving mutation at all. For instance, the high frequency of cystic fibrosis of the pancreas could be maintained if the heterozygote for the mutant gene had a fitness of about 1.7% more than the normal homozygote. There are, however, other explanations for disease frequencies higher than expected on the basis of a balance between mutation and selection. In particular there are genetic heterogeneity and segregation ratio advantage.

Genetic Heterogeneity. When the same clinical disease can be caused by mutants at each of several different loci there is genetic heterogeneity. The more refined our methods of analysis become the more examples are found. For instance, cystic fibrosis can be caused by homozygous mutant alleles at each of at least three different loci. Twenty such loci, each with a mutation rate of 1/60,000, would maintain a disease frequency of one in 3,000.

Segregation Ratio Advantage. If a mutant allele altered the segregation ratio by influencing meiosis or by selective gamete survival, so that the mutant allele was more likely to be passed on to the next generation than its normal partner, this would tend to increase the frequency of the mutant. Examples are known in lower organisms (e.g., the T locus in the mouse) but so far no examples in man have been recognized in which the mutant allele has a segregation ratio advantage.

Genetic Drift. Finally, variations in gene frequency can result from genetic drift, which refers to random fluctuation in gene frequency resulting from small sample size. To take a ridiculous example, suppose that Adam was homozygous for the blood group A gene, that Eve was heterozygous AB, and that all the descendants arose from four of their children. Each child would have an equal chance of being AA or AB. There would be $(1/2)^4$ or one chance in 16 that all children would be homozygous AA. Thus by chance the B gene could have been lost altogether. In populations that arose from small groups of ancestors, quite wide differences in gene frequency may arise simply from this kind of random variation. The high frequency of the Ellis-van Creveld syndrome in the Amish isolate is a well-documented example (see also p. 158).

MEASURING MUTATION RATES

In 1927 the great geneticist H.J. Muller, working with *Drosophila*, showed for the first time that an environmental factor, X-radiation, could cause mutation. Since then a variety of physical and chemical agents have been shown to be mutagenic in a variety of organisms. There is no reason to suppose that man is immune to environmental mutagens, but the difficulty of measuring precisely the spontaneous mutation rate in man has precluded any direct demonstration of mutagenicity in man. How are human mutation rates measured?

The Direct Method. The most obvious method is a direct count. In the case of a disease that shows dominant inheritance, any case that had unaffected parents would presumably represent a fresh mutation. Thus the mutation rate would be estimated directly from the incidence of sporadic cases. This approach assumes that there is no illegitimacy, that there is full penetrance, that there are no phenocopies, and that all cases of the diseases represent mutations at the same locus. It is recognized that these assumptions are not entirely valid. For instance the estimates for conditions such as tuberous sclerosis may be biased upward by reduced penetrance, and the estimates for achondroplasia may be biased upward by the inclusion of cases of recessively inherited chondrodystrophy erroneously diagnosed as achondroplasia. At best, the method will permit only a very rough estimate of the mutation rate. Estimates of rates for a number of dominantly inherited diseases more or less appropriate for this method range from 3 to 68 $\times$ 10⁻⁶ per locus per generation.[3]

The Indirect Approach. Another approach, and the only possible one for recessive mutations in man, makes use of the assumption that, in a population in equilibrium, the input of new mutant genes by mutation is balanced by the loss of genes through selection. As we have seen, the mutation rate for recessive genes is related to disease frequency and fitness according to the formula

$$X = m/(1-f), \text{ or } m = (1-f)X$$

The disease frequency and fitness can be measured, and the mutation rate can be calculated. Thus for a mutant that is lethal in the homozygote, the mutation rate should be equal to the disease frequency. This method also assumes full penetrance,

no phenocopies, and no genetic heterogeneity, and further assumes no effects of the gene on fitness in the heterozygote. This method can also be used for X-linked recessive diseases, using the formula:

$$m = (1-f)X/3$$

Estimates for X-linked recessive and autosomal recessive mutants range from 11 to 95 $\times$ 10⁻⁶ per locus per generation.[3] These are reasonably consistent with those for dominant mutations, which is somewhat reassuring. However, it should be pointed out that the diseases selected for study are those of sufficient frequency to permit reasonably accurate measurements of frequency, and so these figures probably represent the higher ranges of the spectrum of mutation rates.

THE GENETIC LOAD

The burden of disease and death that is created by the effects of our deleterious genes is termed the genetic load. A great deal of effort, stimulated largely by concern over the harmful genetic effects of radiation, has gone into estimating the size and nature of this load. Two concepts relevant to a discussion of the genetic load are "genetic death" and "lethal equivalent."

Genetic Death. A gene that impairs a person's ability to reproduce will eventually fail to be transmitted to the next generation and thus cease to exist, or suffer genetic death. A dominant lethal "dies" in the generation in which it arose. A dominant gene that causes a 20% reduction in fitness may fail to survive after one generation or many, but on the average will survive for five generations. Furthermore there is evidence from *Drosophila* and other organisms that a recessive gene causing severe disease in the homozygote may have a small detrimental effect in the heterozygote. If a gene is rare, it is far more likely to exist in the heterozygous than the homozygous state. Thus small deleterious effects in the heterozygote may actually cause more genetic deaths than a major effect in the homozygote. The main aim of this discussion is to point out that the harmful effects of a mutation may be spread over many individuals and many generations, and to show how difficult it is to predict the extent of mutational damage.

The Lethal Equivalent. To estimate the mutational load by attempting to count the number of mutations at every locus and measure their effects would be an impossible task. The concept of lethal equivalents was developed in an attempt to measure the total impact of recessive mutant genes on mortality, rather than trying to distinguish them individually. A lethal equivalent is a gene or group of genes that, when homozygous, would bring about the death of the individual. Thus, one lethal equivalent could be one recessive lethal mutant, or two recessive genes each of which had a 50% chance of causing death, or ten recessives each of which had a 10% chance of causing death, and so on. Estimates based on the effect of inbreeding on mortality have suggested that the average number of lethal equivalents in man may be about three.

Note that this is not the same as saying that each individual carries an average of three genes causing lethal recessive diseases. Some authors of genetic advice to cousins contemplating marriage have unfortunately made this misinterpretation. If this were so, the frequency of recognizable recessively inherited diseases in the offspring of cousin marriages would be about 10%, but in fact the frequency seems to be much lower than this. The rest of the lethality attributable to increased homozygosity in offspring of cousin marriages is made up by small increases in abortion, stillbirth and mortality from various common diseases.

The Mutational Load. We have already seen that two major factors tend to maintain the frequencies of deleterious genes in the population—mutation and heterozygote advantage. If there were no mutation, there would be less disease and death. The ex-

cess of disease and death due to mutation, above the level expected if there were no mutation, is termed the **mutational load.**

The Segregational Load. On the other hand, some deleterious genes are maintained in the population because they are at an advantage in the heterozygote, but cause disease and death when they segregate into homozygotes. The amount of disease and death due to this kind of gene, in excess of what it would be if there were no heterozygote advantage, is called the **segregational load.**

There has been much discussion and no little argument about the relative importance of the two kinds of genetic load. If the segregation load is the major one, the importance of radiation as a genetic hazard is correspondingly less. Unfortunately the question is still not settled, but it would seem that both components of the genetic load are appreciable.

THE MUTAGENIC EFFECTS OF IONIZING RADIATION

The concern over the genetic effects of ionizing radiation aroused by the advent of the Atomic Age has stimulated a great deal of research on the subject. We have seen that the measurement of mutation rates in man is so subject to error that it would be impossible to detect an increase of the size one might expect from observed exposures to radiation. Almost all our information comes by extrapolation from data on other animals.

The Dose-response Relationship. It is generally assumed that the relation of dose to mutation rate is linear in the low-dose range and that there is no threshold dose, since one "hit" is enough to cause a mutation. However, the picture is complicated by the following features:

1. Different loci may have different mutation rates, and the differences may not be the same for induced as for spontaneous rates.
2. Dose-response relationships vary from species to species, so extrapolations

from lower organisms to man require caution.

3. Both spontaneous and induced mutation rates vary with sex and the stage of gametogenesis.

4. The frequency of induced mutation varies with the dose-rate. Low dose-rates produce much lower mutation frequencies than the same dose at high dose-rates.

The Doubling Dose for Point Mutations. Attempts to predict the effects of exposure to ionizing radiation in man involve estimating the "doubling dose"—that is, the dose of radiation that will increase the mutation rate to double the spontaneous rate, assuming a linear dose-response curve. A permanent doubling of the mutation rate would eventually double the frequency of diseases normally maintained in the population by spontaneous mutation. For dominant lethals the effect would be immediate; for dominant nonlethal mutants and recessives, the final effect would be spread over many generations. For genes maintained by heterozygote advantage the effect would be negligible.

Original estimates of the doubling dose suggested that the probable value for man was about 30 rad per generation. In the light of more recent information, a value of 120 rad is more likely, at least for chronic, low intensity irradiation of male mice. It is somewhat less for females.

The genetically significant (gonadal) exposure of human populations to background and cosmic radiation varies widely, with an average of about 3 rem per generation (a rem is roughly equivalent to a rad). Medical uses of radiation add another 0.5 to 5 rem. Atomic testing may have contributed about 0.05 rem. Thus the contribution of medical practice to our mutation rate is not negligible. For instance, it has been estimated that an exposure of 5r to a population of 100 million people would cause about 40,000 embryonic and neonatal deaths, 16,000 infant and childhood deaths, 8,000 gross mental or physical defects, and 100 cases of achondroplasia in the first generation. The corresponding figure for cases appearing in subsequent generations would be 760,000, 384,000, 72,000 and 20. Obviously every effort should be made to reduce exposure to irradiation to the absolute minimum compatible with good medical care.

Almost nothing is known of the other effects of radiation on the genetic material. At least two studies have suggested that a history of diagnostic or therapeutic pelvic irradiation is found more frequently in parents of children with chromosomal aberrations than in parents of control children. There is no doubt that ionizing radiation causes chromosomal breaks and rearrangements that may persist in the individual for many years. It also increases the frequency of leukemia and other forms of neoplasia. Prenatal diagnostic irradiation increases the risk of the unborn child to develop leukemia or cancer postnatally. It seems likely that the chromosomal breaks are causally related to the neoplasia, but this remains to be clarified. In any case these findings are further good reasons for avoiding as much irradiation as possible.

OTHER ENVIRONMENTAL MUTAGENS

Many environmental agents, including a number of drugs, viruses and food additives, cause chromosomal breaks and rearrangements, particularly *in vitro*. Many of them are mutagenic in lower animals. However, the significance of these findings with respect to genetic damage in man is difficult to evaluate. Although it seems reasonable to suppose that agents that break chromosomes may also be mutagenic, and this has been demonstrated in a number of cases in lower organisms, we have little idea of the quantitative relationships involved. Certainly the fact that an agent will break chromosomes *in vitro* does not necessarily mean that it will do so *in vivo*, or that it will be mutagenic. On the other hand, it would be foolhardy to ignore the possibility. Further data, particularly from the field of somatic cell genetics, may help to resolve some of the uncertainty.

OUR CHANGING GENE FREQUENCIES

A world increasingly concerned about the rapid growth of human populations must also be concerned about the quality of its genes. When widespread family planning becomes a necessary fact of life, parents will want their limited number of children to be free of genetic disease. If there are likely to be changes in the frequency of genetic disorders, public health administrators and others concerned with forecasting the need for health care facilities will want to know ahead of time. What, then, is likely to happen to our gene frequencies?

The frequency of a mutant gene in a population at equilibrium depends on the mutation rate and the strength of selection for or against the gene in the heterozygote and homozygote, as outlined on page 202. This relationship, and particularly the effect of changes in selection pressure, vary with the mode of inheritance.

At present, most diseases caused by mutant genes are rare, as there has been strong selection against them. Nevertheless, they constitute a considerable burden of disease and death. For example, in one North American pediatric hospital, they account for about 7% of admissions and in Great Britain they account for about 11% of pediatric deaths.

Certain genes have a much higher frequency in some populations than in others. There are two possible explanations. In some geographically or ethnically isolated groups (isolates), the present population may have descended from a relatively small group of ancestors. A mutant gene present in the original group may, by chance, either be lost or be transmitted to a relatively high proportion of descendants (genetic drift) and then spread among the descendants, being maintained at a high frequency by lack of outbreeding. In some cases the mutant gene can be traced to a single ancestor, in which case the genetic drift has

been termed the "founder effect." Tyrosinemia in a French-Canadian isolate and the Ellis-van Creveld syndrome in the Amish (recessive) and the South African type of porphyria variegata (dominant) are examples for which the founder has been identified.

There are other examples of an unusually high frequency of a deleterious gene that cannot be accounted for by founder effect, since the populations involved are large and the founder effect depends on small sample variation. Pancreatic cystic fibrosis in Europeans, sickle cell anemia in West Africans, and beta thalassemia in Italians and Greeks are well-documented examples. In the case of sickle cell disease, the high gene frequency resulted from an increased resistance of heterozygotes to falciparum malaria, so that heterozygotes living in a malarial region had a reproductive advantage over those not carrying the gene. Heterozygote advantage is the most reasonable explanation for the other examples too, but the mechanism is not known. Because most mutant genes exist in the heterozygous state a very small heterozygote advantage will exert a relatively large effect on the gene frequency. For instance, it has been estimated that a recessive lethal disease could be maintained at a frequency of one per 1000 births if heterozygotes had about 3% more children than normal homozygotes. This would be virtually impossible to detect.

In populations of intermediate size it may not be possible to establish whether the unusually high frequency of a deleterious gene results mainly from genetic drift or heterozygote advantage or from both—for example, Tay-Sachs disease in Ashkenazi Jews and congenital nephrosis in Finnish populations.

EFFECTS OF RELAXED SELECTION

As we have said, in hereditary disease where the mutant gene is not protected by heterozygote advantage, "natural" selection keeps the gene frequency low by preventing affected individuals from contributing their genes, good as well as bad, to the next generation. Medicine is devoted to the opposite task—that is, ameliorating the effects of our mutant genes, and thus increasing the probability that these genes will be passed on to the next generation. Thus medical care is dysgenic and, in the absence of counter-measures, will lead to an increase in frequency of genetic diseases. Will this increase be large enough to cause concern?[4]

In the case of a lethal (in the sense of preventing reproduction) recessively inherited disease for which a treatment was found that fully restored fertility, the frequency of the gene would slowly increase at a rate equal to the mutation rate. For example, if the original gene frequency was 0.01 (resulting in a disease frequency of one in 10,000) and selection was completely relaxed, it would take 100 generations to double the gene frequency, assuming a mutation rate of 10^{-4}. This would result in a four-fold increase in the disease frequency to one in 2500. The slowness of the rise may be reassuring, but the more diseases for which successful treatments are found, the greater the cumulative effect would be.

For dominant lethals, completely relaxed selection would again lead to an increase in gene frequency equal to the mutation rate, and this will result in a linear increase in disease frequency. If the lethal trait had a frequency of one in 10,000, and selection were completely relaxed, the disease frequency would double in the first generation and rise to 86 in 10,000 after 100 generations (assuming a mutation rate of 5×10^{-5}). There would also, of course, be an increase in the proportion of familial to sporadic cases, and this has already been observed in the case of retinoblastoma, even though the relaxation of selection is far from complete. Thus the effects of relaxed selection would be much more worrisome for dominant than for recessive traits.

Diseases showing X-linked recessive inheritance have an intermediate position, since the gene is exposed to selection in hemizygous males as well as homozygous females. Within four generations of completely relaxed selection the disease frequency would double.

For diseases showing a multifactorial etiology the results of relaxed selection are harder to predict because environmental factors are involved and we know virtually nothing about the nature of the underlying genetic factors and the selective factors acting upon them. In the case of myelomeningocele, for example, improved treatment is allowing many more individuals to reach the reproductive age. The frequency of the malformation in the offspring of affected children is likely to be about 3%, and an increasing number of these affected children will reproduce. It seems likely that, following completely relaxed selection, the frequency of the disease would increase by about 3 to 5% per generation over the next few generations, assuming that there is no change in the relevant environmental factors.[4]

PREVENTION OF GENETIC DISEASE

A program aimed toward reducing the frequency of harmful mutant genes would be termed negative eugenics. Ignoring for present purposes the unpleasant connotations of the term "eugenic," let us consider the possible results of such programs, taking the extreme case in each example and realizing that in practice the theoretic limits are not likely to be met.

For an autosomal dominant gene causing a disease that could be diagnosed before puberty, if all heterozygotes were dissuaded from mating, the frequency of the disease would fall in one generation to twice the mutation rate. Obviously such a program would have no effect on the frequency of a gene that was already lethal (in the sense that it killed or prevented reproduction of the affected individual) since selection would already be maximal. At the other extreme are diseases such as Huntington's chorea, which usually appears after puberty. Assuming a disease frequency of one per 1000 births, a program of prenatal diagnosis and selective termination would reduce the frequency to one per 100,000, assuming a mutation rate of five per million. As there is still no way of diagnosing the disease much before its onset, the only means of reducing the disease frequency is through genetic counseling, and the effect would depend on how successful such a program was in persuading the offspring of affected individuals not to have children.

For achondroplasia, assuming a fertility 20% that of normal, a program of intrauterine diagnosis and selective termination would reduce the frequency to 80% of its original value.

It is more difficult to lower the gene frequencies of autosomal recessive genes, because usually only homozygotes are exposed to selection and the great majority of the genes are heterozygous. The effects of a counseling program would depend on the distribution of family size. Assuming the family size distribution of the United States, a counseling program that persuaded all parents of an affected child to have no more children would reduce the disease frequency by about 15%. Prenatal diagnosis of homozygotes and selective termination of pregnancy would have a similar effect on disease frequency, but the gene frequently would increase slightly because heterozygous pregnancies would not be terminated.

A population with a high frequency of a mutant gene provides the opportunity to screen for heterozygotes premaritally, in the hope that heterozygotes would avoid marrying other heterozygotes. Such programs already exist for sickle disease in populations of West African descent, for thalassemia in Mediterranean races, and for Tay-Sachs disease in Ashkenazi Jews; if completely successful, these programs would result in the disappearance of the diseases altogether. (In the case of Tay-Sachs disease, heterozygotes could marry one another but would have their pregnancies monitored by amniocentesis.) However, we know virtually nothing about the psychologic effects of discovering that one carries a "bad" gene or the kinds of social pressures that may be brought to bear on an individual so identified. Any such program should be accompanied by a well-designed public education campaign, and the early stages of such programs should include intensive study of their psychologic implications.

PREVENTION OF CHROMOSOMAL DISORDERS

Prenatal screening of all pregnancies, with selective termination, would remove a major portion of our load of chromosome disorders, but this would place an impossible burden on our health resources. Screening high-risk populations, however, could be justified in terms of a favorable cost-benefit ratio. For instance, nondisjunctional events are more likely to occur in older mothers; thus the birth frequency of Down syndrome could be reduced by about half by a program of prenatal screening and selective termination in the 10% of pregnancies occurring in women over 34 years of age. The cost of the program would be substantially less than that of institutional care for this fraction of the trisomic population.

In summary, it seems that the means are available for protecting future generations against the dysgenic effects of relaxed selection. We would add our hope that any program for reducing the frequencies of deleterious genes would be by education and voluntary cooperation, not by any form of coercion.

REFERENCES

1. Cavalli-Sforza, L. L., and Bodmer, W. F.: The Genetics of Human Populations. San Francisco, W. H. Freeman, 1971.
2. Levitan, M., and Montagu, A.: Textbook of Human Genetics. London, Oxford University Press, 1971.
3. Report of the United Nations Scientific Committee on the Effects of Atomic Radiation. United Nations, New York, 1962.
4. World Health Organization: Genetic Disorders: Prevention, Treatment and Rehabilitation. WHO Technical Report Series, no. 497, 1972.

Chapter 12

THE GENETICS OF DEVELOPMENT AND MALDEVELOPMENT

Because the human embryo is to a large extent hidden from the investigator and man is not subject to controlled matings, little is known of human developmental genetics and much must be extrapolated from lower organisms. This chapter will touch briefly on what is known of how development is controlled by genes, both normal and abnormal.[6]

Development of an organism has been compared to the building of a ship. The ship starts as a set of plans—specific instructions as to what goes where and in what order. These are analogous to the organism's genes, which are specific instructions on how the amino acids are put into sequences of particular polypeptides at specific places and times. The ship's plans are written on pages of blueprints. The organism's blueprints are its chromosomes—23 pages, in duplicate, for man. The building materials of the ship are put together according to the instructions, and similarly the biologic substrates are put together to form the developing embryo according to the genetic instructions. Then the ship is launched, but development of the ship is not finished. Fitting of the ship continues after launching, and development of the

human organism continues after birth. How well the ship, or baby, does will depend on the accuracy of the instructions and integrity of the blueprints, the accuracy with which they are translated into structure, the quality of the building materials, the quality of the shelter in which it is built, and finally, the rigor of the environmental hazards it meets as it is built and sails, drifts, churns, or is towed through the sea of life.

Errors in development resulting in structural defects or malformations can occur at several levels. There can be errors in the instructions (mutations), errors in the way the instructions are carried out (translational defects), extra or missing or transposed pages of blueprints (chromosomal aberrations), defects in quantity or quality of building blocks (vitamin deficiencies, antimetabolites), or damage from termites, rust and rot (environmental teratogens). Finally the ship can be defective not from any such major reason, but by the interaction of "a lot of little things" such as poor workmanship and inferior materials, no one of which would have caused a major defect, but which do so in combination (the multifactorial group). This analogy provides a useful way of thinking about the etiologies of various groups of diseases, ranging from mental retardation to congenital malformations, in four major categories: diseases resulting from *mutant genes*, from *chromosomal aberrations*, from *environmental pathogens*, and from *multifactorial* causes.

However, our analogy breaks down in some important ways when one thinks about the developmental process. Developing organisms show the phenomenon of **differentiation;** i.e., cells with the same genetic information may turn out quite differently. Secondly, development involves the process of **induction,** whereby a signal from one tissue or organ induces another tissue to begin developing along a new pathway. Thirdly, there is **morphogenesis,** which is the emergence of formed structures from relatively unformed ones and the synchronized integration of various tissues into structured organs.

DIFFERENTIATION

The human organism begins as a fertilized egg. Repeated cell divisions render it multicellular, each cell receiving a replica of the original nucleus and thus an identical complement of genes. Yet many dozens of different cell types occur in the adult organism, migrate, become organs, and interact, virtually all with the same complement of genes. How can the same genome give rise to many different cell types?[10]

A logical model can be developed from the assumption that the same genotype will respond differently to cytoplasms of different compositions and that the cytoplasm of the original egg is not homogeneous; there are regional concentrations of yolk granules, mitochondria and other components, as well as gradients of oxygen, glucose, etc. If this is so then cleavage, which divides the egg cytoplasm into compartments, will result in identical nuclei operating in cytoplasms that differ in the concentration of various components. If the nuclei respond differently to the cytoplasmic differences they will create new differences, and so

differentiation will proceed by a process of progressively more specialized nucleo-cytoplasmic reactions.

Differentiation, then, is the process by which genetically identical cells become functionally different. (**Determination** refers to the point where the progress of a cell line to its differentiated state becomes irreversible.) Differentiation appears to result largely from differential gene activity. All nucleated cells produce certain enzymes necessary for the maintenance of the cell (the "housekeeping enzymes"); a differentiated cell in addition has the enzymes to produce one or more special proteins relevant to its particular function (e.g., a reticulocyte produces hemoglobin and a lymphocyte does not). Thus the genetic system for making hemoglobin molecules is "switched on" in the reticulocyte, but "switched off" in the lymphocyte.

An example of gene activation during development is provided by the isozymes of lactic dehydrogenase (LDH). Isozymes are different forms of the enzyme, similar but not identical in structure and function. In the case of LDH there are five electrophoretically different isozymes. These are made up of varying combinations of two polypeptide chains, alpha and beta. Thus there must be a gene coding for each of these chains. The five isozymes represent varying combinations of the two chains. There may be four alpha, three alpha and one beta, and so on, to four beta chains, five types in all. The proportions of the five isozymes are different in different tissues and in the same tissue at different stages, indicating that the relative activities of the two genes differ from time to time and from place to place. The isozymes vary somewhat in their properties, such as degree of inhibition by lactate, and their varying proportions in different cells presumably has some functional significance. For instance, in striated muscle, lactate resulting from strenuous exercise inhibits the "muscle" type LDH, which weakens the muscle. This would be perilous for heart muscle, which conveniently has more of the isozyme not inhibited by lactate.[12]

Regulation of Transcription. It has been amply demonstrated that regulation of gene activity can occur at the level of transcription—the synthesis of the messenger RNA molecule from the DNA template. The array of messenger RNA molecules produced by one type of cell can be shown, by DNA-hybridization techniques, to differ from the array produced by another cell type. Furthermore, the same tissue may produce different arrays of mRNA's at different stages of development.

Little is known so far about the ways in which the onset and rate of transcription are controlled. It is clear from nuclear transplantation and cell hybridization experiments that the initiation of both DNA replication and transcription may depend on signals (DNA polymerases?) from the cytoplasm. In the ameba the use of radioactive tracers has demonstrated a class of proteins that migrate rapidly from nucleus to cytoplasm and from cytoplasm to nucleus, which seem likely candidates for conveyors of information that will initiate or suppress gene activity.

The Operon. In bacteria, the activity of a certain group of genes (an **operon**) may be regulated by another gene (the **regulator**) by means of a cytoplasmically transmitted **repressor,** probably a protein, that binds to a locus (the **operator**) at one end of the operon. The RNA polymerase that synthesizes the messenger RNA from the DNA template binds to a site, distal to the operator, called the **promoter.** If the repressor is bound to the operator, the RNA polymerase cannot function. A small molecule in the cytoplasm, such as a metabolic substrate (the **inducer**) may combine with the repressor and prevent its binding with the operator. Then the RNA polymerase can begin synthesizing messenger, and the genes of the operon are "turned on" when the appropriate substrate appears. A mutation in the promoter or the operator or regulator gene could prevent the operon from being "turned on" when the inducer appears, so the corresponding enzymes would not appear when needed.[12]

No well-substantiated example of an operon is known in mammals, but there are examples of genes that appear to regulate the activity of other genes. The switch from the production of fetal to adult hemoglobin is an example. Normal adult human hemoglobin consists largely of hemoglobin A, comprising two alpha and two beta polypeptide chains ($\alpha_2^A\beta_2^A$). Fetal hemoglobin (F) consists of two alpha and two gamma chains ($\alpha_2^A\gamma_2^A$). The human fetus makes mostly fetal hemoglobin, but well before birth the production of hemoglobin A in the blood begins to increase and of hemoglobin F to decrease. This "switch" from hemoglobin F to A continues after birth and is virtually complete by the age of one year.

Thus in the fetal red cell precursor the gene for the gamma chain is active and the gene for the beta chain is suppressed, while in the adult the beta chain gene is transcribed and the gamma chain gene is inactive. The nature of the factor responsible for the switch is unknown, but the switch appears to be under genetic control. A mutant gene, "high F," closely adjacent to the beta chain prevents the switch, so that homozygotes for this gene continue to produce hemoglobin F and not A. Heterozygotes produce intermediate amounts of F and A, showing that the high-F gene suppresses only the beta chain gene on the same chromosome, and not that on the homologous chromosome. Thus the normal allele at the high-F locus behaves like an operator. Furthermore, the gene for the delta chain, a component of the minor hemoglobin component A² ($\alpha_2^A\delta_2^A$), is closely linked to the beta chain gene, and its activity is also suppressed by the high-F gene. Perhaps in the normal switch-over from hemoglobin F to A the production of beta or delta messenger suppresses the activity of the gamma chain gene, but so far this is just conjecture.

Learning how to "operate the switch" could have practical benefits. For instance, in a person homozygous for the sickle cell gene ($\alpha_2^A \beta_2^S$), if the switch from gamma to beta chain production could be prevented, the patient would continue to make hemoglobin F (which has no beta chains) and would not suffer from the effects of the mutation.

Heterochromatin. Another example of differential gene activation is provided by the heterochromatin, stretches of chromosome that remain tightly contracted, deeply staining and genetically inactive during interphase, unlike euchromatin which becomes dispersed. The outstanding example is the inactivated X chromosome of the mammalian female, most of which is heterochromatic, but there is heterochromatin in other chromosomes as well. Presumably heterochromatic regions are so compacted that their DNA is not amenable to transcription, but what determines where and when the euchromatin will become heterochromatic remains a mystery.

Chromosomal RNA and Proteins. The activity, or inactivity, of the DNA in being transcribed by messenger RNA seems to depend on the chromosomal proteins. Histones repress messenger RNA synthesis, but lack sufficient specificity to account for regulation of individual loci. However the specificity may be added by a special type of RNA, with a high content of 5-methyl dihydrocytidylic acid, which may bind to specific regions of the DNA and is also bound to chromosomal protein. This histone-RNA complex could bind to specific regions of the chromosome, thus achieving differential gene inactivation.

Hormones. Ample evidence demonstrates that the activity of certain genes is regulated by hormones, but it is still not clear how this is done. There are semispecific proteins in the plasma that bind certain hormones (e.g., for estrogen and testosterone). In the cell cytoplasm there are very specific binding proteins (e.g., an estrogen cytosol receptor complex that somehow facilitates entry of estrogen into the nuclei of the endometrial cells). There, in combination with a specific acceptor protein, the hormone is bound to the chromosome, suggesting that it regulates gene activity at the transcriptional level. However, the hormones appear to be organ-specific and may affect groups of seemingly unrelated enzymes. The mechanism of this coordinate control is still obscure.

Gene Amplification. A special example of differential gene activity has been found in the amphibian oocyte. When the embryo begins to develop, it will need large numbers of ribosomes for the rapid synthesis of proteins. In the maturing oocyte the genes that code for ribosomal RNA are replicated many times. The copies are released from the chromosome and form hundreds of nucleoli which then synthesize ribosomal RNA. Thus the activity of the gene for ribosomal RNA is amplified several hundredfold in apparent anticipation of the need for rapid protein synthesis.

Redundant RNA. Another way in which the activity of a particular kind of gene could be amplified would be to have it exist in many copies in linear sequence. The amount of DNA in a mammalian cell is at least 1000 times as much as needed to code for the actual number of proteins. DNA-annealing techniques have shown that about 70% of the DNA of a haploid genome is present in single copies, and that 30% recurs in copies from 1,000 to 1,000,000 times per cell. Much of the redundancy is accounted for by the ribosomal RNA genes; the function of the remainder of the redundant DNA remains unknown, but may well have something to do with gene regulation.

Polyploidy. One way of achieving cell differentiation would be to alter the number of chromosomes, and there are a number of tissues that are normally polyploid (bladder epithelium) or have a number of polyploid cells (liver), but in these cases it is not clear whether the polyploidy is a cause of the differentiation or merely associated with it. In any case polyploidy does not seem to be important as a cause of differentiation in man.

Regulation of Translation. We have considered a number of examples of differential gene activity through changes in transcription It appears that control at the level of translation (synthesis of polypeptide on the ribosome) may also be an important means of regulating gene activity.

It has been known for some time that a messenger RNA molecule may be transcribed from the DNA long before it begins to synthesize its polypeptide. For example, during oogenesis of the sea urchin egg, messenger is synthesized and stored inactive (the "masked messenger") until fertilization, when there is an abrupt increase in protein synthesis without a concomitant increase in RNA synthesis. In the mouse oocyte the ribosomes (and messenger) are held in a protein lattice that presumably keeps them inactive and disappears shortly after fertilization.[1]

Similarly, the messenger RNA synthesized in the erythroblast is not translated into hemoglobin until the reticulocyte stage, about two days later. In the interval it becomes associated with groups of four ribosomes (polysomes) where it appears to remain stable. Globin synthesis is regulated by the amount of heme present and this appears to occur at the translational level.

Epigenetic Control. Brief mention should be made of regulation beyond the level of translation, the so-called epigenetic level. Enzyme activity can be regulated, for instance, by controlling the rate of degradation of the enzyme, rather than its synthesis. The way the molecule is folded may differ in different cytoplasmic states, resulting in changed activity. Polymerization or addition or deletion of part of a peptide chain are other ways of achieving epigenetic control.

Diseases due to Defective Differentiation. Many genetic defects can be attributed to errors of differentiation in which a specific cell type does not appear, or takes some abnormal form.[7] For instance, in the pituitary dwarf mouse the eosinophils fail to differentiate, resulting in a specific growth hormone deficiency, and various hereditary chondrodystrophies result from failure of specific aspects of cartilage differentiation.

MORPHOGENESIS

Morphogenesis, or the emergence of form in the developing organism, is much more complicated than the activation or inactivation of genes. To account for the migration of cells, their aggregation into tissues, the synchronized spreading, bending, and thickening of tissues, the transfer of developmental instructions from one tissue to another (induction), and in short the whole complexly integrated series of interactions that eventually result in the adult organism seems a superhuman task, yet a beginning has been made. We cannot cover the whole subject of morphogenesis and its genetic control in this book, but will refer to a number of representative examples.

There is no doubt that morphogenetic processes are influenced by genes, since there are large numbers of mutant genes that alter the shapes of organs. Many of these are well described in structural terms, but little is known of their precise modes of action. Mutant genes can be useful in revealing the normal, and there are a large number of mutant genes in the mouse and other animals that produce phenotypes resembling human diseases and malformations.[7,8,14,15]

Induction. Induction, to the embryologist, is the process by which a signal from one tissue initiates a change in the developmental fate of another. For instance, the optic cup, growing out from the brain, induces the ectoderm that lies over it to form a lens, and the two structures integrate with one another to form the eye. Recently the use of mutant genes has shown not only that the induction is under genetic control, but that inductive relations are more complicated than previously suspected. For example, the very early chick limb consists essentially of an ectodermal jacket surround-

ing an apparently undifferentiated mesoderm. Inductive interactions have been analyzed by the use of mutant genes in the
chick causing such things as extra fingers
or winglessness. By combining mutant ectoderm with normal mesoderm, and vice
versa, and seeing how the resulting limb
develops, it has been shown that the overlying ectoderm induces the mesoderm to
organize digits. However, the number of
digits depends on an inductive stimulus
from the mesoderm to the ectoderm. Thus
morphogenesis of the hand depends upon a
series of genetically controlled reciprocal
inductive interactions between ectoderm
and mesoderm. It is likely that some of the
malformations of hands and feet seen in
human babies result from disturbances in
inductive relationships.

In some cases, abnormal development of
an organ results from **failure of induction
due to asynchrony** rather than an abnormal
inductive mechanism. There is a gene that
causes absent or small kidneys in the mouse.
Embryologic studies show that the migration of the ureter is delayed so that it is
late in reaching the kidney precursor tissue. This suggested that the kidney tissue
requires an inductive stimulus from the
ureter bud to initiate its differentiation, and
that the abnormal kidney resulted from a
diminished or absent stimulus. In culture,
when mutant ureter and mutant kidney
precursor were put together, kidney differentiation occurred. Thus the ureter could
induce and the kidney precursor could respond; abnormality resulted from failure to
bring the two together at the right time.

These examples show how a mutant gene
may reveal normal developmental mechanisms, as well as the means by which they
go wrong. Such studies can contribute to
the understanding of human malformations.

Shape and Pattern. The most complex
developmental problem of all is the means
by which genes control the shapes of organs
and the patterns seen in such profusion and
with such beauty wherever one looks in
nature. The influence of genes on pattern

is beginning to be analyzed in higher organisms. The mouse mutant "reeler," for example, deranges the form of the cerebellum
and cerebrum. The various organized layers
are unrecognizable, the various cell types
being intermixed instead of sorted out into
their normal layers, and lack their vertical
orientation. Experiments show that dissoci-
ated isocortical cells from day 18 mutant
embryos will form aggregates normally, but
do not organize themselves into an external
molecular layer and an internal nerve fiber
zone as do aggregates of normal cells of
this age (but not a day earlier or later).
Thus the mutant produces a defect in self-
organization of the mutant brain cells at a
particular stage of development, showing
that this property is under genetic control.[3]

In another example a morphogenetic
change due to a mutant gene has been
traced to a property of the cell membrane.
The mutant gene "talpid[3]" in the chick
causes midline facial defects, fusion of mesenchymal precartilage condensations and
polydactyly. Cell aggregation experiments
demonstrate that these result from increased
adhesiveness and decreased motility of the
mesenchymal cells.[4]

Much of the work on pattern comes from
Drosophila. For instance, the bristles are
distributed on the fly in a very regular pattern. Many mutant genes are known that
change the number or position of specific
bristles. How does a cell in a certain place
on the *Drosophila* thorax "know" that it is
to form a bristle, while the cell right next
to it forms cuticle? Presumably the genetic
machinery of the *Drosophila* cells is programmed so that any cell finding itself in
that particular environment and with that
particular history will respond, so to speak,
by turning on its bristle-making genes. If
so, there must be an underlying system of
gradients of chemical and physical change
making that particular spot different from
any other—a so called "prepattern." Inge-
nious experiments making use of bristle mutants and a technique for producing mosaic
flies containing a mixture of normal and

mutant tissues were able to show that the mutant bristle appears in a different place because its genes have changed its program rather than the distribution of the underlying pattern. Thus we return to the idea advanced at the beginning of the chapter: differential gene activity may result from differences in the cytoplasm in which the genotype resides, and development proceeds by the emergence of more and more specialized kinds of cytoplasm.

GENES AND MALDEVELOPMENT

The Modes of Action of Mutant Genes. Theoretically, for every process involved in normal development one might expect malformations resulting from mutations of each gene affecting that process. Thus one might have malformations resulting from: a mutant structural protein (as in hydrotic ectodermal dysplasia); absent or abnormal enzymes (homocystinuria); defective properties of cell adhesiveness (the "talpid" chick); defective capacity of cells to migrate or orient themselves (the "reeler" mouse); failure to die at the proper time (syndactyly); excessive cell death (the rumpless chick); failure to respond to signals from other tissues either by contact (anophthalmia resulting from failure of the ectoderm to respond to induction by the optic cup) or a humoral inducer (testicular feminization); asynchronies in growth resulting in inductive failure (anophthalmia resulting from delayed growth of the optic cup; the kidneys of the Danforth short mouse); and no doubt many other causes. The wealth of mutant genes in the mouse and other mammals provides a fruitful field for research into the developmental links between mutant genes and phenotype, with the possibility of extrapolation to analogous human syndromes.

Gene-environmental Interactions. Environmental teratogens may also strike at various points in the developmental network or may interact with mutant genes affecting the same developmental processes. A particularly instructive example is the interaction of 5-fluorouracil (FUDR) and the mutant gene "luxoid" (lu) in the mouse.[2] Either a low dose of the teratogen or the mutant gene in the heterozygous condition produces only a minor defect, polydactyly of the hind foot. The homozygous mutant or a high dose of the teratogen produces polydactyly and tibial hemimelia. The combination of a low dose of teratogen plus the heterozygous gene will produce polydactyly and tibial hemimelia even though neither would individually. One wonders whether an analogous situation may exist in man. Why, for instance, does a synthetic progestin produce masculinization of the genitalia in only a minority of babies exposed to it at the appropriate gestational age? Could they be heterozygous for a rare recessive gene, such as one that causes the adrenogenital syndrome in the homozygote?

Our second example illustrates the possibility that malformations can be prevented by prenatal measures. The mutant gene "pallid" in the mouse causes ataxia resulting from failure of the otoliths of the inner ear to form. Maternal manganese deficiency causes a similar condition in the rat. Putting these facts together, it was possible for Hurley and associates[5] to correct the ataxia in pallid mice by giving their mothers large doses of manganese during pregnancy!

Finally, we must recall the numerous examples of gene-environmental interactions involving multifactorial threshold characters. An embryo's genes may place a particular developmental variable near a threshold of abnormality, so that a relatively small additional environmental influence may place that organ beyond the threshold and result in malformation. In another embryo in which the organ is not near the threshold, the same environmental insult will have no effect. An example described in detail in Chapter 13 is cleft of the secondary palate, where the variable is the time at which the embryonic palatal shelves reach the horizontal, so they may fuse, and the threshold is the latest stage of development when they can reach each other when they do become horizontal.

The Developmental Basis of Pleiotropy, Penetrance and Expressivity. *Pleiotropy.* Pleiotropy refers to the fact that a single mutant gene may have several end effects, as in numerous inherited syndromes. The multiple effects of single genes can be explained in several ways.

The several end effects may be secondary, tertiary or even more removed results of the initial defect. Gruneberg[9] coined the term "pedigree of causes" to refer to this phenomenon. Thus in sickle cell disease the basic molecular defect leads to hemolysis, which leads to anemia, pallor and fatigability; to intravascular sickling, which causes leg ulcers, infarcts of various organs and splenic rupture; and to marrow hypertrophy, which causes bone pain and the "tower skull." In phenylketonuria the mental defect, growth retardation, hypopigmentation, skin rash and seizures are all, no doubt, results of the basic enzyme defect, although some of the steps are not yet clear. In many syndromes the developmental connections are entirely obscure. For instance,

what biochemical defect is common to the retinitis pigmentosa and polydactyly of the Laurence-Moon-Biedl syndrome?

Pleiotropy can also occur if the same polypeptide is common to more than one protein. A mutant polypeptide would then result in more than one mutant protein and more than one end effect. We do not know of any relevant example. A great challenge for students of developmental mammalian genetics will be to trace the developmental connections revealed by pleiotropic mutant genes.

Penetrance and Expressivity. Little is known about the developmental basis of penetrance and expressivity. A convenient if oversimplified model is based on the developmental variable-threshold concept. If a group of individuals (such as a particular strain of mice) had a genotype and environment that placed it near the threshold, the effect of a major mutant gene might be to throw all the individuals beyond the threshold, and one would say that the gene had full penetrance (Fig. 12-1). In another group who were far from the threshold, the effect of a mutant gene might place only a

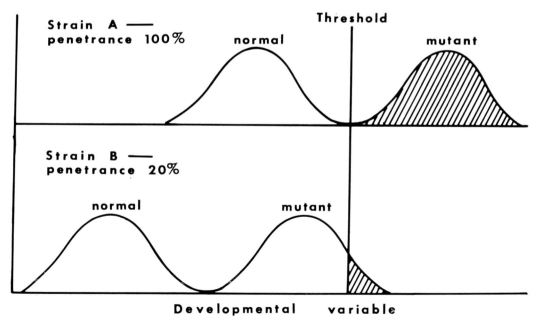

Figure 12-1. Hypothetic model showing penetrance of gene on two different genetic backgrounds.

few individuals beyond the threshold, and the gene would be said to have low penetrance. Similarly, if individuals near the threshold were mildly affected and those far beyond the threshold were severely affected, it is clear that there would be a correlation between penetrance and expressivity, as there often seems to be in experimental animals in which this can be adequately tested.

Phenocopies. Phenocopies are individuals with a mutant phenotype but a nonmutant genotype; that is, some environmental factor has simulated the effects of a mutant gene. Much has been deduced about the mode and time of action of mutant genes by analysis of their phenocopies, but this approach is only just beginning to be applied in man. An interesting example is given by Lenz[11] who showed that, depending on the stage of exposure, the teratogenic effects of thalidomide on the limb could resemble those of the mutant genes for the Holt-Oram syndrome, the Fanconi anemia syndrome, or the radial aplasia with amegakaryocytosis syndrome respectively.

REFERENCES

1. Burkholder, G., Comings, D. E., and Okada, T. A.: A storage form of ribosomes in mouse oocytes. Exp. Cell Res., 69:361, 1971.
2. Dagg, C. P.: Combined action of fluorouracil and two mutant genes on limb development in the mouse. J. Exp. Zool., 164:479, 1967.
3. DeLong, G. R., and Sidman, R. L.: Alignment defect of reaggregating cells in cultures of developing brains of reeler mutant mice. Develop. Biol., 22:584, 1970.
4. Ede, D. A., and Agerback, G. S.: Cell adhesion and movement in relation to the developing limb pattern in normal and talpid[3] chick embryos. J. Embryol. Exp. Morph., 20(1):81, 1968.
5. Erway, L., Hurley, L. S., and Fraser, F. S.: Neurological defect: manganese in phenocopy and prevention of a genetic abnormality of inner ear. Science, 152:1766, 1966.
6. Fraser, F. C., and McKusick, V. A. (eds.): Congenital Malformations. New York, Excerpta Medica, 1970.
7. Green, E. L. (ed.): Biology of the Laboratory Mouse. 2nd ed. New York, McGraw-Hill, 1966.
8. Green, M. C.: Genes and development. In Green, E. L. (Ed.): Biology of the Laboratory Mouse. 2nd ed. New York, McGraw-Hill, 1966. p. 329.
9. Gruneberg, H.: An analysis of the "pleiotropic" effects of a new lethal mutation in the rat (*Mus norvegicus*). Proc. Roy. Soc. Lond., Ser. B., 125:123, 1938.
10. Hamburgh, M.: Theories of Differentiation. New York, American Elsevier, 1971.
11. Lenz, W.: Genetic diagnosis: molecular diseases and others. In de Grouchy, J., Ebling, F. J. G., and Henderson, I. W. (eds.): Human Genetics. Amsterdam, Excerpta Medica, 1972.
12. Markert, C. L., and Ursprung, H.: Developmental Genetics. Englewood Cliffs, Prentice-Hall, 1971.
13. Motulsky, A. G.: Biochemical genetics of hemoglobins and enzymes as a model for birth defects research. In Fraser, F. C., and McKusick, V. A., *op. cit.*, p. 199.
14. Pinkerton, P. H., and Bannerman, R. M.: The hereditary anemias of mice. Hemat. Rev., 1:119, 1968.
15. Sidman, R. L., Green, M. C., and Appel, S. H.: Catalogue of the Neurological Mutants of the Mouse. Cambridge, Harvard University Press, 1965.

Chapter 13

MULTIFACTORIAL INHERITANCE

METRICAL TRAITS

Everyone knows that close relatives tend to resemble each other with respect to a number of quantitative or metrical characters such as height, weight, size of nose, "intelligence," and so on. The question of how closely relatives resemble each other and how much of the familial tendency is due to genes shared in common is one that has received a good deal of attention from mathematical geneticists; there is an extensive literature on the subject.[3] We will review only a few basic principles here.

For any particular metrical character, a first approach to the question of genetic basis is to see whether the frequency dis-

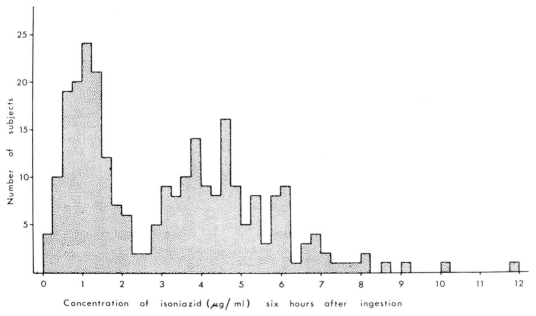

Figure 13-1. Frequency distribution of isoniazid blood levels six hours after a standard dose. The distribution is bimodal, illustrating the presence of two phenotypes—fast and slow inactivators.

tribution of the trait has a single mode (or peak) or more than one mode. A bimodal frequency distribution strongly suggests that a major genetic difference is segregating in the population, as in the case of isoniazid degradation (Fig. 13-1). A unimodal curve (as in the case of blood pressure or intelligence) suggests that no single factor is making a major contribution to the variation in the trait.

Heritability. Many quantitative traits have a distribution that fits the familiar bell-shaped curve known as the normal curve. This is compatible with the assumption that the magnitude of the trait is determined by a number of genes, each adding a small amount to the quantity of the trait or subtracting a small amount from it, and each acting independently of the others (i.e., acting additively, with no dominance or epistasis). This is known as **polygenic** inheritance. There are a few individuals at the extremes of the distribution and many in the middle because it is unlikely for an individual to inherit a large number of factors

all acting in the same direction. For instance, if height were determined by one gene locus with three alleles, one adding two inches to the height (h^+), one subtracting two inches (h^-) and one neutral (h), and if h were twice as frequent as the other two, the expected distribution of heights can be found by calculating the frequencies of pairs of gametes from the available pool, as in Table 13-1 and Figure 13-2. Thus if the mean height was 68 inches, 1/16 of the population would be h^-h^- and 64 inches tall, 1/16 would be h^+h^+ and 72 inches tall, 4/16 would be hh and 68 inches tall, 2/16 would be h^+h^- and also 68 inches tall, and so on.

If we add another locus, also with three alleles in the same proportions, the distribution of heights is beginning to look like the normal curve (Fig. 13-3). Thus a relatively small amount of genetic variation can produce a distribution that is fairly normal. In this case only 1/256 individuals would inherit all four $-$ alleles or $+$ alleles and be at the extremes of the distribution. Harris[7] has shown, for example, that the enzyme red

TABLE 13-1. Frequencies of Genotypes for Height if Determined by Three Alleles at a Single Locus*

	Sperm		
	1 h⁺	2 h	1 h⁻
1 h⁺	1 h⁺h⁺ 72"	2 h h⁺ 70"	1 h⁺h⁻ 68"
2 h	2 h⁺h 70"	4 h h 68"	2 h h⁻ 66"
1 h⁻	1 h⁺h⁻ 68"	2 h h⁻ 66"	1 h⁻h⁻ 64"

(Eggs)

h = average   h⁺ = plus 2 inches   h⁻ = minus 2 inches

* After Carter, C. O.: Human Heredity. Baltimore, Penguin Books, 1970.

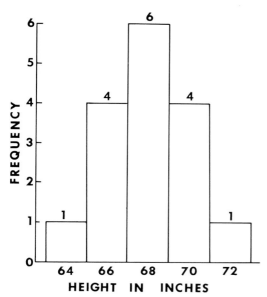

Figure 13-2. Frequency distribution of heights from Table 13-1.

cell acid phosphatase exists in three electrophoretically different forms, varying in their enzymatic activities, and that the apparently normal distribution of enzyme activities in the general population comes from various combinations of these alleles, very much as in the theoretic height model.

Of course, a number of environmental factors, each adding or subtracting a small amount to the final result, will also result in a normal distribution even without any genetic variation. In most cases the variation in the populaton results from a number of genes and environmental factors acting together to determine the final quantity. This can be termed multifactorial inheritance. The proportion of the total variation in the trait that results from genetic variation is the **heritability** of the trait.

The problem then is to determine how much of the variation in the multifactorial trait is due to segregating genes and how

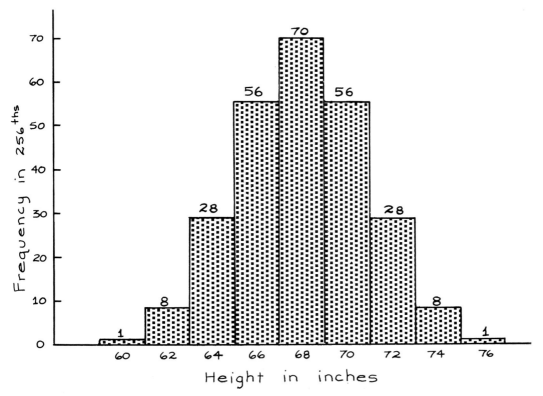

Figure 13-3. Frequency distribution of heights assuming two loci each with three alleles.

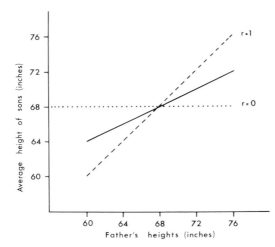

Figure 13-4. Regression toward the mean of son's on father's phenotype for a polygenic character. For any father's value, the mean value for sons is halfway between father's value and the mean of the population (assuming no assortative mating).

much to environmental factors. One can reason as follows: If all the variation were due to environmental factors (which did not themselves show a familial tendency), there would be no tendency for relatives to resemble one another—i.e., the correlation between relatives would be 0. What would it be if the inheritance was polygenic, with no environmental variation? Consider, for instance, the correlation between father and son. The son gets half of his father's genes, so if the father's genes for the trait in question are such that he deviates from the mean, the son on the average should deviate by half as much. For a series of such pairs this would lead to a father-son correlation (and regression of son on father) of 0.5. A similar situation exists for pairs of brothers, who have half of their fathers genes in common (Fig. 13-4).

. This relationship was first formulated by Sir Francis Galton as the "law of filial regression"—the mean value of the sons would be halfway between the mean of the fathers and the mean of the population (assuming

there was no assortative mating). In other words, the mean of the sons "regressed" from the mean of the fathers toward the mean of the population. Obviously the more environmental, nonfamilial variation there is the lower the correlation will be. Conversely, the less important environmental factors are (i.e., the higher the heritability), the closer to 0.5 will be the correlation between first-degree relatives. Note however that familial environmental factors will also increase the correlation between relatives. Some attempt to measure these can be made by comparing, for instance, similarities between pairs of unrelated children raised in institutions and raised in different foster homes, respectively, but the practical difficulties are great. Furthermore, it was postulated that the genes act additively; nonadditive interactions such as dominance or epistasis would modify the correlations in a complicated way. They will, for instance, lead to parent-child correlations being different from sib-sib correlations.

Finally, it should be emphasized that heritability estimates are made on specific populations in a specific range of environments and should not be extrapolated uncritically to other populations and environments. For instance, an estimate of heritability of skin color based on a Swedish population would be misleadingly low if applied to the population of the United States where there is much more genetic variation.

A variety of statistical techniques have been developed to estimate the various components of the variation in a trait from, for instance, comparisons between monozygotic and dizygotic twin pairs, twins reared together and reared apart, correlation between child and biologic parents and between child and foster-parents (see Jensen[8]). Estimates of heritability have been made for many quantitative human traits, but in most cases these should be regarded as no more than indications of whether the role of genes in determining the trait is relatively large or small.

THRESHOLD CHARACTERS

A number of relatively common defects and diseases that are clearly familial cannot be made to fit all the expectations for mendelian inheritance, in spite of enthusiastic attempts to do so, sometimes by statistical methods more vigorous than rigorous. It was first recognized by Wright[13] that the inheritance of a discontinuous character (polydactyly in the guinea pig) could be accounted for by multifactorial inheritance of a continuously distributed variable, with a **developmental threshold** separating the continuous distribution into two discontinuous segments—polydactylous and not-polydactylous. Gruneberg[6] showed that a number of discontinuous but seemingly nonmendelian traits in mice fitted this model and called them "quasi-continuous variants."

Developmental Thresholds. A well-documented example of a developmental threshold is cleft of the secondary palate. In order to close, the palatal shelves must reorient themselves from a vertical position on either side of the tongue to a horizontal plane above the tongue, where their medial edges meet and fuse. During the time of reorientation the head continues to grow, carrying the base of the shelves farther apart. If the shelves become horizontal late enough the head will be so big that they will be unable to meet and a cleft palate will result. The latest point in development when the shelves can reach the horizontal and still meet can be considered a threshold; all embryos in which the shelves become horizontal earlier than this will have normal palates, and all embryos in which the shelves become horizontal later than this will have cleft palates. Other thresholds may involve (1) other developmental asynchronies, such as neural tube closure; (2) physiologic characteristics, such as renal tubular reabsorption; or (3) mechanical relationships, such as the degree of occlusion of the pyloric canal necessary to cause the signs of pyloric stenosis or the pressure at which a blood vessel ruptures. To return

to the palate, the important point is that a continuous, multifactorial variable (stage at which self movement occurs) is separated into discontinuous parts (normal and cleft palate) by a threshold. If the continuous variable involves a postnatal process (e.g., blood pressure), it is possible to place any given individual on the distribution. For a prenatal process, it is possible to tell only whether or not the individual fell beyond the threshold.

However, it is possible to make some deductions about how such a trait will be distributed in the population and in the relatives of affected persons. Furthermore, for traits that fit the predictions, one can then estimate the heritability of the underlying variable from the observed frequencies in families.

Models of Quasi-continuous Inheritance. Several mathematical models have been proposed, from which estimates of heritability of liability to the disease can be calculated.

According to Falconers model,[4] the term **liability** represents the sum total of genetic and environmental influences that make an individual more or less likely to develop a disease. The liabilities of individuals in a population form a continuous, normally distributed variable. A person develops overt disease if his liability reaches a certain threshold.

In the case of cleft palate, for instance, many things influence the stage at which the shelves move to the horizontal—the intrinsic shelf force, tongue size, forward growth of the mandible, and so on—and each of these is influenced by genetic and environmental factors. This, then, is a multifactorial model. Figure 13-5 represents palate closure as a multifactorial threshold character. The stage at which the shelves reach the horizontal would represent the liability to cleft palate (the later the more liable) and the latest stage at which they can still bridge the gap would be the threshold. Note that genes and environmental factors can also influence the threshold, in

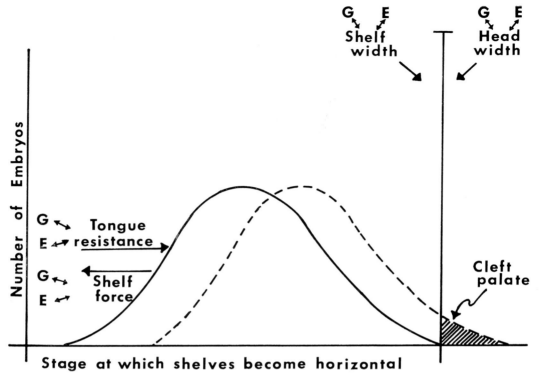

Figure 13-5. Diagram of factors influencing palate closure, illustrating its multifactorial threshold nature.

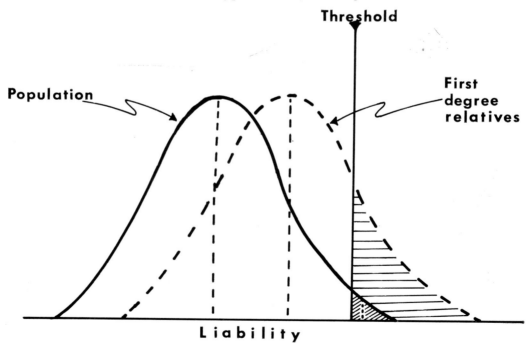

Figure 13-6. Hypothetic frequency distribution for a threshold character, showing the distribution of the population (solid line) and that of first-degree relatives (dotted line).

this case by altering the size of the gap through changes in shelf width and head width.

Figure 13-6 illustrates a population in which liability for a given disease is normally distributed (solid curve), and all individuals beyond a certain threshold (T) actually have the disease (diagonal hatching). Thus the affected individuals have a mean liability near the tail of the distribution. The usual family study ascertains a series of such individuals as probands and measures the frequency of affected individuals in the near relatives. What will the frequency be in the proband's sibs and children?

The dotted line in Figure 13-6 illustrates the distribution of liabilities for first-degree relatives, assuming that all the variation is genetic (a heritability of 1). By the law of filial regression it will have a mean halfway between the mean of the probands and the mean of the population, and the frequency of the disease will be higher than that in the general population (horizontal hatching). How much higher?

If liability is normally distributed, an estimate can be deduced from a property of the normal curve, which is that there is a fixed relationship between the distance from the mean (measured in standard deviations) and the number of individuals that lie under the curve beyond that distance. For instance, from the normal curve area table, we can see that if a threshold were set two standard deviations from the mean, 2.27% of individuals would lie beyond the threshold and be affected, and at three standard deviations from the mean 0.13% would be affected. Thus we can estimate, from the frequency in the population, how far the threshold is from the mean. For a frequency of one per 1,000 the table tells us that the threshold is 3.1 standard deviations from the mean. If we assume that all the variation is genetic, the mean of the distribution of liabilites for first-degree relatives should be intermediate between that of the affected probands (e.g., 3.3 standard

deviations) and that of the general population, or at about 1.65 standard deviations. If so we would expect (from the normal curve) that about 5% of the first-degree relatives would be affected. If the heritability is less than 1, the observed frequency in the relatives would be correspondingly lower, so it is possible to estimate the heritability by the difference between the observed figure and that expected if the heritability were 1. Mathematical details and appropriate tables can be found elsewhere.[4,11,12] It turns out that even for defects with a rather low recurrence risk the heritability can be quite high.

Edwards' model[2] assumes that the liability is continuously distributed and that the probability of being affected increases exponentially as the liability increases. This has some advantages, both conceptual and mathematical, over Falconer's model, but for practical purposes such as predicting recurrence risks, it does not seem any more useful. Finally, Morton[9] proposes a model in which the disease is determined by rare genes in a small number of cases and small effects of many genes in others, and shows that the three models predict about the same recurrence risks in conditions for which there is no evidence of recessive genes with major effects.

Family Features of Multifactorial Threshold Diseases. Nevertheless, there are features of the family distributions of certain common congenital malformations that are most easily explained by the multifactorial threshold model, as first pointed out by Carter for pyloric stenosis.[1] Some of the features are explained equally well by other models, but some are not.

Relation of Recurrence Risk to Population Frequency. With the aid of a number of reasonable mathematical approximations it has been shown that, for a threshold character with high heritability, the frequency of occurrence of the trait in first-degree relatives of affected individuals is approximately the square root of the frequency in the population.[2] This relation-

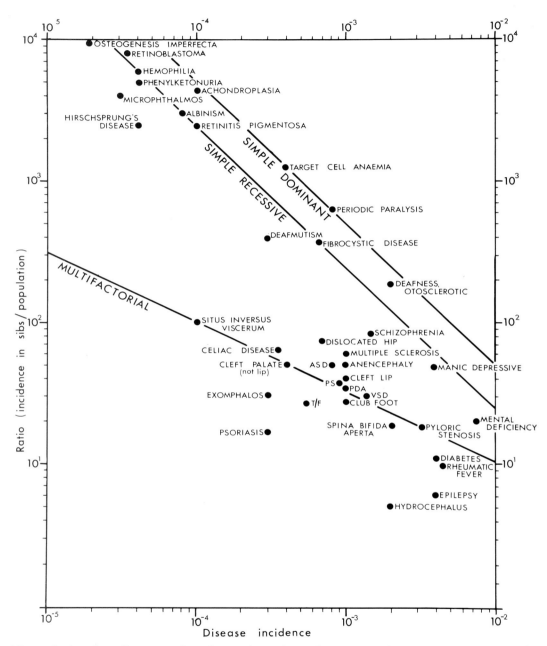

Figure 13-7. Chart illustrating the relation of population frequency to frequency in first-degree relatives for a multifactorial threshold character. (Modified from Newcombe, H. B., Second International Conference on Congenital Malformations. International Medical Congress, New York, 1964. p. 345.)

ship holds for a number of common congenital malformations and not for diseases known to show mendelian inheritance or diseases with a known major environmental component (Fig. 13-7), which suggests that the former are indeed multifactorially determined threshold characters.

Nonlinear Decrease in Frequency With Decreasing Relationship. We have already seen that the distribution of the underlying variable in first-degree relatives of affected individuals will have a mean halfway between the mean of the affected relatives and the mean of the population. For second-degree relatives the mean will be between the mean for the first-degree relatives and that of the population, and so on. Thus if the distance between the curve for the first-degree relatives and the curve for the population is 1, the distance for the second-degree relatives will be 1/2, and for the third-degree relatives 1/4, and so on. However, the proportion of affected relatives will be represented not by these ratios but by the area under the curve beyond the threshold for the respective distributions (Fig. 13-8). Since the tail of the curve becomes progressively flatter, the drop in frequency should be greater between first- and second-degree relatives (on the steep part of the curve) than that between second- and third-degree relatives (on the flatter

part of the curve). This has been shown for several common congenital malformations including pyloric stenosis, dislocation of the hip, talipes equinovarus and cleft lip ± cleft palate.[1] In the case of cleft lip, for instance, the frequency of the defect is about 40 per 1,000 for first-degree relatives, seven for second-degree relatives and three for third-degree relatives.

Increased Risk of Recurrence After Two Affected. As we have said, with threshold characters one cannot tell where a given individual is on the distribution of liability. However, parents who have an affected child must have contributed a relatively large number of genes for liability to the child and are therefore likely to be carrying more than the average number of such genes themselves. That is, they will tend to lie between the population mean and the threshold. Thus their future children will have a greater than average risk of being affected. If they do have a second affected child they can be assumed to carry still more predisposing genes and lie still closer to the threshold, so the recurrence risk will be even greater than it was after one affected and lie still closer to the threshold. This has been shown to be true for cleft lip and palate and for spina bifida aperta, where the recurrence risk after one affected child is about 4% and after two affected children, about 10%.

Increased Recurrence Risk With Increased Severity of Defect. It is reasonable to suppose that, for a threshold character, a person with a severe form of the defect would be nearer the tail of the distribution of liability than a person with a mild form. If so, the risk of recurrence should be higher in patients with the more severe defects. In the case of cleft lip, for instance, the recurrence risk is about 2.6% for probands with unilateral cleft lip and 5.6% for bilateral cleft lip and palate,[5] and for Hirschsprung's disease the risk of recurrence varies with the length of aganglionic segment. This feature does not require a threshold, but does suggest multifactorial inheritance.

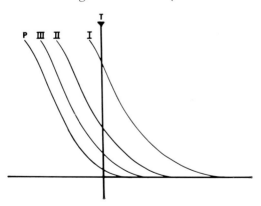

Figure 13-8. Relation of the tail of the frequency distribution to the threshold for the population (P) and the first (I), second (II), and third (III) degree relatives of affected individuals.

Recurrence Risk and Sex of Proband. In defects that occur more frequently in one sex than the other it must be assumed that the threshold is nearer the tail of the distribution in the sex less often affected. For instance, if the defect appears less often in females than males, females must have more genes for liability in order to fall beyond the threshold and be affected. If so, the recurrence risk should be higher for the relatives of female patients. This was first shown by Carter for congenital hypertrophic pyloric stenosis, which affects about five times as many males as females. In this case the risk is about 20% for sons of affected females as compared to 5% for sons of affected males. Similar though less striking differences occur in the case of cleft lip and palate and isolated cleft palate. In each case *the recurrence risk is higher when the proband is of the least frequently affected sex.*

CONCLUSION

These features suggest that a number of familial relatively common diseases and defects fit the multifactorial threshold model. Admittedly, it is difficult to distinguish critically between this model and that of Morton, in which there is a mixture of "sporadic" cases with low recurrence risk and a smaller number of cases with a strong genetic component. The nonlinear decrease in risk with decreasing relationship and the variation in recurrence risk with sex of proband (if there is a sex difference in frequency) are difficult to account for by Morton's model, but appropriate data are often not available. The difference is important. If Morton's model is correct, one should concentrate on attempting to identify the genetic cases by looking for biochemical differences. If the multifactorial threshold model is correct, there will be no major identifiable biochemical factor, and one might be better off to concentrate on identifying the underlying variable and its threshold. In any case one should resist the temptation to invoke the concept, as some have done, for familial conditions that have not

been tested by the above criteria. Neither should the term be used to refer to etiologic heterogeneity—that is, when different cases of the disease have different causes.

From a counseling point of view, it may be useful to develop with the parents of an affected child the idea of susceptibility being the result of the adding up of "a lot of little things," none of which is in itself abnormal, so that the parents should not feel guilty about having "bad genes" or having unknowingly exposed the baby to a prenatal insult.

What can be done to reduce the frequency of such conditions? One approach is to try to identify the individual components contributing to susceptibility, for instance, familial joint laxity with congenital hip dislocation, differences in face shape with cleft lip, or blood group O and nonsecretor status with duodenal ulcer. The more components that can be identified, the better the identification of susceptible individuals, although being a near relative of an affected person will probably be the best indicator for some time to come. The other approach stems from the observation that multifactorial threshold characters often vary in frequency with season of birth, socioeconomic class, geographic region and other environmental differences. This shows that extrinsic factors may shift the relationship of underlying distribution and threshold; we must now learn to identify these factors. The preventive approach would then be to protect genetically susceptible individuals from all possible precipitating factors.

REFERENCES

1. Carter, C. O.: Genetics of common disorders. Brit. Med. Bull., 25:52, 1969.
2. Edwards, J. H.: Familial predispositions in man. Brit. Med. Bull., 25:58, 1969.
3. Falconer, D. S.: Introduction to Quantitative Genetics. Edinburgh, Oliver and Boyd, 1960.
4. ———: The inheritance of liability to diseases with variable age of onset, with particular reference to diabetes mellitus. Ann. Hum. Genet., 31:1, 1967.
5. Fraser, F. C.: The genetics of cleft lip and

cleft palate. Amer. J. Hum. Genet., 22:336, 1970.

6. Gruneberg, H.: Genetical studies on the skeleton of the mouse. IV. Quasi-continuous variations. J. Genet., 51:95, 1952.

7. Harris, H.: The Principles of Human Biochemical Genetics. Neuberger, A., and Tatum, E. L. (eds.): Frontiers of Biology. Vol. 19. New York, American Elsevier, 1970.

8. Jensen, A. R.: How much can we boost IQ and scholastic achievement? Harvard Educ. Rev., 39:1, 1969.

9. Morton, N. E., Yee, S., Elston, R. C., and Lew, R.: Discontinuity and quasi-continuity:

alternative hypotheses of multifactorial inheritance. Clin. Genet., 1:81, 1970.

10. Price Evans, D. A., Manley, K. A., and McKusick, V. A.: Genetic control of isoniazid metabolism in man. Brit. Med. J., 2:485, 1960.

11. Smith, C.: Discriminating between different modes of inheritance in genetic disease. Clin. Genet., 2:303, 1971a.

12. ———: Recurrence risks for multifactorial inheritance. Amer. J. Hum. Genet., 23:578, 1971b.

13. Wright, S.: An analysis of variability in number of digits in an inbred strain of guinea pigs. Genetics, 19:506, 1934.

Chapter 14

MALFORMATIONS AND DISEASES DETERMINED BY MULTIFACTORIAL INHERITANCE

All interest in disease and death is only another expression of interest in life.

Thomas Mann

A frequently accepted point of division between common and uncommon diseases is a population frequency of one in 1,000. Among the genetically determined disorders, multifactorial diseases are, in general, common and diseases caused by mutant genes are uncommon. Diseases in the third major category of genetic diseases, chromosomal anomalies, fall on either side of this division. There is an increasing number of disease entities for which there is data consistent with multifactorial inheritance; a selection of these will be presented in this chapter. Certain other diseases conforming to multifactorial inheritance are discussed in their appropriate chapters (e.g., Chapter 23).

The genetic counseling of families having diseases determined by multifactorial inheritance may be more difficult than for single mutant gene disorders, since the risks given are usually average risks rather than precise probabilities. Empiric recurrence risks are becoming increasingly available, but are often incomplete for a given disease even if the multifactorial etiology is reasonably well established. For example, although recurrence risks after one affected first-degree relative may be known, the recurrence risk after two or three affected first-degree relatives may not be established. Under these circumstances, it is reasonable to apply generalizations from experience with multifactorial diseases in which such empiric risks have been established to multifactorial diseases for which there are no established risks. Smith[15] provides a useful theoretic model for calculating such risks (Table 14-1).

From the theoretic model and from experience with cleft lip and palate, spina bifida/anencephaly and some congenital

TABLE 14-1. Recurrence Risks (%) for Multifactorial Diseases According to Number of Affected First-degree Relatives and Heritability

Population Frequency (%)	Heritability (%)	Affected Parents 0			Affected Parents 1			Affected Parents 2		
		Affected Sibs 0	1	2	Affected Sibs 0	1	2	Affected Sibs 0	1	2
1.0	100	1	7	14	11	24	34	63	65	67
	80	1	6	14	8	18	28	41	47	52
	50	1	4	8	4	9	15	15	21	26
0.1	100	0.1	4	11	5	16	26	62	63	64
	80	0.1	3	10	4	14	23	60	61	62
	50	0.1	1	3	1	3	7	7	11	15

This table, adapted from Smith,[15] provides theoretic recurrence risks for a multifactorial threshold character. It can be used as a guide when no empiric figures are available. For instance, to estimate the risk for the next child of diabetic parents who have a diabetic child, the frequency is close to 1%, heritability is, say, 80%, so the risk would be about 47%. For a parent with cleft lip and palate who has two affected children the frequency is about 0.1, the heritability is 80%, and the risk would be about 23%. The risk decreases with each unaffected child, but not very much.

heart lesions, the recurrence following the birth of two affected first-degree relatives would be two to three times greater than that after one. Beyond two affected first-degree relatives there are little data for any diseases, but the experience with some congenital heart lesions suggests that the risk becomes quite high and the predictions may well be based on the frequency already appearing in such a family. (See Capter 23, type C families with congenital heart defects.)

Clinical Example. This couple appeared for genetic counseling because their second-born child, an eight-month-old boy, had spina bifida, meningomyelocele and hydrocephalus. The baby had paraplegia and an expanding head size despite surgical intervention with a shunting procedure. The couple also had a normal three-year-old daughter. They were aware that their infant son would not survive much longer and hoped to have another child, yet they felt they could not readily withstand the emotional and financial stress of having another child with spina bifida.

No other child on either side of the family was known to have spina bifida (Fig. 14-1). There was a first cousin with cleft lip and palate and an aunt who was a "blue

baby" and was considered to have had a congenital heart lesion, but there was no autopsy performed to confirm this clinical suspicion. This family, which had moved to our city recently from Boston, was third-generation Irish-American.

The mother had a "virus" during the second month of her pregnancy and took dextroamphetamine to "initiate a diet," also during the second month. This young woman was slightly overweight and admitted that two or three times a year she had to diet for a week or so and always got her diet off to a successful start with three or four days of dextroamphetamine.

In counseling, we usually discuss in some detail the background information we have on diseases like the spina bifida-anencephaly complex—the hereditary predisposition and the environmental triggers. Our major source of data is the extensive work of Carter and his associates. We began by discussing the hereditary predisposition in this Irish family, which was interesting in that there had been no outbreeding with other Boston populations. There is evidence to suggest increased genetic liability in those of wholly Irish ancestry, whether they remain in Ireland or move to Boston. With outbreeding the predisposition seems to

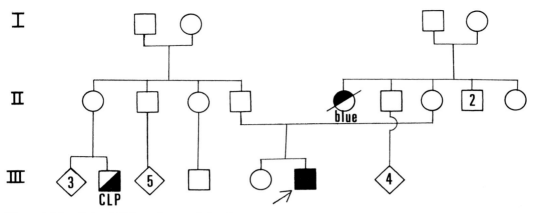

Figure 14-1. Spina bifida pedigree of family in case history.

diminish. This is not to cast aspersions on the Irish; it is only a way of making the point about the genetic predisposition to the lesion.

We then discussed the possible environmental triggers and mentioned that "clusters" of spina bifida cases have been reported on a number of occasions. This may mean, although there is no proof, that certain viruses may act as environmental triggers on individuals with hereditary predisposition to spina bifida. We also discussed what is known or suspected about dextroamphetamine—the suspicion of some investigators that dextroamphetamine may be implicated in some cases of spina bifida in the human, and our own experience with this drug in the production of exencephaly in the mouse. Again we emphasized that we were discussing suspicions, not proof.

We told the parents that the risk of having another child with spina bifida was of the order of 5%. To some families this is considered an enormous risk and not worth undertaking. Other families think of this as quite a small risk, as did this family. The couple expressed a desire to consider a future pregnancy. Because they had been reading about amniocentesis they wondered whether this technique could be used to identify spina bifida in utero. We explained that it could not, although radiologic or ultrasound visualization might detect the

more severe forms of the condition. We had no trouble in convincing the mother of the inadvisability of dextroamphetamine ingestion during pregnancy (or for that matter any other time). We told her that although we could not assure her that avoidance of dextroamphetamine would reduce the recurrence risk below 5%, we felt that it would be prudent to eliminate as many potential environmental triggers as possible.

The affected child in this family died of sepsis at 14 months of age, when the mother was three months pregnant. She eventually delivered a normal eight pound baby boy.

ANENCEPHALY-SPINA BIFIDA

These disorders are generally accepted as related. It is not necessary to discuss the anatomic defects in detail. Spina bifida is a failure of fusion of spinal lamina, most often in the lumbar region. In **spina bifida occulta** the defect is limited to the bony arch. In **spina bifida aperta** the bony defect is accompanied by meningocele or meningomyelocele; hydrocephalus may also occur, with an associated Arnold-Chiari malformation. This has led to some confusion in family studies reported in the literature, through a tendency to combine family data from cases of isolated hydrocephalus and hydrocephalus with spina bifida. Hydrocephalus associated with spina bifida should

TABLE 14-2.   Recurrence Risks for Sibs of Children with Various Multifactorially Inherited Malformations

	Sex of Proband	Sex of Sib	Anencephaly*	Spina Bifida*	Cleft Lip ± Palate	Cleft Palate	Talipes Equinovarus	Dislocated Hip† Neonatal Diagnosis in Proband	Dislocated Hip† Late Diagnosis in Proband	Hirschsprung Disease	Legg-Perthes Disease	Pyloric Stenosis
Population frequency /1000			0.2-5	0.2-4	1	0.4	1.2	4	1	0.2	7‡	3
Sex ratio M:F			0.6	0.8	1.6	0.7	2.0	3.1	1.5	3.7	5.2	5
% risk for sib after one affected — sib—parents normal	male	male	1.9	5.1	3.9	6.3	2.0	6(0)	0	2.6	5.9	5
	male	female						20(16)	9(7)		1.4	2.5
	female	male	6.5	7.2	5.0	2.3	6.0	—	2(1)	7.2	7.3	18
	female	female						26(9)	8(5)		1.6	
	either	either	4.1	6.1	4.3	2.9	2.9	14(6)	5(3)	3.6	3.8	8
% risk for sib after two affected — sibs—parents normal				10	9							

Risks for offspring are expected to be and (where measured) are of similar magnitude.

*Risk for either anencephaly or spina bifida.

†Risk for late diagnosis dislocation is given in parentheses.

‡Attack rate to age 15.

be considered a secondary manifestation of the spinal defect; hydrocephalus without spina bifida should be considered separately. **Anencephaly** is an absence of skin, skull, overlying membranes, forebrain and midbrain, which produces stillbirth or death shortly after birth. Embryologically and genetically, spina bifida aperta and anencephaly appear to be variations of the same basic defect.

The usual findings in patients with spina bifida with meningomyelocele are paresis of the lower extremities and urinary and fecal incontinence. Progressive hydrocephalus may be arrested by neurosurgical intervention, but the course has usually been one of progressive deterioration with an infection often being the terminal event. Recent improvements in surgical management are improving the outlook, however.

The population frequency of this group of disorders is variable. The incidence is high in Ireland, Wales, Alexandria and Bombay, and low in Mongolians and Africans in the Sahara. The population frequency ranges from a low of about two per thousand for all lesions in the spina bifida-anencephaly group to a high of over 1% in Ireland. An intermediate figure would represent the frequency in North America (five per thousand is the approximation we currently use).

A recurrence risk of 3 to 6% in first-degree relatives has been derived from a number of European and North American studies.[9] Whether the proband has anencephaly or spina bifida aperta, the sibs are at risk for either one or the other or both. The frequency in first-degree relatives is about seven times the population frequency and the recurrence risk after two affected first-degree relatives is about 10% (Table 14-2).

The sex ratio in this group of lesions reveals an excess of females: the male/female ratio being 0.89 for spina bifida and 0.34 for anencephaly. There is also a small excess of first-born infants and infants in which the maternal age exceeds 40 years.

That environmental triggers are probably involved in the production of these lesions was suggested in the preceding case presentation. The striking variations with season of birth, socioeconomic class, geographic region and from year to year certainly suggest environmental factors. However, there is no convincing evidence yet that specific teratogens play major etiologic roles in this group of malformations, although potato blight has recently been suggested as an etiologic consideration.

CLEFT LIP AND CLEFT PALATE (FIG. 14-2)

The evidence that congenital clefts of the primary and secondary palate are multifactorially determined threshold characters has been discussed in Chapter 13. The secondary palate closes later in development than the primary palate, which forms the gum and lip, and the genetic and environmental factors that influence its closure are different from those that influence closure of the primary palate. On the other hand, abnormal development of the primary palate, leading to a cleft lip, may interfere secondarily with secondary palate closure. Thus, on both embryologic and genetic grounds, congenital cleft lip (CL) and cleft lip with cleft palate (CLP) appear to be etiologically related [in data

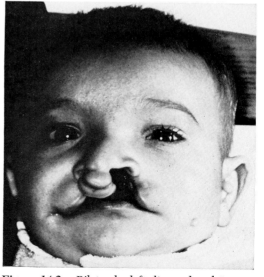

Figure 14-2. Bilateral cleft lip and palate.

combining the two they may be designated CL(P)]. Isolated cleft of the secondary palate (CP) is an etiologically independent entity.

There are a large number of syndromes in which CL(P) or CP may be one of the features. For most of these the cause is unidentified, a few are associated with recognizable chromosomal aberrations, and about a third are caused by major mutant genes. Each of these syndromes is rare, and together they may account for perhaps 5% of all cases, most of the rest being multifactorially determined. For counseling it is important to distinguish cases associated with syndromes from the multifactorial type, as the recurrence risks are different. Inclusion of unrecognized cases of syndromes in family studies may account for the fact that the recurrence risk for sibs of patients with CL(P) is reduced from 4% to 2% if the proband has an additional malformation.

Table 14-3 lists a number of inherited syndromes in which cleft lip ± cleft palate, or cleft palate are a feature.[7] Oddly enough, some genes will cause cleft lip and palate in some individuals and cleft palate in others. The embryologic basis remains obscure.

Cleft Lip With or Without Cleft Palate —CL(P). Most cases of CL(P) or CP without associated malformations appear to be multifactorially determined, although even in this group there is almost certainly genetic heterogeneity.[5] More males than females are affected with CL(P). There are striking differences in frequency between races: Orientals have relatively high frequencies (1.7/1,000 births), Caucasians are intermediate (1/1,000) and Africans tend to have low frequencies (0.4/1,000). These differences persist in different geographic regions, suggesting that they do not result from environmental alterations, and we find it tempting to think that they may be associated with differences in face shape.[6]

As expected for multifactorial traits, the risk for relatives of affected persons drops off sharply from first- to second-degree relatives. Thus it is about 4% for sibs and children, 0.7% for uncles, aunts, nephews and nieces, and 0.4% for first cousins. Occasionally these figures are useful for counseling; for instance, the sib of a person with CLP can be advised that the chance of having an affected child is about 0.7% or one in 140.

The recurrence risk is somewhat higher in the sibs of female probands (5.0%) than of male probands (3.9%), in the sibs of patients with a severe defect than in those with a mild form (5.6% when the proband has a bilateral cleft lip and palate, but 2.6% when the proband has a unilateral cleft lip only), and after two affected sibs (9.0%) than after one (4%) (Table 14-2). There are little data on the risk for sibs of an affected child with an affected parent. The available figures suggest a figure of about 15%, but the numbers are small.

Experimental findings in the mouse predict that the shape of the embryonic face influences the predisposition to cleft lip. If so, one should be able to detect indications of these differences in the near relatives. Preliminary evidence suggests that this is so; parents of children with CLP tend to have less prominent maxillae, an increased bizygomatic diameter and more rectangular or trapezoid-shaped faces than controls.[6]

In spite of many attempts to demonstrate environmental factors associated with CL(P), no association has been convincingly demonstrated between CL(P) incidence and such things as seasonal trend, geographic location (except when there are differences in racial groups), social class, maternal age or parity, or paternal age. A number of prenatal factors have been tentatively implicated, such as pernicious vomiting of pregnancy, antiemetics and other drugs (antiepileptic drugs are currently under suspicion), maternal bleeding, toxemia of pregnancy, and toxoplasma, but none are firmly supported.

Cleft Palate (CP). Isolated cleft palate

TABLE 14-3. Syndromes Involving Cleft Lip (CL), Cleft Lip and Palate (CLP), or Cleft Palate (CP)*

I.   *Autosomal Dominant Syndromes:*
   1. Acrocephalosyndactyly (Apert syndrome)
   2. Ankyloblepharon filiforme adnatum with CL and/or CP
   3. Arachnodactyly of Marfan and CP
   4. Clubfoot, camptodactyly and CP
   5. Deafness, white forelock, dystopia canthorum (Waardenburg syndrome) and CL, CLP or CP
   6. Ectodermal defects (thin wiry hair, hypohidrosis, nail dystrophy) and CLP
   7. Lip-pits with CL, CLP or CP
   8. Lobster-claw defect, dacrocystitis, hypodontia (EEC syndrome)
   9. Mandibulofacial dysostosis and CP
  10. Myopia, retinal detachment, joint disease and CP (Stickler syndrome)
  11. Neuroblastoma with CL, CLP or CP
  12. Nevoid basal cell carcinoma, multiple, with CL, CLP or CP
  13. Popliteal pterygium syndrome with CL, CLP or CP
  14. Spondyloepiphyseal dysplasia, congenital, with CP

II. *Autosomal Recessive Syndromes:*
   1. Chondrodystrophia calcificans congenita with CP
   2. Cryptophthalmia with CL, CLP or CP
   3. Diastrophic dwarfism with CP
   4. Multiple dislocations with CP (Larsen syndrome)
   5. Microtia, ocular hypertelorism with CLP
   6. Orofaciodigital syndrome II, with CP (Mohr syndrome)
   7. Phocomelia, penile or clitoral enlargement, with CLP
   8. Polycystic kidneys, exencephalocele, polydactyly, microcephaly, microphthalmia, etc., with CL, CLP or CP (Meckel syndrome)
   9. Pterygium, multiple, with CP
  10. Radial and ulnar deficiency, joint contractures, cloudy cornea, etc., with CLP
  11. Smith-Lemli-Opitz syndrome, with CP

III. *X-linked Syndromes:*
   1. Micrognathia, clubfoot, atrial septal defect, persistent left superior vena cava, with CP
   2. Orofacial digital syndrome I with CL (median), CP
   3. Otopalatodigital syndrome

IV. *Syndromes of Unclear or Nongenetic Etiology:*
   1. Anencephaly with CL, CLP or CP
   2. Buccopharyngeal membrane with CP
   3. Heart defect, congenital, with CL, CLP or CP (miscellaneous)
   4. Constrictions, ring, of limbs, with CLP
   5. de Lange syndrome with CP
   6. Encephalomeningocele with CL, CLP or CP
   7. Forearm bone aplasia, other malformations, with CLP
   8. Frontonasal dysplasia (median cleft face) with CL, CLP or CP
   9. Glossopalatine ankylosis with CP
  10. Holoprosencephaly with CL or CLP
  11. Robin syndrome
  12. Proboscis, lateral, with CLP
  13. Teratoma, oral, with CP

V.   *Chromosomal Syndromes:*
   1. 4p—
   2. 5p—
   3. Trisomy C mosaicism
   4. Trisomy 13, 18, 21
   5. Dp—
   6. 14q—
   7. 18p—
   8. 18q—
   9. XXXXY syndrome
  10. Monosomy G
  11. Triploidy

* Modified from Gorlin, R. J., Cervenka, J., and Pruzansky, S.: Facial clefting and its syndromes. Birth Defects: Original Article Series, 7:3, 1971. New York, The National Foundation.

is rarer than CL(P), with an average frequency in Caucasians of about 0.45 per 1,000 births. More females than males are affected. There is little, if any, racial variation. The frequency appears somewhat higher than average in older mothers of high parity and (for those with associated malformations) with increasing parental age.

Where available, the recurrence risks for CP are similar to those for CL(P) except that the risk is higher for sibs of male probands (6.3%) than for sibs of female probands (2.3%), as expected for a multifactorial threshold character (Table 14-2). The rather low rate in MZ co-twins (23.5% vs. 10% in DZ co-twins) suggests that the environmental contribution to causation is larger than it is for CL(P).

CONGENITAL DISLOCATION OF THE HIP (CDH) (FIG. 14-3)

It is difficult to establish reliable figures for the prevalence of this defect either in populations or families because of variations in diagnostic efficiency. A recent survey by Wynne-Davies[17] provides the most appropriate information. Subluxation and dislocation of the hip may be demonstrated by appropriate examination in the first few

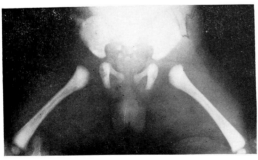

Figure 14-3. Bilateral congenital dislocation of hips.

days of life (the **neonatal diagnosis group**). An unknown fraction of these cases, if untreated, would go on to frank dislocation at the time of weight-bearing, and the rest would correct themselves spontaneously.

Those diagnosed only after the first few weeks are referred to as the **late diagnosis group**. The more effectively patients are diagnosed in the neonatal period, fewer cases will appear in the late diagnosis group. Effective neonatal screening has been introduced only recently, and family data will include varying proportions of the two types, depending on the age group involved. The following discussion presents figures for the neonatal diagnosis group with corresponding figures for the late diagnosis group in parentheses. The true figure lies somewhere in between. Further details may be found in Table 14-2.

For probands with early diagnosis CDH and normal parents, the risk is about 3% (1%) for brothers and 24% (11%) for sisters, or a risk for all sibs of 13% (6%)—a strong indication for careful screening at birth. No data are available for offspring in this group. For probands with late diagnosis CDH and normal parents, the risk is about 2% (1%) for brothers and 8% (5%) for sisters, or an overall sib risk of 5% (3%). For children of CDH patients, the risk is about 6% (−) for sons and 17% (4%) for daughters, or an overall risk of 12% (2%) for all children.

The data are consistent with a multifactorial etiology. Susceptibility varies with the degree of acetabular dysplasia, which appears to be polygenically inherited, and with the degree of laxity of the joint capsule. Thus a dominantly inherited joint laxity is frequently found in the families of patients with CDH, particularly in the neonatal diagnosis group. A number of associations with environmental factors have also been identified. There is an excess of first-born children and of breech births. CDH occurs more often in babies born in the winter than summer months (perhaps because tight swaddling may elicit frank disease in a predisposed baby) and also (at least in Edinburgh) in the upper socioeconomic groups.

Closed reduction and immobilization in a hip spica cast is recommended, but the success of this treatment depends on early diagnosis and prompt therapy.

DIABETES MELLITUS

It is becoming increasingly apparent that diabetes mellitus fulfills the expectations for multifactorial inheritance.[10] A development of this point of view and equal time for contrary opinions will not be provided here. The condition is undoubtedly heterogeneous, and recurrence risk estimates vary widely from study to study, depending, no doubt, on the degree of bias in ascertaining families, the diagnostic criteria used, and the statistical methodology. Since the most relevant event in counseling situations is usually the advent of juvenile diabetes, figures will be given for onset before age 20. It is clear that the risk in near relatives is greater if the proband has juvenile rather than late-onset diabetes, and the risk increases with the number of affected relatives. No doubt the risk will also vary with the diet and other environmental factors. The following estimates are presented as rough guides to the counselor.

The frequency of diabetes in the general population is about 0.15% for individuals less than 20 years old, 0.6% for those under 40, 2.25% for those under 60 and 6% for those under 80. For normal parents, the sibs of an early-onset (under 20) diabetic themselves having early-onset diabetes is about 2 to 5%, and would be expected to double for sibs of two affected children.

The risk of a child having early-onset diabetes is about 10% if one parent has early-onset diabetes and about 6% if a parent has late-onset diabetes. For an affected parent and child the risk for subsequent sibs should be higher than this, perhaps double, but there are very little data.

Information on offspring of two diabetic parents is also sparse, and estimates range from 20% to 70% or more. In any case it seems well below the figure (close to 100%) expected on the basis of recessive inheritance postulated by some workers.

So far there is no reliable test for detecting those individuals who will later develop diabetes, though the presence of an insulin antagonist in the plasma albumin, and/or impaired glucose tolerance curve with or without previous glucocorticoid "stress" can be demonstrated in near relatives more often than in the general population. There is undoubtedly genetic heterogeneity.

EPILEPSY, GENERALIZED[1,10]

This textbook began with a quotation of Hippocrates on the subject of the heritability of epilepsy. It is therefore appropriate to include a discussion (however brief) of current thinking about the genetics of epilepsy. There has been some progress in our understanding of the hereditary aspects of this disease since the time of Hippocrates, but less than one would hope to find over a period of 2500 years.

Most workers put epilepsy in the multifactorial inheritance category, although a minority of investigators favor mendelian inheritance. One must be cautious about discussing epilepsy in broad terms and should speak of specific types of epilepsy. This discussion is limited to the most common forms of epilepsy, often categorized as generalized epilepsy. Within this grouping there is room for mendelian types, but mendelian interpretations have been offered to encompass the entire category. A certain amount of debate cannot be avoided, especially with respect to the clinical features one will accept as diagnostic of epilepsy (seizures? abnormal electroencephalogram?).

Recent twin studies having careful documentation of zygosity have not been found, but a high concordance rate among presumed monozygotic twins and a low concordance rate among dizygotic twins have been reported.

Apart from convulsions associated with diseases of known mendelian causation, the only category of the epilepsies for which there are reasonably reliable figures on recurrence risk is that of subcortical or centrencephalic epilepsy. Even here the problem is complicated by variable age of onset and the fact that the characteristic EEG abnormality, which may be the only indication of predisposition, may disappear with increasing age. The following figures, taken from the studies of Metrakos and Metrakos,[10] may provide a rough guide for counseling. A child who has a parent or sib with centrencephalic epilepsy has a basic risk of about 8% of being similarly affected. This is increased to 10% if the onset in the relative occurs before 2½ years of age. If both a parent and sib are affected the risk for a sib is about 13%. The risk decreases the longer the child remains free of seizures and if the EEG is negative after five years of age.

HIRSCHSPRUNG DISEASE (CONGENITAL AGANGLIONIC MEGACOLON)

This disorder, with a population frequency of about one in 5000 and an M:F sex ratio of about 6 to 1, recurs in approximately 3.5% of sibs. If the proband is male, the recurrence risk is 2.6%; if the proband is female, the recurrence risk is 7.2%.[12] The hereditary predisposition is clearly consistent with multifactorial inheritance. The clinical picture varies from severe constipation to acute obstruction of the bowel. Roentgenographic study reveals a dilated and hypertrophied colon proximal to a narrowed segment that lacks normal ganglion cells in Auerbach's plexus (Fig. 14-4).

LEGG-PERTHES DISEASE

This disease, aseptic necrosis of the capital femoral epiphysis, has recently joined the group of multifactorial threshold diseases.[8] It occurs five times as often in males as in females. The annual incidence in children under 15 years is at least 3.1 per 100,000, with an attack rate of 1:1,400. As expected for a multifactorial threshold character with a high sex ratio, the recurrence rate is higher for sibs of female probands (7.3% for brothers, 1.6% for sisters) than for sibs of male probands (5.9%, 1.4%), though the difference is not significant and not as striking as in pyloric stenosis. The frequency is 1:26 for siblings, 1:340 in second-degree relatives, and 1:350 for third-degree relatives. Finally, the square root of the population frequency is 2.6%, reasonably close to the sib frequency of 3.8%.

MENTAL RETARDATION[13]

The distribution of "intelligence" in the general population is more or less normally distributed as one would expect for a character with a polygenic hereditary component influenced by a number of subtle environmental factors. Thus if one arbitrarily decides that anyone with an I.Q. of less than 70 is retarded, some individuals will be retarded simply because they received an assortment of genetic and environmental factors, each detracting a small amount from the level of intelligence, that placed them in the lower tail of the normal distribution without any one of these factors being in itself abnormal. In addition a child

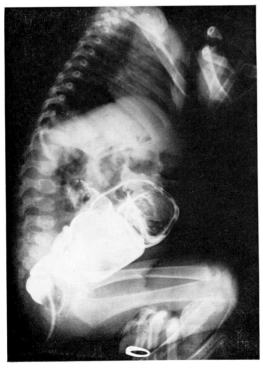

Figure 14-4. Grossly dilated bowel proximal to aganglionic segment in Hirschsprung disease.

may be retarded because of a major insult to the brain, which may result from a chromosomal anomaly, an inborn metabolic error, or an environmental cause such as birth trauma, prenatal viral damage or postnatal meningitis. These cases, which are relatively rare, form a small hump near the lower tail of the distribution of intelligence; i.e., the curve is "skewed to the left."

Thus the causes of mental retardation fall into the same four categories as do congenital cleft lip, heart malformations and other common, familial disorders: those due to major mutant genes, to chromosomal aberrations, to major environmental insults and to a multifactorial etiology. As one might expect, children with specific causes of mental retardation, as in the first three groups, tend to be more severely retarded than those in the multifactorial group, since the damage in the former groups results from an insult that is likely to be major. Also consistent with this concept is the following seemingly paradoxic fact: The intelligence of the near relatives of children with specific and therefore severe types of retardation (excluding those similarly affected) is like that of the general population, whereas the intelligence of near relatives of children with nonspecific and therefore milder mental retardation tends to be lower than average.

When dealing with a case of mental retardation, the genetic counselor first strives to place the child in one of the four etiologic categories by a thorough family prenatal and perinatal history, physical examination, and appropriate chromosomal and biochemical screening. If a specific cause is found, counseling is based on the appropriate estimate of recurrence risk. If no specific cause can be found, the child is assumed, by exclusion, to fall in the multifactorial group. On the average, then, the intelligence of the sibs will be midway between that of the two parents. The empiric risks presented in Table 14-4 taken from the large study of Reed and Reed[13] will serve as a rough guide in the appropriate family situation.

The growing evidence for an X-linked nonspecific type of mental retardation, based on an excess of brother-brother pairs in sibs with mental retardation, would suggest a somewhat higher risk if the proband is a boy, particularly if the family history suggests a sex-linked recessive pattern.[16]

THE MAJOR PSYCHOSES

The genetics of the major psychoses is too vast a subject to be dealt with adequately here. There is strong evidence for a genetic basis for susceptibility, particularly in the case of schizophrenia; concordance rates are much higher for monozygotic than for dizygotic twins, and there is an increased frequency in children of schizophrenic parents reared in adoptive or foster homes. The population frequency of schizophrenia is about 1%, and the risk for the sib or child of a schizophrenic developing the disease is estimated in various studies as about 10%. For the offspring of two affected parents estimates vary from 30 to 70%, in the same range as the risk for monozygotic co-twins. The figures are considerably higher if "schizoid" relatives are included. Whether these figures are interpreted as reflecting polygenic inheritance or an autosomal dominant gene with modifiers is a question that may be solved only when (and if) the genetic predisposition is defined in biochemical terms. Childhood autism seems to have a low recurrence risk and does not behave genetically as a form of schizophrenia.

TABLE 14-4. Risk of Mental Retardation in Children and Sibs of Retardates*

Number of Retarded:			
Parents	Children	Risk for	Risk (%)
0	—	child	1
1	—	child	11
2	—	child	40
0	1	sib	6
1	1	sib	20
2	1	sib	42

*I.Q. less than 70.

For the affective psychoses the picture is also unclear, though most studies report higher recurrence risks than for schizophrenia, approaching the expectation for a dominant major gene in some studies. On the average, for probands with cyclic depression the risk for parents and sibs has been estimated as about 20%, and for recurrent depression about 13%. For a recent review of this confused and confusing subject, consult Erlenmeyer-Kimling[4] and Rosenthal.[14]

PYLORIC STENOSIS[3] (FIG. 14-5)

This, the first of the multifactorial threshold characters, is a disorder in which projectile vomiting, undernutrition, dehydration and electrolyte imbalance result from a muscular hypertrophy of the pylorus. A Rammstedt procedure, incising the hypertrophied pyloric muscle, permanently relieves the condition. The frequency in North American and European populations is about three per thousand.

The M:F sex ratio is 5:1. Carter's observation that the recurrence risks are much higher to the first-degree relatives of affected females than to the first-degree relatives of affected males was the clue to its multifactorial threshold nature. As discussed in the preceding chapter, if a disease is found more frequently in one sex (in this case males), then individuals of the other sex (females) require a greater genetic predisposition in order to develop the disease, since they are, on the average, farther from the threshold. If a greater number of "liability genes" are required for the disease to become manifest in the female, it follows that her first-degree relatives would also have greater genetic liability and a higher frequency of the disorder than the first-degree relatives of a male patient, with less genetic predisposition.

While the overall recurrence risk to first-degree relatives of patients with pyloric stenosis is about 6%, it is preferable to use the more specific risks as shown in Table 14-2, which take into account the greater genetic liability of affected females. Empiric risk figures after two affected first-degree relatives are not available, but one would predict a two- to threefold increase in risk.

TALIPES EQUINOVARUS (CLUBFOOT)[18]

There is more than one type of "clubfoot," but the most common type is talipes equinovarus, in which there is plantar flexion and adduction at the midtarsal joint, the forefoot is supinated and the heel is inverted. There may be associated malformations such as generalized joint laxity (10%), inguinal hernia (7% of affected boys), and minor deformities of the extremities (4 to 5%). About one to two infants per thousand live births have this anomaly and twice as many males as females are affected. If postural talipes equinovarus, talipes calcaneovalgus and metatarsus varus are included,

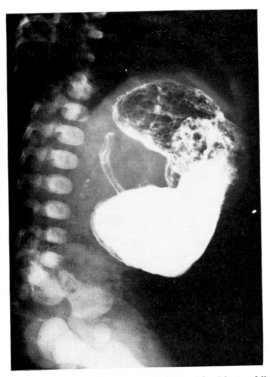

Figure 14-5. Pyloric stenosis. Note "double track" sign revealed by upper G.I. series.

the prevalence increases to four per thousand live births.

The recurrence risk is 2.9% in first-degree relatives or 24 times the frequency in the general population. As expected for a multifactorial threshold character, the recurrence risk for talipes calcaneovarus appears higher for the sibs of female probands (6%) than for the sibs of male probands (2%). There is an additional risk for sibs of about 1% for having metatarsus varus, suggesting a common factor in the etiology of these conditions. (Similarly, for the sibs of patients with metatarsus varus, there is about a 4% risk of metatarsus varus and an additional 2.5% risk for talipes equinovarus.) Patients with talipes equinovarus and talipes calcaneovarus have a somewhat increased frequency of congenital dislocation of the hip, possibly because familial joint laxity predisposes to all three conditions.

REFERENCES

1. Beaussart, M., and Luiseau, P.: Hereditary factors in a random population of 5200 epileptics. Epilepsia, 10:55, 1969.
2. Carter, C. O.: Multifactorial inheritance revisited. *In* Fraser, F. C., and McKusick, V. A. (eds.): Congenital Malformations. New York, Excerpta Medica, 1970. p. 227.
3. Carter, C. O., and Evans, K. A.: Inheritance of congenital pyloric stenosis. J. Med. Genet., 6:233, 1969.
4. Erlenmeyer-Kimling, L. (Ed.): Genetics and mental disorders. Int. J. Mental Health, 1:8, 1972.
5. Fraser, F. C.: The genetics of cleft lip and cleft palate. Amer. J. Hum. Genet., 22:336, 1970.
6. Fraser, F. C., and Pashayan, H.: Relation of face shape to susceptibility to congenital cleft lip. A preliminary report. J. Med. Genet., 7:112, 1970.
7. Gorlin, R. J., Cervenka, J., and Pruzansky, S.: Facial clefting and its syndromes. Birth Defects: Original Article Series, 7:3, 1971. New York, The National Foundation.
8. Grey, I. M., Lowry, R. B., and Renwick, D. H. G.: Incidence and genetics of Legg-Perthe's disease (osteochondritis deformans) in British Columbia. Evidence of polygenic determination. J. Med. Genet., 9:197, 1973.
9. Laurence, K. M.: The recurrence risk in spina bifida cystica and anencephaly. Develop. Med. Child Neurol., 20(Supp. 1):23, 1969.
10. Metrakos, J. D., and Metrakos, K.: Childhood epilepsy of subcortical ("centrencephalic") origin. Clin. Pediat. 5:536, 1966.
11. Neel, J. V.: Current concepts of the genetic basis of diabetes mellitus and the biological significance of the diabetic predisposition. Supplement to Proceedings of VI Congress of International Diabetes Federation, p. 68, 1967.
12. Passarge, E.: Genetics of Hirschsprung's disease. New Eng. J. Med., 276:138, 1967.
13. Reed, R. W., and Reed, S. C.: Mental Retardation: A Family Study. Philadelphia, W. B. Saunders, 1965.
14. Rosenthal, D.: Genetic Theory and Abnormal Behaviour. New York, McGraw-Hill, 1970.
15. Smith, C.: Recurrence risks for multifactorial inheritance. Amer. J. Hum. Genet., 23:578, 1971.
16. Turner, G., Turner, B., and Collins, C.: X-linked mental retardation without physical abnormality; Renpenning syndrome Devel. Med. Child Neurol., 13:71, 1971.
17. Wynne-Davies, R.: A family study of neonatal and late-diagnosis congenital dislocation of the hip. J. Med. Genet., 7:315, 1970.
18. ———: Family studies and aetiology of club foot. J. Med. Genet, 2:227, 1965.

Chapter 15

DISORDERS AND SYNDROMES OF UNDETERMINED ETIOLOGY

When we began to write this book, we felt that this would be the longest chapter. It now appears that it will be one of the shortest. One reason for this turn of events is that new information on a number of disorders originally classified as being of undetermined etiology has encouraged us to place them in "known" categories. Another reason is that we excluded a great many disorders of undetermined etiology because they were so lacking in information useful for counseling. What remains is a selection of syndromes that have diagnostic interest or have been observed to recur in families, but whose genetic aspects are not yet clearly defined.

Clinical Example. A four-year-old boy was referred to our cardiology service because of a heart murmur. In his letter the referring physician commented on the patient's peculiar facies: "like the boy on Mad magazine." The patient was submitted to cardiac catheterization and found to have a gradient across the supravalvular aortic area of 60 mm Hg, a 40-mm gradient across the supravalvular pulmonic area, and gradients across the pulmonary arteries totaling 25 mm. Serum calcium and phosphorus deter- minations were within normal limits. A psychometric evaluation placed him in the dull normal range. The diagnosis was supra- valvular aortic stenosis with hypercalcemia syndrome.

From the cardiovascular evaluation no surgical intervention was recommended. The genetic work-up revealed that the pro- band had no relatives in the family with similar phenotypic findings. The parents' question was: what would be the risk of having another child with the same condi- tion? The answer was that the majority of patients we had seen (and the majority of patients reported in the literature) who had the full expression of the syndrome with peculiar facies, supravalvular aortic steno- sis and mental retardation were sporadic. However, we had in our clinic examples of recurrence in siblings without affected par- ents, and patients in whom there had been direct transmission of the fully or partially expressed syndrome. We emphasized the possible role of vitamin D in the pathogen- esis of the disorder and suggested that vita- min D supplementation in the form of multivitamins and enriched milk be discon- tinued.

Polycythemia, diaphragmatic eventration, cryptorchism, linear fissures of the ear lobes and varying degrees of mental retardation are occasional features. Some of the problems detailed above may be responsible for neonatal death. The cause of the syndrome is not yet firmly established, but recurrence in sibs has been reported several times and autosomal recessive inheritance is not unlikely.

BLACKFAN-DIAMOND PURE RED CELL ANEMIA[4]

The onset of anemia is usually evident by two to six months of age. The bone marrow examination characteristically shows a deficiency of red cell precursors associated with normal myeloid and megakaryocyte production. There seems to be an increased number of chromosome breaks in the nuclei of peripheral lymphocytes. The child usually has no other associated congenital anomalies.

A genetic basis for this disease has been suggested because of its familial occurrence, but the specific mode of inheritance is still unclear. Both males and females are affected equally. Although an abnormality in tryptophan metabolism has been reported in some patients, the biochemical basis remains uncertain.

The clinical course is one of progressive anemia leading to heart failure and ultimately death unless blood transfusions and other therapy are given. Symptomatic treatment with packed red cells is administered as needed. Prednisone in the therapeutic dosage range, 2 to 4 mg per kg per day, is often beneficial if started early.

DE LANGE SYNDROME[5]

This disorder, although first recognized almost 40 years ago by a Dutch pediatrician, Cornelia de Lange, has not been widely appreciated until the past decade. The characteristic midline meeting of the eyebrows (synophrys) and thin, down-turning, upper lip is usually apparent in early infancy but may not be diagnostic until a later age. When skeletal anomalies such as micromelia, phocomelia or oligodactyly are present, the diagnosis may be entertained immediately. Mental and growth retardation are consistent features, as is a low-pitched cry.

A large number of other features are commonly found including long, curly eyelashes, anteverted nostrils, micrognathia, hirsutism, and congenital heart defects. These patients rarely reach adult age; congenital heart defects, aspiration and infections are frequently implicated in their deaths.

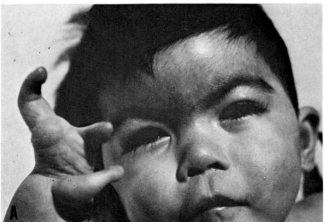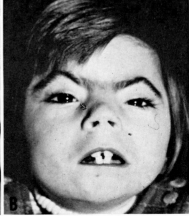

Figure 15-3. Characteristic facies in two children with de Lange syndrome. (Note the hand anomaly, a frequent feature.)

The etiology must still be classified as unknown. Opitz has suggested that the frequent association of chromosomal anomalies of different types may be secondary to a point mutation, recessively transmitted, that causes many chromosome breaks early in gestation and is therefore semilethal, with only a few homozygotes surviving. Whatever the cause, the recurrence risk appears to be low, probably less than 5%. (Etiologic clues from our own cases suggest that a profound teratogenic influence may produce the anomalies of this syndrome.)

DI GEORGE SYNDROME (THYMIC APLASIA)[6]

In this disease the thymus is absent and the parathyroids are rudimentary or absent. The affected infant has neonatal tetany, hypoparathyroidism and, within a few weeks or months, recurrent respiratory tract infections, diarrhea, moniliasis and failure to thrive. There may be associated malformations of the mouth (fish-mouth deformity), ears and esophagus. When the disease has been diagnosed in life it has been because of the cardiovascular anomalies, which most often involve the great vessels. A newborn wtih interrupted aortic arch and no thymic shadow on x-ray (or absent thymus at surgery) has Di George syndrome until proved otherwise and should be treated accordingly. (A teratogenic exposure has been recognized in our recent cases.)

KARTAGENER SYNDROME[7]

This syndrome of mirror-image dextrocardia with abdominal situs inversus, bronchiectasis and sinusitis recurs occasionally in sibs. Claims that the recurrence risk fits the expectation for recessive inheritance were based on failure to exclude sibs when calculating the recurrence risk. Some observers have suggested a dominant mode of inheritance. It may be best to continue to classify the etiology as unknown, and the recurrence risk appears to be relatively low.

KLIPPEL-FEIL SYNDROME (BREVICOLLIS)[8]

Since its first description, this syndrome has accumulated a large number of associated defects. The core anomaly is fusion and reduction in a number of cervical vertebrae, resulting in a short, usually webbed neck that appears to rest on the chest with diminished mobility of the head.

Other anomalies sometimes associated include low posterior hairline, spina bifida, Sprengel's deformity, various axial skeletal anomalies, deafness, facial asymmetry, synkinesis and congenital heart defects. Mental retardation may occasionally occur. The congenital heart abnormalities (which had been largely ignored until the last decade, possibly because of the state of the art of diagnosis and the tendency to focus on the more obvious anomalies) may be present in as many as 50% of these patients. The critical point is that many of these patients develop pulmonary hypertension and could become inoperable from the cardiovascular

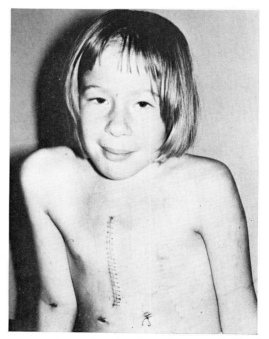

Figure 15-4. Klippel-Feil syndrome with "head resting on chest" and thoracotomy scar from recent surgery for commonly associated congenital heart disease.

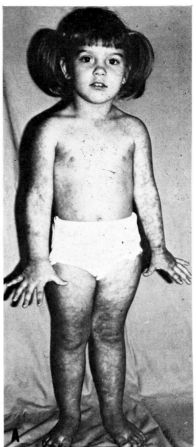

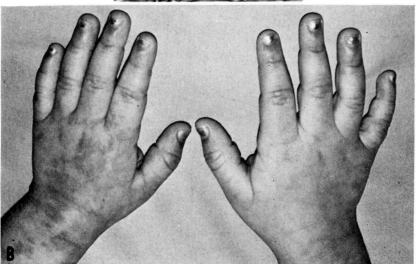

Figure 15-5. Full view of girl with Klippel-Trenaunay-Weber syndrome showing hemangiomata and that the right arm and left leg are larger than the contralateral limbs. View of hands hands showing disparity in size.

point of view while the physician is directing his attention to the other defects.

The genetic basis of this syndrome is not firmly established. Most of the cases are sporadic, but there are some familial cases in which parent-child transmission occurs and others in which affected siblings with unaffected parents occur.

KLIPPEL-TRENAUNAY-WEBER SYNDROME[9]

The major features of this syndrome are hemangiomata associated with underlying bony and soft tissue hypertrophy. Often the patient with this disorder will have one leg larger than the other and perhaps the contralateral hand or arm larger (unlike the Silver syndrome in which the hypertrophy of the extremities always occurs on the same side and there is no accompanying hemangioma formation). Facial hemangiomata are common and this disorder may be considered in the differential diagnosis of the Sturge-Weber syndrome (there have been reports of the association of the two syndromes in families). Mental retardation is not a feature. Familial cases have been recognized, but a pattern of inheritance has not been confidently proposed. (Recent family studies of our own are consistent with an autosomal dominant mode of inheritance with variable expressivity.)

McCUNE-ALBRIGHT SYNDROME[10]

This syndrome, also called osteitis fibrosa cystica, has as its core features sexual precocity, café au lait spots (mainly on the back and buttocks) and progressive thickening of bone (fibrous dysplasia) that may be deforming and result in fractures of long bones. The fibrous dysplasia of the skull may lead to blindness and deafness. Because of the sexual precocity and early closure of the epiphyses, ultimate height attainment is often significantly reduced. Diabetes mellitus, hypercalcemia and hyperthyroidism are occasionally encountered. There are no reported familial cases of this syndrome (which should not be confused with the Albright syndrome, hereditary

osteodystrophy). The counseling for this disorder is that recurrences should not be anticipated.

OCULO-AURICULO-VERTEBRAL SYNDROME (GOLDENHAR SYNDROME)[11]

This syndrome is similar in many ways to the Treacher Collins syndrome. Malformed ears, frequent deafness and mandibular and malar hypoplasia are common to both syndromes. The Goldenhar syndrome has the additional features of epibulbar dermoids and notching of the upper, rather than the lower lid, and there is a higher frequency of vertebral anomalies (cervical and thoracic vertebral fusions and hemivertebrae). Dental malocclusion is frequent; cleft lip and palate and congenital heart diseases (transposition of the great vessels) are occasionally encountered. Intelligence is usually normal and if development of speech is delayed, hearing loss should be the first etiologic consideration. Although the facial defects may be profound, plastic surgery provides reasonably satisfactory restoration.

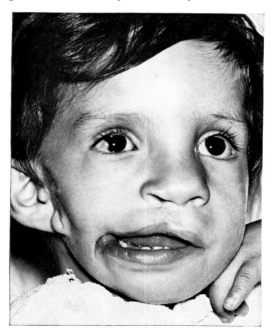

Figure 15-6. Facies in oculo-auriculo-vertebral syndrome. Note the epibulbar dermoid in right eye.

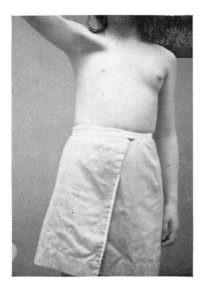

Figure 15-7. Absence of pectoralis major muscle in patient with Poland syndrome.

Almost all cases are sporadic. The hemifacial syndrome (unilateral microtia, macrostomia and aplasia of the mandibular ramus and/or condyle) may be a variant.

POLAND SYNDROME[12]

The key features of this syndrome are absence of the pectoralis muscles associated with syndactyly and shortening of the fingers on the same side of the body. Rib defects and hypoplasia of the entire hand or arm may be found. Congenital heart defects have been observed. To date, reported cases have all been sporadic, so the chances of recurrence are considered to be remote. (An important teratogenic exposure has been documented in the cases of David.[12])

PRADER-WILLI SYNDROME[13]

This syndrome of obesity, mental retardation, small hands and feet, hypotonia in

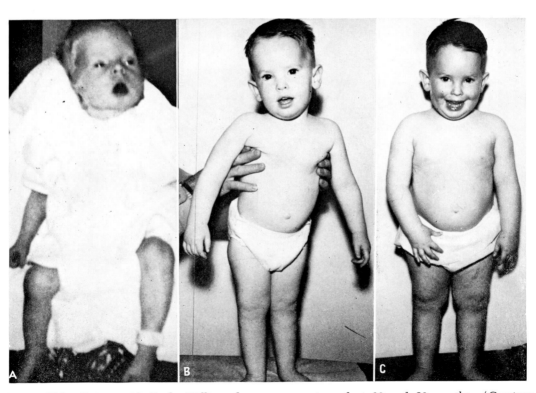

Figure 15-8. Patient with Prader-Willi syndrome as neonate and at 20 and 30 months. (Courtesy D. W. Smith. From Hall, B. D., and Smith, D. W.: Prader-Willi syndrome. J. Pediat., 81:286, 1972.)

infancy and hypogenitalism has not been described as recurring in families. For counseling, it should be distinguished from the autosomal recessive Laurence-Moon-Biedl syndrome, which is not characterized by small hands and feet and usually has the additional features of polydactyly and retinitis pigmentosa.

PRUNE-BELLY SYNDROME[14]

This vividly descriptive name emphasizes one aspect of a syndrome that consists of absence of abdominal muscles, urogenital malformations, and intestinal malrotations. The urogenital anomalies include obstructions of the urinary tract and undescended testes. Affected sibs have been reported but a clear genetic mode of transmission has not been established.

ROBIN SYNDROME[15]

In this syndrome (often incorrectly designated as the Pierre Robin syndrome), severe micrognathia, glossoptosis and marked respiratory distress in the newborn are often associated with feeding difficulties and aspiration. It may be considered necessary to suture the tongue forward until the lower jaw develops sufficiently to accommodate the tongue.

Within a few months the jaw develops to a physiologically satisfactory size and some

adults who had significant problems with the Robin syndrome as infants do not have striking facial deformity. However, a characteristic appearance of the mandible is still apparent on radiographs. Microphthalmia and cataracts occasionally occur. The syndrome is sometimes confused with the dominantly inherited Treacher Collins syndrome, because of the micrognathia shared by the two disorders, but the eye and ear abnormalities of the Treacher Collins syndrome should permit clear distinction.

The genetic basis of the Robin syndrome is not clear, but recurrences in sibs have been observed, as have partial manifestations in parents. The recurrence risk is low, however, probably less than 5%.

RUBINSTEIN-TAYBI SYNDROME[16]

This syndrome of unknown etiology has as its features broad thumbs and broad great toes, shortness of stature, mild to severe mental retardation and a characteristic facies (narrow maxilla, beaked nose, antimongoloid slant to the palpebral fissures, epicanthic folds). Other features include cryptorchism in the male, congenital cardiovascular lesions, ptosis, strabismus, low-set ears, dermatoglyphic abnormalities, syndactyly and polydactyly. All of the cases reported in the literature have been sporadic except for one example of recurrence in

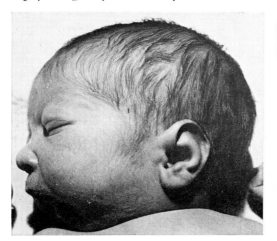

Figure 15-9. Severe micrognathia of Robin syndrome.

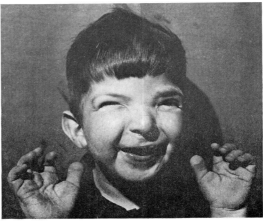

Figure 15-10. Facies and broad thumbs of Rubenstein-Taybi syndrome.

sibs. We have also seen a family in which there was a recurrence in sibs, after having assured the then-pregnant mother only a few months before that the risk of having another affected child was remote. Such disconcerting events are to be expected occasionally when the counselor is dealing with diseases of low but finite recurrence risk.

SILVER SYNDROME[17]

This syndrome of unknown etiology has as its most striking feature a skeletal asymmetry involving the ipsilateral extremities and the head, sometimes referred to as hemihypertrophy. Shortness of stature and variations in sexual development (elevated urinary gonadotrophins, precocious puberty) are the other core features stressed by Silver. The face is characteristically triangular in shape. Delayed osseous matura-

tion, clinodactyly, syndactyly, down-turned mouth, café au lait spots and moderate mental retardation are frequently found.

STURGE-WEBER SYNDROME[18]

Hemangiomata most often following the course of the trigeminal nerve and confined to one side of the face are associated with hemangiomata of the meninges, cerebral cortical atrophy, seizures and mental re-

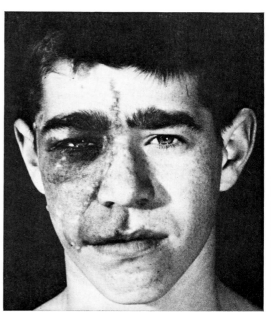

Figure 15-12. Facial hemangioma in patient with Sturge-Weber syndrome.

tardation in this syndrome. X-ray films of the skull reveal a "double-contour," calcification of the convolutions of the brain. Mental retardation and seizures are not invariable, but over half of these patients are so affected, and about one-third have paresis. Almost all cases are sporadic, but recurrences within families have been observed.

REFERENCES

Aortic Supravalvular Stenosis With Hypercalcemia Syndrome

1. Black, J. A., and Bonham-Carter, R. E.: Association between aortic stenosis and facies of severe infantile hypercalcemia. Lancet, 2:745, 1963.

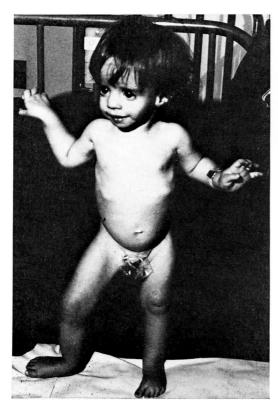

Figure 15-11. Striking right-sided hemihypertrophy in child with Silver syndrome.

2. Beuren, A. J., *et al.*: The syndrome of supra-valvular aortic stenosis, peripheral pulmonary stenosis, mental retardation and similar facial appearance. Amer. J. Cardiol., 13:471, 1964.

Beckwith Syndrome (Wiedemann-Beckwith Syndrome)

3. Wiedemann, H. R.: Complexe malformatif familial avec hernie ombilicale et macroglossie un "syndrome nouveau"? J. Genet. Hum., 13:223, 1964.

Blackfan-Diamond Pure Red Cell Anemia

4. Diamond, L. K., Allen, D. W., and Magill, F. B.: Congenital (erythroid) hypoplastic anemia: a 25 year study. Amer. J. Dis. Child., 102:403, 1961.

de Lange Syndrome

5. Ptacek, L. J., *et al.*: The Cornelia de Lange syndrome. J. Pediat., 63:1000, 1963.

Di George Syndrome (Thymic Aplasia)

6. Di George, A.M.: Congenital absence of the thymus and its immunologic consequences: concurrence with congenital hypoparathyroid-ism. *In* Good, R. A. (ed.): Immunologic Deficiency Diseases. New York, National Foundation, 1968. p. 116.

Kartagener Syndrome

7. Holmes L. B., Blenner-hassett, J. B., and Austin, K. F.: A reappraisal of Kartagener's syndrome. Amer. J. Med. Sci., 255:13, 1968.

Klippel-Feil Syndrome (Brevicollis)

8. Nora, J. J., Cohen, M., and Maxwell, G.: Klipple-Feil syndrome with congenital heart disease. Amer. J. Dis. Child., 102:858, 1961.

Klippel-Trenaunay-Weber Syndrome

9. Brooksaler, F.: The angioosteohypertrophy syndrome (Klippel-Trenaunay-Weber syndrome). Amer. J. Dis. Child., 112:161, 1966.

McCune-Albright Syndrome

10. Samuel, S., *et al.*: Hyperthyroidism in an infant with McCune-Albright syndrome: Report of a case with myeloid metaplasia. J. Pediat., 80:275, 1972.

Oculo-auriculo-vertebral Syndrome (Goldenhar Syndrome)

11. Gorlin, R. J., and Pindborg, J. J.: Oculoauriculovertebral dysplasia. *In* Syndromes of the Head and Neck. New York, McGraw-Hill, 1964.

Poland Syndrome

12. David, T. J.: Nature and etiology of the Poland anomaly. New Eng. J. Med., 287:487, 1972.

Prader-Willi Syndrome

13. Hall, B. D., and Smith, D. W.: Prader-Willi syndrome. J. Pediat., 81: 286, 1972.

Prune-belly Syndrome

14. Burke, E. C., Shin, M. H., and Kelalis, P. P.: Prune belly syndrome: clinical findings and survival. Amer. J. Dis. Child., 117:668, 1969.

Robin Syndrome

15. Smith, J. L., and Stowe, F. R.: The Pierre Robin syndrome (glossoptosis, micrognathia, cleft palate). A review of 39 cases with emphasis on associated ocular lesions. Pediatrics, 27:128, 1961.

Rubenstein-Taybi Syndrome

16. Rubenstein, J. H., and Taybi, H.: Broad thumbs and toes and facial abnormalities. A possible mental retardation syndrome. Amer. J. Dis. Child., 105:588, 1963.

Silver Syndrome

17. Silver, H. K.: Asymmetry, short stature, and variations in sexual development. A syndrome of congenital malformations. Amer. J. Dis. Child., 107:495, 1964.

Sturge-Weber Syndrome

18. Chao, D. H. C.: Congenital neurocutaneous syndromes of childhood. III. Sturge-Weber disease. J. Pediat., 55:635, 1959.

Section II.
Special Topics

Chapter 16

ANTENATAL DIAGNOSIS OF GENETIC DISEASES

Diseases desperate grown
By desperate appliances are relieved
Or not at all.

Shakespeare

It is emphasized throughout this book that certain more or less orderly steps are taken in the diagnosis, treatment and counseling of patients who have a genetically determined disorder. The first step is accurate diagnosis of the presenting disease. This is followed by careful assessment of the familial nature of the disorder as recognized from previous experience and as manifested in the specific family under consideration.

The questions that are always uppermost are: why did this happen and what is the chance that it will happen again? In the recent past, if a single-mutant-gene disorder or chromosomal translocation were diagnosed, the genetic counseling could be based only on mendelian ratios and empiric recurrence risks. This is still true for the majority of genetically determined diseases. However, for an increasing number of disorders a new dimension has been added to

genetic counseling and risk determination —antenatal diagnosis. Antenatal diagnosis is the detection, prior to delivery, of a harmful condition of the fetus. This is mainly determined by the study of amniotic fluid samples, although certain problems may be recognized through the analysis of maternal blood (e.g., hemolytic disease of the newborn) and maternal urine (e.g., methylmalonic aciduria) or radiographically (e.g., anencephaly).

AMNIOCENTESIS

Amniocentesis has been employed as a diagnostic aid since the 1930's. In the mid-1950's a number of authors demonstrated the feasibility of determining the nuclear sex of the fetus from amniotic fluid cells. However, only during the last several years has there been a significant clinical and investigative emphasis on this method beginning with its use in hemolytic disease of the newborn. Before presenting current applications of amniocentesis,[1-3] certain background information should be provided, and it should be pointed out that the number of fetuses identified by this method as having genetic abnormalities is still quite small.

Amniocentesis is performed almost exclusively by a transabdominal uterine puncture with a hypodermic needle, withdrawing 5 to 10 ml of amniotic fluid which contains cells of fetal origin, mainly skin and amnion. In theory any disease that may be diagnosed through fibroblasts obtained by skin biopsy and culture should be diagnosable by culturing fetal skin cells shed into the amniotic fluid. The supernate of the amniotic fluid itself is of diagnostic value in hemolytic disease of the newborn and a few inborn errors of metabolism. However, the majority of diseases diagnosed by amniocentesis require cells. The cells may be utilized directly (uncultured) for sex determination by Barr and fluorescent Y bodies and for some enzyme assays or, more commonly, are cultured for chromosomal and biochemical studies. Examples of the use of uncultured cells for sex chromatin determination are in families with X-linked disorders such as hemophilia A and Duchenne type muscular dystrophy. Although the actual presentation of these diseases cannot yet be determined by amniocentesis, the information regarding the sex of the fetus provides a basis for genetic counseling (0% risk for females; 50% risk for males). The addition of the fluorescent Y body to the Barr body increases the reliability of sex determination by uncultured cells; however, in practice a confirmation of sex by chromosomal culture is recommended before a final decision regarding therapeutic abortion is made.

Because the viability for culture of the desquamated cells is greatest early in the pregnancy and also because termination of the pregnancy may be under consideration, it is recommended that the procedure be performed as early as possible and certainly before 20 weeks gestation. The amniotic fluid has been reported as being adequate as early as eight to ten weeks gestation. Therefore, the range of time for performing amniocentesis for cell culture is theoretically ten to 20 weeks. However, in practice it is difficult to perform a successful amniocentesis before 14 weeks gestation. A preliminary procedure to amniocentesis is ultrasonic localization of the placenta. An anterior placenta overlying the prospective route of amniocentesis is a contraindication.

If Rh disease is the indication for amniocentesis, the procedure is performed during the third trimester. Colorimetric measurements of bilirubin in the amniotic fluid provide a more accurate guide to the severity of the erythroblastosis than measurements of a rising anti-Rh titer in maternal blood. The goal of periodic bilirubin determinations from amniotic fluid samples is the prevention of damage to the unborn infant. If rising bilirubin levels in the late weeks of pregnancy represent a significant threat, early delivery of the baby is recommended. On the other hand, if high levels of bilirubin are discovered at a period too early in the third trimester to permit delivery of an infant mature enough to survive, then *in utero* blood transfusions may be appropriate. The latter therapeutic option is not undertaken lightly.

In the first chapter we stated that there are three major categories of genetically determined disorders (mutant gene, chromosomal and multifactorial) and one minor category (maternal-fetal interaction). Presently there are applications of antenatal diagnosis by amniocentesis for all categories except multifactorial inheritance.

Some of the current practical problems connected with amniocentesis require emphasis. First, there is the concern of risk to the mother and the baby. Mortality and maternal morbidity by the transabdominal approach is essentially zero in experienced hands. However, leakage of amniotic fluid and induction of abortion are not uncommon. Although a few centers claim almost invariable success from each first attempt at amniocentesis on given patients, second and third attempts are required more frequently than the literature would lead one to conclude. The next problem is whether the study can yield the desired result. As far as cell cultures are concerned, the best record of success in growing the cells is about 80%; this means obtaining the cells before 20 weeks gestation to ensure acceptable viability. Once cells are obtained for culture to detect a biochemical abnormality, the length of time required to reach a decision is often four to six weeks. Clearly, one must meet a very tight schedule if antenatal diagnosis is to be successful.

How many diseases can one really diagnose in this manner? At the time of this writing, in addition to hemolytic disease of the newborn and chromosomal disorders, over 40 genetic diseases are eligible for prenatal diagnosis because they are detectable by somatic cell cultures. We elected not to list these diseases because such a list would certainly be out of date by the time of publication. Earlier we suggested that any disease that could be diagnosed in fibroblast culture should also be confidently diagnosable by amniocentesis. This is presently far from the case. Table 16-1 lists the 15 mutant-gene diseases that currently may be diagnosed by amniocentesis with reasonable confidence. However, we anticipated that this list will be enlarged. Cystic fibrosis does not appear on the list in spite of claims that cultured fibroblasts from patients develop characteristic metachromatic granules. There is more than one form of

this disease, including an orthochromatic form that would not be detected in cultures of fetal cells. Furthermore, the diagnostic test is positive in heterozygotes. Thus, at this time, it cannot be confidently stated that cystic fibrosis is or is not present in the fetus on the basis of the results of the culture of amniotic fluid cells. There are many more diseases diagnosed in somatic cell culture that are genetically heterogeneous like cystic fibrosis. These include: cystinosis, homocystinuria, OTC deficiency, galactosemia, G6PD deficiency, maple syrup urine disease, beta galactosidase deficiency, adrenogenital syndrome, orotic aciduria, hyperlysinemia and lactic acidosis. These diseases appear with cystic fibrosis on lists of diseases eligible for prenatal diagnosis, but caution must be exercised in their diagnosis because of their heterogeneity.

Before illustrating this subject with a clinical example, it is important to emphasize that until more experience is gained, antenatal diagnosis by amniocentesis is to be considered an experimental procedure except in Rh disease. In the case of sex determination studies (Barr and fluorescent Y body and cell culture), the answer as to whether or not the fetus has the suspected X-linked disease is not provided, but only that the fetus is a female with 0% risk or a male with 50% risk. Most families, however, will desire therapeutic abortion for a known 50% risk situation, especially if the mother has taken the step of undergoing amniocentesis. Indeed, the amniocentesis should not be done unless the parents have considered this option. With regard to the biochemical

TABLE 16-1. Disorders in Which Amniocentesis is of Diagnostic Value (Partial List)

Adrenogenital syndrome	Maple syrup urine disease
Chromosomal aberrations	Metachromatic leukodystrophy
Fabry disease	Methylmalonic aciduria
Galactosemia	MPS I (Hurler syndrome)
Gangliosidosis, generalized, GM(1)	MPS II (Hunter syndrome)
Glycogen storage disease Type II (Pompe)	Niemann-Pick disease
Hemolytic disease of the newborn	Sandhoff disease
Lesch-Nyhan syndrome	Sex determination for X-linked diseases
Lysosomal acid phosphatase deficiency	Tay-Sachs disease

abnormalities studied in amniotic fluid cell cultures, the pitfalls (e.g., orthochromatic cystic fibrosis) are still significant even in expert hands and reliable studies are not yet available at "neighborhood hospitals."

Although biochemical studies are becoming more widely performed, the major application of amniotic fluid cell cultures is in the study of chromosomal aberrations. Even here there remain serious pitfalls, such as the cloning out of an unrepresentative cell line.[4]

Clinical Example. A 23-year-old mother delivered a female infant who had the classic stigmata of 13 trisomy. A karyotype of the infant, who survived only one month, revealed an unbalanced D/D translocation, 46,XX,–D,+t(DqDq) (Fig. 16-1). The parents and their one living child were studied. The mother was found to be a balanced D/D translocation carrier, 45,XX,–D,+t (DqDq) (Fig. 16-2) and the father and sister were normal. In the course of investigating this family (Fig. 16-3), a number of balanced translocation carriers were identified through four generations.

Although the mother was cautioned about future pregnancies, she was also informed about the possibility of antenatal diagnosis by amniocentesis should she become preg-

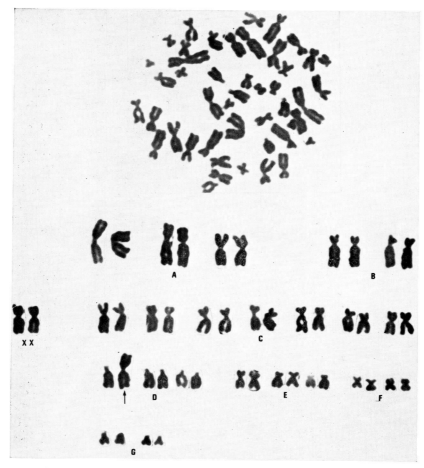

Figure 16-1. Proband in clinical example with unbalanced D/D translocation. Note that there are 46 chromosomes and 6 chromosomes in the D group, but that one D group chromosome has essentially all of the genetic information possessed by the long arms of two D chromosomes and therefore has a D chromosome in triplicate and the stigmata of 13 trisomy.

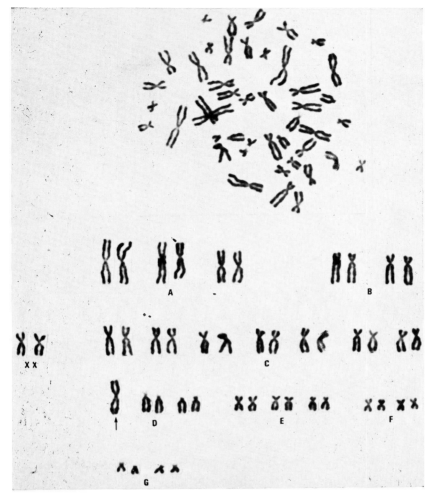

Figure 16-2. Patient with balanced D/D translocation from family in clinical example. Note that although there are only 45 chromosomes, one D chromosome has the equivalent genetic material of two chromosomes and the patient is normal.

nant. While the karyotyping of the various family members was still in progress, the mother informed her physician in the genetics clinic that she was eight weeks pregnant. An attempt at amniocentesis was made at 12 weeks but did not provide diagnostic information. Another attempt at 14 weeks was also unsuccessful. The amniocentesis performed at 16 weeks was diagnostic. The fetus was determined to be a female carrier of a balanced D/D translocation. The mother elected to continue the pregnancy. A healthy female infant was delivered and

confirmation of the balanced D/D translocation was made from peripheral blood cells.

In this family the D/D translocation has been transmitted through four generations. Although the family has not been completely studied, approximately one-half of the living members investigated so far are balanced D/D translocation carriers. In generation III, there are an equal number of living members and spontaneous abortions. The proband has the only confirmed unbalanced D/D translocation, but one

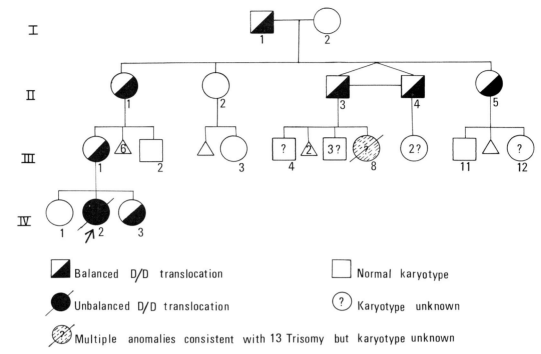

Figure 16-3. Family with D/D translocation transmitted through four generations.

other infant is known to have died at two days of age with multiple anomalies consistent with 13 trisomy.

The recurrence risk for unbalanced D/D translocation within this family appears to be of the order of 10%, and the risk of balanced D/D translocation approximates 50%. As was mentioned in Chapter 3, D/D translocation is one of the most common autosomal errors and the vast majority are balanced. The risk of 1% of unbalanced translocation to offspring of a balanced D/D translocation carrier is mentioned in the literature. This family and others we have studied lead us to believe that the risk is higher and that amniocentesis is certainly fully justified.

FETOSCOPY

Progress is being made in visualization of the fetus directly or by radiographic and ultrasonic techniques, which may be of value in detecting gross structural malformations.

REFERENCES

1. Nadler, H. L., and Gerbie, A. B.: Role of amniocentesis in the intrauterine detection of genetic disorders. New Eng. J. Med., 282:596, 1970.
2. Milunsky, A., et al.: Prenatal genetic diagnosis (three parts). New Eng. J. Med., 283:1370, 1441, 1498, 1970.
3. Bergsma, D., and Motulsky, A.G. (eds.): Symposium on Intrauterine Diagnosis. Birth Defects: Original Article Series, 7, (No. 5) 1971. New York, The National Foundation.
4. Kardon, N. B., et al.: Pitfalls in prenatal diagnosis resulting from chromosomal mosaicism. J. Pediat., 80:297, 1972.

Chapter 17

GENETIC ANALYSIS BY FAMILY AND TWIN STUDIES

How does an investigator determine whether or not genetic factors are important in a disease whose etiology is unknown? Several tools are available.

First, if a disease has a genetic basis, it will occur in familial aggregates. This does not mean that all diseases found in more than one member of a family are necessarily genetic: take, for example, an epidemic of chickenpox or a bout of food poisoning. How then can one distinguish between familial environmental causes and genetic causes? One may begin by testing the data to see whether they fit the expectation for mendelian or multifactorial inheritance. If they do, a nongenetic cause is unlikely.

Second, twin studies measuring the differences in concordance between monozygotic and dizygotic twins with respect to a given disease offer a means to determine whether the familial distribution results from genetic factors and to assess the contribution of these genetic factors to the disorder.

Finally, animal homologies are used to aid in the understanding of etiologic mechanisms in the human subject.

FAMILIAL AGGREGATES

Prior to 1954, there were seven published cases of the Ellis-van Creveld syndrome in the world literature. In no instance was there more than one affected individual in a family. In 1954, seven more patients with this syndrome were reported: two sets of siblings, a concordant set of dizygotic twins and a "sporadic" case. Thus, of 14 patients in the world literature, six were first-degree relatives. These were familial aggregates that could not be dismissed and that required a genetic analysis.

It will be remembered that an individual with an autosomal dominant disease has an affected parent (unless he represents a fresh mutation), and that a patient with a rare autosomal recessive disease characteristically does not have an affected parent but may have affected sibs, with a one-in-four expectation for each sib. In none of the 14 patients with the Ellis-van Creveld syndrome was there an affected parent. Obviously dominant transmission was not involved, but what about recessive inheritance? The ratio of affected to unaffected sibs was compatible with the expected one-in-four ratio, although the numbers involved were too small to be reliable. Both males and females were affected, which was against X-linked recessive transmission. Further support for an autosomal recessive mode came from the fact that in four of 11 families for which information was available, there was parental consanguinity. Consanguinity increases the likelihood of homozygosity for rare recessive genes. Conversely, when children with a rare disease have consanguineous parents more often than expected in the general population, this fact strongly suggests recessive inheritance.

On the basis of the simple genetic analysis presented above, Metrakos and Fraser[7] suggested an autosomal mode of inheritance for the Ellis-van Creveld syndrome. Subsequent studies including the large inbred pedigree reported by McKusick and co-workers[6] have confirmed the autosomal recessive inheritance of this syndrome.

It should be emphasized that occurrence in parent and child or in siblings of normal parents is not enough to prove dominant or recessive simple mendelian inheritance respectively. For instance, in the case of atrial septal defect (ASD), some reports in the literature claimed autosomal dominant inheritance and others autosomal recessive inheritance. That is, there were pedigrees in which the defect appeared in parent and child, and other pedigrees in which sibs were affected but not parents. However, an analysis of 100 families ascertained through a proband having ASD failed to meet the expectation for either autosomal dominant or recessive inheritance (Table 17-1).[9]

There was evidence of direct parent to child transmission in seven families ascertained through an affected child (3.5% of parents); a fully penetrant autosomal dominant disorder would have direct transmission in all 100 families (50% of parents) excluding fresh mutations, and this option is eliminated by data collected on the offspring of parents with ASD in which only 2.6% were affected. Also, in autosomal dominant disorders, the expectation is that one-half of the sibs would be affected. The empiric data fall far short ($p < 0.001$) of the expectation for dominant inheritance. Only 3.7% of sibs, 3.5% of parents and 2.6% of offspring of patients with ASD also had congenital heart lesions, most often ASD.

The expectation for autosomal recessive diseases (in a random-mating population) is that 25% of the offspring will be affected and none of the parents. This differs strikingly ($p < 0.001$) from the actual finding that only 3.7% of the sibs and 3.5% of the parents were affected.

Are the data significantly different from what one would expect if no genetic factors were at work—if these were merely random recurrences? The data show that the recurrences of ASD in these familial aggregates do not occur by chance alone ($p < 0.001$). The expectation for recurrence of ASD in sibs and offspring by chance would be the population frequency, about 0.1%. The observed recurrence rates were 3.7% and 2.6% respectively.

Thus, the data suggest that there may be genetic factors at work, but the mode of transmission does not meet the expectation for single mutant gene inheritance on the

TABLE 17-1. Frequency of ASD in First-Degree Relatives of Probands

Relationship	Total	Number Affected	% Affected	Predicted by $\sqrt{p}$
Sibs	279	10	3.7	3.2
Parents	200	7	3.5	3.2
Children	190	5	2.6	3.2

(From Nora, J. J., et al.: Hereditary factors in atrial septal defect. Circulation, 35:448, 1967. By permission of The American Heart Association, Inc.)

basis of family studies. A gross chromosomal aberration underlying ASD could be ruled out on the basis of several large investigations of chromosomal anomalies in patients with congenital heart lesions. This leaves multifactorial inheritance as the alternative genetic hypothesis to account for the aggregates found in these families. As has been emphasized throughout this volume, the investigator cannot prove an hypothesis; he can only disprove or fail to disprove it.

As outlined in Chapter 13, there are criteria for multifactorial inheritance just as there are for mendelian inheritance. Wright, in 1934, recognized that a trait or disease may appear in parent and child in one pedigree and in sibs in another without being either simple dominant or recessive. This simulation of mendelism in multifactorial inheritance was further elucidated by Edwards, who suggested that the recurrence risk in a first-degree relative of an individual having a disease determined by multifactorial inheritance was roughly the square root of the population frequency ($\sqrt{p}$).

The population frequency of ASD (by most recent estimates) is 0.1% (0.001) and the square root of the population frequency is 3.2% (0.032). The empiric risk data as displayed in Table 17-1 approximate closely this expectation of multifactorial inheritance. It may be noted in Figure 13-7 that ASD falls almost precisely on the line for multifactorial inheritance.

It is obvious that this test (as well as population frequency data) is only an approximation. However, on the basis of this test, it is not possible to disprove the multifactorial inheritance of ASD. In fact, the family data are precisely what one would expect. It will be difficult to obtain enough data of sufficient reliability to apply some of the other tests for multifactorial inheritance outlined in Chapter 13.

In summary, family studies may give evidence of genetic predisposition through the demonstration of familial aggregates. If there is direct transmission from parent to child, with about 50% of the offspring affected, a mendelian dominant mode is indicated. If there is no affected parent but about 25% of the siblings have the disorder, a mendelian recessive is considered; an increased parental consanguinity rate provides further support for this conclusion. If the pedigrees consistently show that the affected individuals are males and the disease is transmitted through unaffected females, the inheritance is probably X-linked recessive. Finally, if the disease is directly transmitted by males to all their daughters and none of their sons, and by females to half of their sons and half of their daughters, the pattern of inheritance is X-linked dominant.

Diseases determined by multifactorial inheritance are often common diseases, i.e., diseases found in the population more frequently than one per thousand. They may appear in parent and child in one pedigree, in siblings in another pedigree and sporadically in yet another, but this should not be taken to mean that they show mendelian dominant, recessive, or no inheritance in the respective families. When analyzing a sizeable number of families having such a disease, several features become clear. The recurrence risks in first-degree relatives are not 50% or 25% as in recessive or dominant diseases, but some lower figure, usually between 1% and 10%. The frequency in first-degree relatives approximates $\sqrt{p}$. Other features are described in Chapter 13. These diseases also may give evidence of responding to the influences of genetic "background," such as sex of the patient, or environmental factors, such as socioeconomic class, geographic area and maternal exposure to drugs, infections, chemicals and radiation. Further confirmation may be obtained through twin studies.

TWIN STUDIES

Galton, in 1874,[5] pointed out the importance of twin studies to weigh the effects of "nature and nurture"—heredity and environment. The basic concept is that if ge-

netic factors play a role in the etiology of a
disease, that disease will be concordant
(i.e., affecting both members of the pair)
more often in **monozygotic (identical)** than
in **dizygotic (nonidentical or fraternal)**
twins. Identical twins are assumed to have
the same heredity in similar environments
while nonidentical twins have different heredity in similar environments. Of course, it
is not true that the intrauterine environment is the same for both members of a
twin pair, whether they are monozygotic or
dizygotic, since there may be differences in
vasculature, crowding, position, and so on.
While the postnatal environments of twins
raised together may be similar, they also
are not entirely the same. One way of distinguishing the postnatal influences of nature and nurture is the study of identical
twins raised apart.

Monozygotic or Dizygotic? Monozygotic
(MZ) twins, as the name implies, arise
from a single fertilized ovum, or zygote. At
an early stage the zygote develops into two
embryos. Dizygotic (DZ) twins, who are
no more genetically similar than sibs, are
produced when two ova are extruded during the same cycle and fertilized by two
separate sperms.

Normally both members of an MZ twin
pair have identical genotypes and the various laboratory and clinical tests of genotype will be the same in both. The higher
the number of identical gene markers in

members of a twin pair, the greater the
likelihood that the twins are identical,
whereas a single well-established difference
is enough to prove dizygosity. Skin grafts
between MZ twins are not rejected, but between DZ twins they usually are rejected.
Statistical methods for calculating the exact
probability of dizygosity are available.[12]

The most important clinical finding is
that MZ twins usually have facial and other
somatic features that look very much alike.
The mother will usually tell the physician
whether or not her twins are identical, and
her judgment will be quite accurate (unless distorted by having been told they are
dizygotic because they had two placentas!).
Occasionally, however, one MZ twin may
be considerably larger than the other, or
may have a malformation that alters facial
features, such as cleft lip, or influences nu-
trition, such as a congenital heart defect.
In these cases, or if one is engaged in a research project or planning a kidney transplant, the judgment as to monozygosity or
dizygosity requires more than a mother's
opinion. Then laboratory evidence such as
blood groups and other clinical findings are
called into service. Blood groups—ABO,
Rh, MN, Lutheran, Kell, Duffy and a number of others—are commonly used as genetic "markers" (see Chapter 21). Histocompatibility antigens (see Chapter 20)
and serum proteins such as haptoglobins
are also useful.

The precise color-shading and speckling
of the iris is controlled by many genes but
is strikingly similar in MZ pairs. Any obvious difference between the pairs favors
dizygosity. Dermatoglyphic patterns and
ridge counts are more similar in monozygotic than in dizygotic twins. Comparison
of features on the right side of the body of
a twin with features on the right side of a
co-twin (and left with left) is frequently
helpful, but in the case of mirror-imaging,
opposite sides should be compared. The
shade of hair color, the form of hair and
the shape of nose, lips, eyes and teeth are
virtually identical in MZ twins.

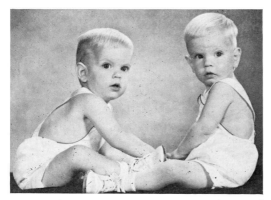

Figure 17-1. Monozygotic twins with atrial
septal defect.

TABLE 17-2. Placentas and Fetal Membranes in Twins

Placenta	Chorion	Amnion	MZ	DZ
1	1	1	Rare	—
1	1	2	± 75%	—
1 (or fused)	2	2	± 25%	± 50%
2	2	2	Rare	± 50%

The report of the appearance of placenta, amnion and chorion is potentially of value, especially if one twin does not survive, but in practice adequate information is seldom provided (Table 17-2). Both MZ and DZ twins may have separate placentas or placentas that are single or appear to be single due to fusion. So simply counting the placentas is of no value. Both types of twins may have separate chorions and amnions with separate placentas. The situation that occurs in MZ twins alone is a single chorion with a single placenta, but this must be carefully distinguished from secondarily fused chorions and placentas.

Frequency of Twins. In the North American Caucasian population, twins occur in approximately one birth in 87 (11.5 per 1000). The frequency of MZ twins in almost all populations of the world is about 3.5 per 1000 births. MZ twins are, of course, always of the same sex, whereas DZ pairs are just as often of opposite sex as of the same sex. Therefore, in North American whites there is an approximately equal distribution of monozygotic to like-sex dizygotic to unlike-sex dizygotic pairs. This sort of information is sometimes used to draw conclusions about concordance rates from twin studies that lack accurate zygosity data. It is not recommended for this purpose, however.

The differences in frequency of twin births from population to population are almost all due to differences in the frequency of dizygotic twins. The range varies from low in Oriental races (6 per 1000 in Japan) to intermediate among Caucasians (11.5 per 1000 in North America) to a high of over 30 per 1000 in certain West African populations.

With increasing maternal age and parity there is an apparent increase in the frequency of DZ twins (but not MZ twins). There also appears to be a tendency for DZ twins to run in families. Contrary to previous claims of paternal as well as maternal transmission of this tendency, more recent data suggest that the familial tendency to twinning is limited to dizygotic twins and maternal transmission.

Application of Twin Studies. The major uses of twin studies are in the evaluation of diseases for which an estimate of the role of genetic factors is being sought and (for MZ pairs) comparison of the results of different treatments on the same genotype. The relevant mathematics and possible applications are well reviewed by Bulmer.[2]

Concordance rates can be expressed as the proportion of affected twin pairs in a series of twins in which both members are affected (the pairwise concordance rate), or as the proportion of affected co-twins of previously defined index cases (the proband concordance rate). Methods of calculating concordance rates must also take ascertainment bias into account.[1]

In single mutant gene diseases with full penetrance, if one member of an MZ twin pair has a disorder, the co-twin will also have it, whether the transmission is dominant or recessive (100% concordance). In dizygotic twins, if one member of the pair has a mendelian trait, the chance that the co-twin will be affected is the same as it is for a sib. If penetrance is incomplete it can be estimated from the difference between observed and expected concordance rates.

In chromosomal disorders, the essential etiologic test is the examination of karyotypes, not pedigree analysis or twin studies. The concordance in MZ twins would be expected to be 100%, but there are reports of twins who, by careful analysis of genetic markers, should be monozygotic but are discordant for 21 trisomy or the XO Turner syndrome. This discordance may be explained on the basis of postzygotic nondisjunction; i.e., the chromosomal anomaly developed in one twin after the first cleavage division of the egg.

It is in multifactorial inheritance and diseases in which the etiologic influence of both heredity and environment are being investigated that twin studies prove most useful. In Table 17-3, typical rates of concordance in MZ and DZ twins are presented in four disease categories, including disorders considered to be determined by multifactorial inheritance. The usual finding is that the concordance in MZ twins is five to ten times as great as in DZ twins.

If no genetic factors were operating, the concordance in MZ and DZ twins would be expected to be the same. On the other hand, if genetic factors were the exclusive basis for the disorder, then the concordance in MZ twins would be 100%, as in single gene diseases. However, in multifactorial inheritance both genetic and environmental factors play a role, which is what the twin studies seem to reflect. Concordance in MZ twins is not 100%, as if heredity were the only consideration, but concordance is much higher in MZ than DZ twins, showing that heredity is playing an important part. Statistical methods have been developed for multifactorial threshold characters in order to estimate heritability from concordance rates, and concordance rates of 50% or less for MZ twins are compatible with relatively high heritability.[11]

Limitations of Twin Studies. Caution must be exercised in interpreting twin data present in the literature as well as in collecting new twin data. Case reports of twins are much more likely to be concordant than discordant. This is to be expected: there is not much interest in publishing a report of twins discordant for a disease.

Many twin studies in the literature are imprecise in both the diagnosis of the disease under consideration and the determination of zygosity. It is unfortunate but true that there has been a good deal of guesswork as to whether twins were identical or not and whether they did in fact have the malformation or disease being studied. This was particularly true in twin studies of congenital heart diseases. The imprecision in this area is generally related to the limitations of diagnostic methods at the time of the study. Cardiac catheterization and mul-

TABLE 17-3. % Concordance in Twins

Diseases	MZ	DZ
Rare single gene (dominant)	100	50 (sib. freq.)
Rare single gene (recessive)	100	25 (sib. freq.)
Chromosomal	100	rare (sib. freq.)
Multifactorial and miscellaneous		
Congenital dislocation of hip[3]	40	3
Cleft lip ± cleft palate[4]	38	8
Club foot[3]	35	3
Congenital heart diseases[8]	25	5
Rheumatic fever[3]	20	
Rheumatoid arthritis[3]	34	3
Hypertension[3]	25	11
Stroke[3]	22	11
Coronary occlusion[3]	26	14

tiple blood group determinations have only recently become established in the diagnostic armamentarium.

The relative strengths of the environmental influences on identical and nonidentical twins cannot be assumed to be equivalent. Atrial septal defect, for example, is found predominantly in females, illustrating the importance of the factor of sex in determining the expression of the disease. It is therefore recommended that comparisons of concordance should be made between MZ pairs and DZ pairs of like sex.

Finally, twin studies do not provide specific etiologic answers. However, the investigator usually does not expect to discover specific etiology from a twin study; rather, he looks to the twin study merely for clues to the existence and magnitude of genetic factors.

Clinical Example. Are genetic factors operating in the etiology of atrial septal defect? From the earlier discussion of family studies, the trait appears to be familial and conforms to at least one criterion for a multifactorial threshold character, but we have not ruled out the possibility of an environmental factor that clusters in families. However, in data obtained from a study of congenital heart diseases in twins,[9] there is clearly a difference in concordance between MZ and like-sex DZ twins: three of seven (43%) of the MZ twins are concordant for ASD compared with no concordance within the eight sets of DZ twins.

This difference is statistically significant and indicates that genetic factors underlie the development of this defect. If genetic factors were not operating one would expect concordance to be similar for both MZ and DZ twins. On the other hand, if genetic factors were almost entirely responsible for ASD, as in single gene disorders, then concordance would be 100% in MZ twins instead of 43%, and considerably lower in DZ twins. The conclusion is that genetic factors are playing a role but are not exclusively responsible for ASD. The concordance of less than 100% in MZ twins

is what one would expect in multifactorial inheritance. For DZ twins one might expect concordance to be somewhat higher than the sib frequency, to the extent that the uterine environment is more similar for DZ twins than for sibs. However the situation is complicated by the mechanical interactions of two embryos sharing the same space and by the occurrence of vascular anastomoses in some cases.

A certain amount of insight into the role of the environment and the genetic-environmental interaction may be gained by looking at one pair of identical twins. Both of the particularly handsome twins pictured in Figure 17-1 had atrial septal defect, but the twin on the right has had additional lesions repaired in infancy: coarctation of the aorta and patent ductus arteriosus. Are the additional lesions coincidental? Or do all three lesions result from the same genetic predisposition, with the environment exerting sufficient influence to prevent additional maldevelopment in one of the twins? Further such observations may help to answer these questions.

ANIMAL HOMOLOGIES

One further method for testing genetic or developmental hypotheses about diseases of complex etiology is the analysis of their homologies in experimental animals. Atrial septal defect has been studied in the A/J inbred strain of mice.[10] ASD is the cardiac anomaly to which the A/J strain is predisposed. In a control group of 233 fetuses sacrificed at day 18 of gestation, three (1.3%) had ASD spontaneously. ASD may be considered to be the heart lesion "running in the family" but clearly the genotype is not the only etiologic factor, since the mice have virtually identical genotypes.

On day 8 of gestation a single intraperitoneal injection of dextroamphetamine sulfate (50 μg per gm of body weight) was given and 24 (13.1%) of the 183 liveborn fetuses were found on histologic examination to have cardiac anomalies, usually ASD.

These data are not consistent with mendelian inheritance. Assuming that the inbred A/J strain is truly isogenic, then a defect caused by a single mutant gene should appear in all offspring rather than 1% as found in the control group. There is also clear evidence that the frequency of ASD in the A/J strain is greatly increased by exposure to environmental teratogens, in this case dextroamphetamine.

What is found in this animal homology reflects what is found in the human. There appears to be an hereditary predisposition to atrial septal defect that is nonmendelian and is made manifest by the environmental milieu. This is consistent with a multifactorial mode of inheritance.

REFERENCES

1. Allen, G., Harvald, B., and Shields, J.: Measures of twin concordance. Acta Genet., 17:475, 1967.
2. Bulmer, M. G.: The Biology of Twinning in Man. Oxford, Clarendon Press, 1970.
3. Carter, C. O.: Multifactorial inheritance revisited. Congenital malformations. Fraser, F. C., and McKusick, V. A., (eds.): Proceedings of the Third International Conference. New York, Excerpta Medica, 1970. pp. 227-231.
4. Fraser, F. C.: The genetics of cleft lip and palate. Amer. J. Hum. Genet., 22:336, 1970.
5. Galton, F.: English Men of Science: Their Nature and Nurture. London, Macmillan, 1874.
6. McKusick, V. A., et al.: Dwarfism in the Amish I. The Ellis-van Creveld syndrome. Bull. Hopkins Hosp., 115:306, 1964.
7. Metrakos, J. D., and Fraser, F. C.: Evidence for a hereditary factor in chondroectodermal dysplasia (Ellis-van Creveld syndrome). Amer. J. Hum. Genet., 6:260, 1954.
8. Nora, J. J., et al.: Congenital heart disease in twins. New Eng. J. Med., 277:568, 1967.
9. Nora, J. J., McNamara, D. G., and Fraser, F. C.: Hereditary factors in atrial septal defect. Circulation, 35:448, 1967.
10. Nora, J. J., Sommerville, R. J., and Fraser, F. C.: Homologies for congenital heart diseases: murine models influenced by dextroamphetamine. Teratology, 1:413, 1968.
11. Smith, C.: Heritability of liability and concordance in monozygous twins. Ann. Hum. Genet., 34:85, 1970.
12. Smith, S. M., and Penrose, L. S.: Monozygotic and dizygotic twin diagnosis. Ann. Hum. Genet., 19:273, 1955.

Chapter 18

TERATOLOGY

. . . a substantial collection of the monstrosities of nature, well examined and described . . . Francis Bacon: Advancement of Learning.

Bacon advocated the importance of the negative instance, the exception to the rule —the monstrosities of nature. This Baconian approach is a cornerstone of genetics, medicine and indeed of all biology. It is the mutation that illuminates our understanding of gene function. It is the study of the diseased organ system that helps define normal structure and function. Thus, the above quotation and concept could be used to introduce any chapter in this text.

Teratology (literally translated, the study of monsters) has so evolved that most workers would consider teratology to be the study of abnormal development, especially as it is influenced by environmental agents (teratogens) such as drugs, viruses, chemicals and radiation.

Our interest is in the human subject, but the difficulties of making controlled observations on naturally occurring events in humans and the ethical interdiction against performing any experiment in the human that could be harmful to the subject necessitates the use of animal models for experimental teratology. The assumption of a phylogenetic continuum from single-celled organisms to the human underlies biologic experimentation. The exponential growth of the biologic sciences in the past few decades may in large part be traced to the inductive inferences gained from looking at the similarities in different organisms and processes while de-emphasizing the traditional taxonomic approach of cataloguing differences.

Yet, as Pope has pointed out: "The proper study of mankind is man." Facts gained from animal teratologic studies cannot be assumed to apply to the human. The ease with which thalidomide causes malformations in man and the difficulty in reproducing these malformations in animal models emphasize this point. Animal studies may help establish the teratogenic *potential* of a drug and define teratologic mechanisms, but the final proof that a drug is teratogenic in man must be demonstrated in man. In this connection, the distinction between a **teratogen** and a **mutagen** should be made (although the same agent, such as radiation, may have both teratogenic and mutagenic effects). **A teratogen acts on the somatic cells of the developing organism. A mutagen acts on the germ cells and alters the genetic material.**

Experimental teratogenesis and the ways that teratogens may be used to alter embryonic processes in animal models have been reviewed extensively in the literature.[3,4] From animal studies and from observations in the human, a number of principles have emerged.

PRINCIPLES OF TERATOLOGY

Fetal Susceptibility. The developing embryo is not a "little adult." The requirements for making a heart, a brain, a bone or an eye are quite different from those for maintaining these structures. One dose of thalidomide, which effectively accomplishes its purpose of tranquilizing the mother without having any damaging effect on her, may horribly malform her unborn child. A corollary of this principle, first documented by the classic work of Warkany in the 1940's, is that the fetus is not as well protected by the uterus as had previously been assumed.

Periods of Vulnerability and Exposure. Teratogens act at vulnerable periods of embryogenesis and organogenesis. There is no demonstrable teratogenic effect prior to implantation (one week in the human). The type of exposure is more likely to be a short-term one (one or a few doses of thalidomide rather than months of chronic thalidomide ingestion). Long-term exposures generally cause the death of the embryo or may have a much lower degree of teratogenicity, presumably because of induction of detoxifying enzymes. Taking the effect of thalidomide on the human heart as an example, the teratogenic exposure occurs about two weeks before the completion of the developmental event. That is, a thalidomide exposure in the fifth week causes a ventricular septal defect, although ventricular septal closure does not occur until the seventh week. Dextroamphetamine exposure also appears to have its teratogenic effect about two weeks prior to the completion of the embryologic event. From mouse studies, antiheart antibody must be given later in gestation than dextroamphetamine to cause ventricular septal defect. In general, however, the teratogenic exposure occurs a considerable time before the developmental event. This is what is treacherous about teratogenic insults: many organ systems, such as the heart, are vulnerable at a time when the mother is just becoming convinced she is truly pregnant and not "just a week or two late." She then decides to stop taking dextroamphetamine for her "diet," but this may already be too late.

Which Agents are Teratogenic? Although relatively few agents have been identified that are potent teratogens capable of causing malformations in a significant proportion of individuals exposed at a vulnerable period of embryogenesis, probably hundreds of agents are teratogenic within a given set of circumstances, such as hereditary predisposition to a malformation and hereditary predisposition to respond adversely to a drug or virus or some interacting environmental factor such as a nutritional deficiency. Rubella and thalidomide, which are discussed later in this chapter, are probably less representative of teratogens than Coxsackie virus or dextroamphetamine.

Relationship to Dose. In experimental animals the teratogenic dose usually overlaps the dose that will kill some of the embryos. There are exceptions, however. Some agents that will kill embryos do not seem to be teratogenic at sublethal doses. Conversely, teratogenic effects may occur at doses well below the embryo-lethal dose, thalidomide being an outstanding example.

There is an additional dosage relationship. In experimental animals, the dosage of drugs on a milligram per kilogram basis required to produce a malformation is usually many times the normal dosage in the human. One assumption is that large doses in experimental animals may mimic the effect of "normal" doses in humans who have a predisposition (such as delayed clearance, abnormal metabolic response, etc.). Pharmacogenetics, an entire subdiscipline of genetics, addresses itself to related problems.

Hereditary Predisposition to the Effects of a Given Teratogen. Clearly, there are species and individual differences in response to the teratogenic effects of an agent. The malformations so readily produced by thalidomide in the human could not be reproduced in a number of traditional animal models, and not all pregnant women who ingested thalidomide during vulnerable periods of embryogenesis produced malformed infants. There is ample experimental evidence of genetic differences that influence the embryo's response to a teratogen, and these may be single gene or polygenic differences.

Interaction of Teratogens and Other Agents. Drugs in combination with other drugs may produce malformations when the drugs taken singly would have no teratogenic effect. It is the usual case that not one but several drugs are consumed by a pregnant woman for a given disorder. Furthermore, a given drug may be teratogenic only through interaction with another environmental factor, such as a virus or nutritional deficiency. From the clinical point of view, this is another pitfall in the path of safe drug administration, and from the research point of view, a further obstacle in defining specific teratogens.

Specificity of Teratogens. Certain drugs and viruses cause malformations and patterns of malformation that are characteristic (e.g., phocomelia from thalidomide; patent ductus arteriosus, pulmonary branch stenosis, deafness and cataracts from rubella virus). These patterns must be related to special properties of the teratogens: in the case of drugs, specific metabolic effects; in the case of rubella virus, the fetal and neonatal immunologic tolerance to the virus with consequent continued proliferation interfering with the host's normal processes of growth and development.

Hereditary Predisposition to the Malformation. This brings us back to the concept of multifactorial inheritance and allows us to summarize the *three components of a typical teratogenic exposure* leading to a malformation: (1) hereditary predisposition to a malformation; (2) hereditary predisposition to the effects of a given teratogen; and (3) administration of the teratogen at a vulnerable period of embryogenesis. The latter two components have been discussed in preceding paragraphs.

Using animal models, about 1% of C57 Bl/6 mice "spontaneously" have a ventricular septal defect. Exposure of the pregnant female to a single large dose of dextroamphetamine at day 8 of gestation produces ventricular septal defects in 11% of offspring. Exposure to antiheart antibody on day 8 produces ventricular septal defects in 20% of C57 Bl/6 offspring. The A/J strain has a low spontaneous frequency of atrial septal defect. Similar exposures of female A/J mice to dextroamphetamine and antiheart antibody on day 8 of gestation produce atrial septal defects in 13% and 22% of offspring respectively. Thus, the C57 Bl/6 strain appears to have a hereditary predisposition to ventricular septal defect, and the A/J strain, a predisposition to atrial septal defect.[10] The same teratogens cause different lesions in the two strains of mice. The predisposition to a rather specific heart defect is seen in human studies in which affected members of a family have the same anomaly: ventricular septal defect in one family, atrial septal defect in another (see Chapter 24).

From experience with humans and experimental animals, it would appear that in the majority of instances in which maldevelopment is produced by a teratogen, there is a hereditary predisposition to the specific malformation that results. The defect occurs when exposure to one or more of any number of teratogens occurs at a vulnerable period of embryogenesis. There are probably few teratogens like thalidomide and rubella virus, which are capable of producing such a high frequency of malformations following maternal exposure in the first trimester. Even in some of these cases there is evidence of a hereditary predisposition to the malformation, as will be discussed in the section on the rubella syndrome.

ROLE OF TERATOGENS IN HUMAN MALFORMATIONS

Even before the thalidomide disaster and rubella pandemic of the past decade, parents of children with birth defects were deeply concerned about the effects of drugs, illnesses, radiation and other environmental triggers on their unborn children. This concern has become intensified by continuing publicity surrounding documented and potential environmental hazards.

The question of teratogens in human malformations may be looked at from two perspectives: that of the patient and his family and that of the research investigator. As in other sections of this text, we will use a clinical (and investigative) example to illustrate the problem.

Clinical Example—Dextroamphetamine and Congenital Malformations. An unusually large and handsome newborn male infant was observed on the second day of life to have cyanosis. A cardiac catheterization revealed that the infant had transposition of the great vessels; since this was before the era of the Rashkind septostomy procedure, a Blalock-Hanlon atrial septectomy was performed. The mother volunteered that she had been taking dextroamphetamine sporadically during the first two months of her pregnancy and regularly during the last trimester to curb her appetite and control her weight gain. She asked directly whether this drug could have caused her baby's heart disease.

This proved to be a more provocative question than the mother had anticipated, because she was the third mother in two weeks to present with this history of having a child with transposition of the great vessels and a first-trimester exposure to dextroamphetamine. To the first mother in this series of cases we had responded with the confident assurance that her baby's heart disease and the dextroamphetamine exposure were unrelated. To the second we had said that there was no evidence in the literature implicating dextroamphetamine as a teratogen. But to the third mother we had to confess that, although there was no evidence, our suspicions were now aroused and we would have to investigate the problem.

The parents of a child with a birth defect usually have some feelings of guilt. If the etiology is clearly genetic, they still feel some guilt regarding the contribution of "bad genes," however vague this concept may be. However, when a readily avoidable environmental exposure such as an unnecessary drug comes under suspicion, the cause-and-effect relationship becomes less vague to the parents, more easily understood and more guilt-producing. To this mother, the sense of guilt became very great indeed. "If only I had possessed more willpower I could have dieted without dextroamphetamine and my baby would have been normal," she said. We argued that there was still no evidence for an etiologic relationship, but the mother had already reached her own conclusions. In subsequent visits she began to seek for those who should share her guilt. The parents went as far as employing legal counsel with the aim of bringing a suit against the physician who prescribed the dextroamphetamine and the company that manufactured it. We were eventually successful in dissuading the parents from pursuing this course. Although different families react in different ways to the birth of a child with a serious defect, the reaction in this case is by no means uncommon. Guilt and transference of guilt are all too frequently encountered and must be handled with considerable sensitivity.

The next problem was to try to discover whether dextroamphetamine really had the potential to produce human malformations, specifically congenital heart disease. The ultimate answer would be gained from studies in humans, so prospective and retrospective clinical studies were instituted. As a collateral investigation, experimental studies were undertaken in other animal species. This sequence, a clinical observation arousing suspicion and leading to investigations in humans and in animal models, is rather typical of studies in this area. Large multicenter surveillance studies have theoretic value, but in practice have produced very little useful information. One would assume that some of the more sophisticated statistical analyses could effectively sort out teratogens if the input is sufficiently comprehensive and accurate. However, the original input of data depends on the interest and motivation of those obtaining the primary data, and when these are busy physicians the input is likely to be incomplete.

Retrospective studies are studies that begin after the event and take as the index case a patient with the disorder under investigation. The retrospective protocol employed in the study of dextroamphetamine required an extensive teratogenic history, developed after trying out several history forms and selecting questions that seemed to provide maximal information and minimal bias. The questions did not explore just dextroamphetamine exposure, but exposure to over 100 teratogens and potential teratogens, viruses, radiation and chemicals as well as drugs. Many questions were asked more than once in alternative forms, and often the second reworded question elicited a positive answer. Positive answers were verified from records in most cases.

With this form, a genetic history form was also completed, patiently repeating questions and, in an unhurried fashion, drawing the complete pedigree. The minimal time required for completion of an initial teratogenic and genetic history was two hours at the beginning of the study and, as the study progressed, no less than one hour

(by an experienced history-taker) even for a small family. A single history-taking session was rarely sufficient for either the genetic or the teratogenic history. Family members had to be contacted who were more familiar with "the cousin who died in infancy and may have been blue." Autopsy records had to be obtained when possible. Physicians had to be contacted regarding prescriptions and a search undertaken of medicine cabinets for nonprescription items.

Without elaborating on all the pitfalls a few points should be made. Maternal memory bias is an enormous obstacle. In the first report of our data we admitted into the study only patients who were less than two years of age at the time the history was taken on the assumption that the mother's memory of events during a pregnancy more distant than two years would be unreliable. (For our second report, no patient more than one year of age was included because we felt that our earlier histories were still biased.) This applies to teratogenic exposures in which a physician has not been involved (mild infections, nonprescription drugs, toxic chemicals, etc.). One would think that prescription items at least would be easy to verify. Some physicians are very cooperative; surprisingly, others are not. Even the most adept contacts by mail and by phone from investigating physicians or social workers with permits signed by parents and a comprehensive explanation of the nature of the study will not pry information from some physicians. Fear of lawsuits must be playing a role here.

All the impediments to obtaining the primary data notwithstanding, one must make the best of what one has and analyze what has been obtained. All known etiologic possibilities and interactions must be considered. A control group *matched* for as many factors as possible must be utilized. Age, race, socioeconomic level, place of residence and type of employment are some of the considerations in matching. The control proband should have some defect, not environmentally induced, to reduce maternal memory bias.

The influence of inheritance was estimated from the genetic histories. The vulnerable period of cardiac development was placed within what we considered at the time to be rather broad limits. Data were then obtained on maternal dextroamphetamine exposure from probands under two years of age with congenital heart defects and a matched control group without heart lesions. A statistically significant difference was not detectable between the two groups in maternal dextroamphetamine exposure, but a highly significant difference was noted regarding positive family history for congenital heart lesions.

The study was continued after the first publication of no statistical difference and data collected during subsequent years were analyzed. For the follow-up study only infants one year of age were admitted and the period of vulnerability was increased to coincide with recent evidence regarding the time of closure of the ventricular septum during embryonic development. This time a statistically significant difference was obtained between the congenital heart and control groups with respect to maternal exposure to dextroamphetamine at the vulnerable stage of cardiac development and with regard to positive family history for congenital heart lesions.[11]

Thus two studies conducted by the same investigators produced conflicting evidence. While it was the opinion of the investigators that the second study provided the more accurate input and profited from the mistakes of the first study, the fact remains that the studies did conflict. This brief recapitulation illustrates how difficult it is to conduct retrospective studies to confirm or disprove a clinical clue regarding the teratogenic effects of a given agent on the human subject.

A **prospective study** on the teratogenic effects of maternal exposure to dextroamphetamine was initiated at the same time as the retrospective study. The obstetric service of a large private multispecialty group from which a number of patients with congenital heart defects had recently originated (including one of the infants with transposition) agreed to allow our investigative team to obtain teratogenic histories from their patients. This looked like a promising arrangement because we had discovered that dextroamphetamine was commonly, almost routinely, prescribed by this group. However, one of our medical students involved in chart review at the group clinic mentioned that we were most interested in dextroamphetamine. The obstetricians immediately stopped prescribing the drug and lost their enthusiasm for our reviewing their charts. Although we obtained a small number of prospective patients and a larger number of retrospective patients, the opportunity to find the answers we sought from this group was lost.

In this particular study the investigative team was hampered by working in a medical center where the vast majority of obstetric patients were private and the interest of their obstetricians in the study was difficult to arouse. The one large clinic service was made up of patients from a low socioeconomic level in which interest in prenatal care was so sporadic and histories so unreliable as to make any conclusions suspect. The final chance to conduct a prospective study among patients who were reasonably good historians and who had a satisfactory period of prenatal care was afforded by a clinic at one of the private hospitals within the medical center. Shortly after the prospective study was instituted, the clinic was discontinued and this last group of patients was lost to the study. Needless to say, many fewer than the total number of prospective patients required by the research protocol were obtained.

It should not be assumed that the logistic difficulties encountered by one investigative team in carrying out a prospective study on the relationship of teratogens to human malformations will impede the efforts of other teams. However, from this review some insight may be gained as to why there is so little information on the role of teratogens in human maldevelopment.

The studies in experimental animals of the teratogenic effects of dextroamphetamine were relatively easy by comparison. The pertinent results and inferences from these studies have been discussed on page 273. Although no "proof" regarding human teratogenic effects could be derived from the animal studies, our thinking was greatly influenced about how teratogens produce cardiac malformations, about predisposition to lesions, and about vulnerable periods of cardiogenesis. This is really a great deal of information and just about what one should hope to gain from studies in experimental teratogenesis.

SYNDROMES PRODUCED BY TERATOGENS

Only two teratogens have been established as being responsible for widespread disability: rubella virus and thalidomide. Other agents, including folic acid antagonists and androgenic steroids, have proved to be teratogenic to the human but on a much smaller scale; still other drugs are strongly suspected of teratogenic effect, including anticonvulsants, amphetamines, hypoglycemics, alkylating agents and aspirin.[12] The possibility that hundreds of agents may be somewhat teratogenic has been suggested. That thalidomide and rubella virus *are* teratogenic has been documented beyond question.

Rubella Syndrome. The rubella pandemic of 1964-5 had a medical, sociologic and economic impact that is still being measured. Estimates of the costs of medical care and rehabilitation have been in the billions of dollars. Far exceeding this is the loss and tragedy experienced at the level of the individual family.

The rubella virus was first recognized as a cause of birth defects by the Australian ophthalmologist, Gregg, in 1941.[5] Cataracts, hearing loss and cardiac disease (mainly patent ductus arteriosus) were recognized as the early triad of abnormal-ities resulting from maternal rubella infection during the first trimester of pregnancy. Following the pandemic of 1964-5, additional features were recognized and referred to by some authors as the "expanded" rubella syndrome. These features include neonatal purpura, hepatosplenomegaly, hepatitis, bone lesions, psychomotor retardation and anemia.

Congenital Heart Disease. The most common manifestation of the rubella syndrome in most series is congenital cardiovascular disease. Personal experience with the series in Houston revealed that 71% of patients with congenital rubella had some form of cardiovascular disease. Peripheral pulmonary branch stenosis (with or without pulmonary valve stenosis) was the most common, being present in 55% of patients, while patent ductus arteriosus was present in 43%. A variety of other lesions was found in 8% of patients, including ventricular septal defect, atrial septal defect, tetralogy of Fallot and aortic stenosis. Some patients had more than one lesion.

There was no positive family history of pulmonary branch stenosis and a nonsignificant familial history of patent ductus arteriosus in patients having these lesions. The teratogenic mechanism here is unusual, if not unique, in that the rubella virus may still be recovered from the ductus at the time of surgery or from the pulmonary artery branches. The living virus appears to participate in a progressive disease process for months or years. Indeed, mild pulmonary branch stenosis determined at cardiac catheterization at one month of age may be quite severe at a subsequent catheterization two years later.

With regard to other heart lesions, such as ventricular septal defect and tetralogy of Fallot, the teratogenic insult appears to interact with a hereditary predisposition, as visualized in multifactorial inheritance and as developed in Chapter 24. A positive family history for these heart lesions could be elicited in about the same percentage (38%) of patients with rubella syndrome as in our earlier survey of genetic factors in congenital heart disease (34%).

Deafness. Generally, the next most common manifestation of the rubella syndrome is deafness (56% of patients). Several levels of involvement have been observed: central, organ of Corti and middle ear. The usual defect results from damage to the organ of Corti. Hearing loss is permanent, may be unilateral or bilateral and may be progressive. Vestibular function may also be impaired. Interestingly, from the Houston series, among those rubella patients being followed in our heart clinic who also had deafness, a significant number had a family history of deafness. A similar positive family history for deafness in patients with deafness associated with the rubella syndrome was found in Stockholm.[1] Is the rubella virus capable of producing deafness in certain genotypes and not in others? Is this another example of a genetic-environmental interaction? More firm conclusions would require a study of the types of deafness in the index cases and in affected family members.

Cataracts, Glaucoma and Retinopathy. Cataracts were the lesions calling initial attention to the entire rubella syndrome. Eye defects are present in 40% of patients with congenital rubella. The vast majority of lesions are cataracts and/or a patchy retinopathy. A small percentage of patients have transient cloudy cornea or progressive glaucoma.

Psychomotor retardation was found in varying degrees in about 40% of patients in the 1964-5 pandemic. The rubella virus has frequently been isolated from the spinal fluid in surviving infants, as well as those autopsied and found to have evidence of chronic encephalitis and meningitis. Early symptomatology varies from lethargy to hyperactivity and hypotonicity to hypertonicity. Poor feeding is common; seizures and opisthotonus are uncommon and indicate a poor prognosis. At least one neurologic abnormality persists in the majority of survivors who had evidence of central nervous system involvement in infancy. The degree of discrete intellectual deficit has been difficult to assess in the presence of sensory deprivation in children with multisystem involvement.

Neonatal Purpura. Approximately 30% of patients with congenital rubella have a thrombocytopenic purpura characterized by small discrete macules ("blueberry muffin lesions"), sometimes limited to a few petechiae and occasionally associated with large purpuric lesions. The purpura usually resolves in a few weeks, but serves as a signal that there are likely to be serious associated problems of the "expanded" rubella syndrome.

Other Neonatal Manifestations. Hepatosplenomegaly and, less often, hepatitis and hemolytic anemia are found in neonates with congenital rubella. Characteristic x-ray findings in the long bones include poorly defined and irregular zones of calcification with metaphyseal radiolucencies (Fig. 18-1). A bulging anterior fontanelle and prominent metopic suture may be present.

Immunologic Considerations. During the height of the pandemic, a number of pregnant nurses caring for these sick infants contracted rubella and in turn delivered infants with the birth defects of the rubella syndrome. Through longitudinal observation it became obvious that these infants could shed virus for months and in some rare cases even years.

At a time when our index of suspicion was high following the pandemic, we examined a five-year-old boy in cardiac clinic who had stigmata of rubella syndrome (patent ductus arteriosus, pulmonary artery branch stenosis, deafness and glaucoma). However, his mother and two older siblings also had pulmonary branch stenosis, deafness and cataracts or glaucoma. There was no history of any member of the family having had rubella. We were unable to isolate rubella virus from the index case or the mother although both had positive hemagglutinin inhibition (HI) antibody tests

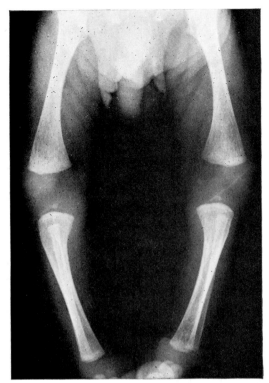

Figure 18-1. "Expanded" congenital rubella syndrome. Metaphyseal radiolucencies of long bones with irregular zones of calcification.

without rising titers to suggest recent infection. A recent publication documented viruria in a 29-year-old woman with the congenital rubella syndrome.[9] This woman had no serologic evidence of a recent rubella infection. It was postulated that an intercurrent infection led to increased shedding of congenitally acquired rubella virus. This finding confirmed our suspicion about our family and illustrates how long (in rare instances) rubella virus may persist in the human host.

This is an example of immunologic tolerance. The viral invasion takes place before the fetus is immunologically mature enough to recognize the virus as being "nonself." Thus, for varying lengths of time, there is tolerance to the virus until the host mounts an immunologic attack of sufficient strength to destroy the invader.

Prevention. Rubella as a cause of birth defects is now a problem for which there is a reasonable solution.[2] A vaccine that offers a seroconversion rate of 95% is available and being used in women of the reproductive age (who have no serologic evidence of past infection and who are not pregnant at the time of immunization) and in school children.

Thalidomide Syndrome. In late 1960, the first cases of a new syndrome were recognized in West Germany, and through 1961 amelia, phocomelia and other anomalies became "epidemic" not only in Germany but in other western European countries, Canada and Australia. In Australia, McBride[8] in 1961 gained the clinical insight into the relationship between maternal thalidomide ingestion and the new syndrome. In West Germany, Lenz and Knapp[7] painstakingly developed the evidence that led to an irrefutable indictment of thalidomide in 1962. But the damage was already widespread. Again, as with the rubella syndrome, the cost of medical care and rehabilitation of these patients on a worldwide scale has been enormous, and the tragedy at the level of the individual has been incalculable.

The thalidomide syndrome has been associated with certain characteristic malformations, but there has been involvement of many systems depending on the stage in embryogenesis at which exposure occurred. Limb anomalies are perhaps the most characteristic stigmata of thalidomide embryopathy. These malformations range from mild dysplasia of the thumbs to complete absence of all limbs (Fig. 18-2). A typical "thalidomide baby" would have some combination of the following: absent or markedly underdeveloped and hypoplastic arms, ranging from phocomelia through absence of radius and thumb to triphalangeal thumb; capillary hemangioma of the midface; aplasia or hypoplasia of the external ear with atresia of the canal; a congenital heart defect; a stenotic or atretic lesion somewhere in the gastrointestinal tract; and

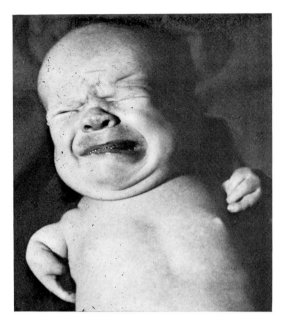

Figure 18-2. Phocomelia in infant with thalidomide syndrome.

malformed legs, ranging from phocomelia through tibial absence to club feet.

Lenz, through careful analysis of almost 800 patients with thalidomide embryopathy, was able to devise a timetable specifying at which stages of embryogenesis thalidomide exerted its teratogenic effect on which developing structures. This has proved useful in studying the effects of other potential teratogens on organogenesis. For example, no malformations occurred when thalidomide was taken before 34 days *after the onset of the last menstrual period.* This coincides with the general expectation of relative resistance to teratogenic effect during the first weeks of gestation, the period before implantation and shortly thereafter. The vulnerable period was essentially from the 34th to the 50th day after the last menstrual period, a 16-day period from three to five weeks of gestational age. For hypoplasia or absence of the arms, thalidomide exposure must occur between the 39th and 44th days; for similar malformations of the legs, between the 42nd and 48th days; for tetralogy

of Fallot, truncus arteriosus and anomalies of truncoconal maldevelopment, between the 41st and 43rd days.[6]

In general, the teratogenic exposure to thalidomide precedes the completion of the developmental event by about two weeks. Studies of comparable developmental stages in animal models suggest that many teratogens would have to be administered on about the same timetable as thalidomide to produce malformations (e.g., dextroamphetamine in the mouse), while other teratogens may have somewhat different timetables (e.g., antiheart antibody).

These and many other insights derived from the tragic experience of thalidomide have contributed significantly to our understanding of human teratology and have followed the Baconian admonition regarding "monstrosities, well-examined and described."

ATTEMPTED ABORTION, TERATOGENS AND MALFORMATIONS

It is not uncommon that a newborn with multiple congenital anomalies is the first-born child of a very young mother, often unwed or wed after conception. A careful history based on good rapport between the mother and genetic counselor frequently will reveal an attempted abortion with a variety of drugs taken in large doses. Two important requirements for teratogenesis are met under these circumstances: the drugs are taken at the most vulnerable period of organogenesis (just at the time the mother first realizes she is pregnant), and the dose of the drug is very large, not large enough to kill mother or embryo, but large enough to malform. (In experimental teratogenesis it is customary to give dosages of drugs many times higher on an mg/kg body weight basis than the therapeutic dosage for the human.) However, except for aminopterin, there is no well-documented relation between attempted abortion and malformations.

VACTERL ASSOCIATION

This acronym has been progressively lengthened to encompass a number of co-existing anomalies: V = vertebral; A = anal; C = cardiac; T = tracheal; E = esophageal; R = renal; and L = limb. In general, we use this designation when three or more of these malformations are found in the same patient. Only within the past decade have these anomalies been described as occurring together in a syndrome. Actually the structures involved recapitulate those affected in the thalidomide syndrome, although the pattern of presentation differs somewhat. Presently, an important teratogenic input is suspected in the etiology, and exposure to progestogen/estrogen has been implicated in a preliminary study.[10] The influence of other teratogens interacting or acting discretely is subject to further investigation.

REFERENCES

1. Anderson, H., Bengt Barr, E. E., and Wedenberg, E.: Genetic disposition—a prerequisite for maternal rubella deafness. Arch. Otolaryng., 91:141, 1970.
2. Cooper, L. Z.: Rubella: a preventable cause of birth defects. *In* Intrauterine Infections. Birth Defects: Original Article Series, 4:23, 1968. New York, The National Foundation.
3. Fraser, F. C.: The use of teratogens in the analysis of abnormal developmental mechanisms. *In* First International Conference on Congenital Malformations. Philadelphia, J. B. Lippincott, 1961. p. 179.
4. ———: Experimental teratogenesis in relation to congenital malformations in man. *In* Second International Conference on Congenital Malformations. New York, International Medical Congress Ltd., 1964. p. 277.
5. Gregg, N. M.: Congenital cataract following German measles in the mother. Trans. Ophthal. Soc. Aust., 3:35, 1941.
6. Lenz, W.: Chemicals and malformations in man. *In* Second International Conference on Congenital Malformations. New York, International Medical Congress Ltd., 1964. p. 263.
7. Lenz, W., and Knapp, K.: Thalidomide embryopathy. Arch. Env. Health, 5:100, 1962.
8. McBride, W. G.: Thalidomide and congenital abnormalities. Lancet, 2:1358, 1961.
9. Menser, M. A., *et al.*: Rubella viruria in 29-year-old woman with congenital rubella. Lancet, 2:797, 1971.
10. Nora, J. J., and Nora, A. H.: Birth defects and oral contraceptives. Lancet, 1:941, 1973.
11. Nora, J. J., Sommerville, R. J., and Fraser, F. C.: Homologies for congenital heart diseases: Murine models influenced by dextroamphetamine. Teratology, 1:413, 1968.
12. Nora, J. J., *et al.*: Dexamphetamine a possible environmental trigger in cardiovascular malformations. Lancet, 1:1290, 1970.
13. Wilson, J. G.: Present status of drugs as teratogens in man. Teratology, 7:3, 1973.

Chapter 19
DERMATOGLYPHICS

TERMINOLOGY

Dermatoglyphics are the dermal ridge configurations on the digits, palms and soles. They begin to develop about the 13th week of prenatal life[7] as the fetal mounds on the digit tips, interdigital, thenar and hypothenar areas of the hand and the corresponding areas of the foot begin to regress. The pattern formation is complete by the 19th week.

Certain syndromes include unusual combinations of dermatoglyphic patterns. These can help to establish a probability index for a particular diagnosis, as first demonstrated by Walker in the case of Down syndrome. This approach has been extended to a number of other syndromes,[5] but there are now so many invalid claims for associations of dermatoglyphic patterns with syndromes and diseases that the literature must be approached with caution.

Finger Patterns. The patterns on the finger tips are of three main types, classified by the number of triradii present (Fig. 19-1). The simplest pattern is the arch (A). A simple arch has no triradius; a tented arch has a central triradius. The loop has a single triradius and is called ulnar (U) or radial (R), depending on the side to which it opens. The whorl (W) has two or more triradii and may be a double loop or, more commonly, a circular type of pattern.

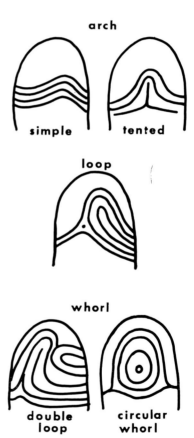

Figure 19-1. The three basic finger patterns. The arch has no triradius or central triradius. The loop has a single triradius and opens to one side. The whorl has two or more triradii.

287

The frequency of these patterns for Caucasians is shown in Table 19-1. Conventionally the digits are numbered from thumb to little finger. Arches and radial loops have the lowest overall frequency; when present they occur most often on digit 2, especially in the case of radial loops. Whorls occur most often on digits 4, 1 and 2. Ulnar loops occur more frequently than any other pattern type. The most frequent combination of patterns is ten ulnar loops. Another common distribution is shown in Figure 19-2.

The pattern frequencies vary somewhat with side and with sex, females having slightly more arches and fewer whorls than males. There are also racial differences in pattern frequencies. Orientals, for example, have a higher frequency of whorls than European-Americans.[2]

Palmar Patterns. The palm can be divided into the hypothenar, thenar and four interdigital areas (I_1, I_2, I_3 and I_4) (see Fig. 19-2). The normal palm has a triradius at the base of the palm between the thenar and hypothenar areas. This is the axial triradius (t). A variety of patterns (loops and whorls) may be found in the hypothenar area, which are classified by the location and number of triradii. A pattern in either I_3 or I_4 is common and a pattern in the thenar/I_1 and the I_2 area is less common. The mainline from the a triradius us-

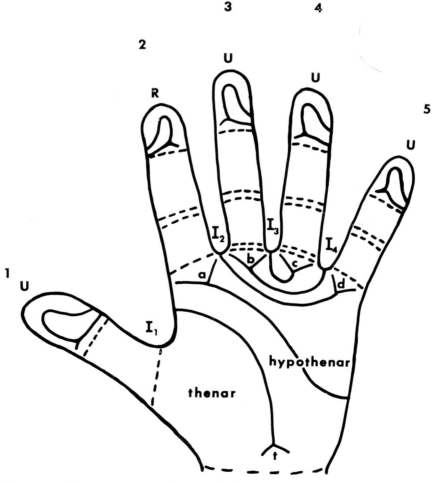

Figure 19-2. One of the more common finger and palm patterns.

ually exits in the hypothenar area, that from b in I_4, that from c in I_3 and that from d in I_2. The axial triradius t is usually proximal, but may be displaced distally. Its height from the base of the hand can be measured as a percentage of the height from the distal wrist crease to the proximal crease at the base of the third digit; t is defined as a height of 0-14%, t' as 15-39% and t" as greater than 40% of the total height. This method of classification is less age-dependent than the alternative method, measuring the atd angle. Since both methods are used in the literature we have established approximate values from our data for converting the angle measurements to t, t' or t". We define t as less than 46° and t" as greater than 63°.

Soles. Because of the difficulties in printing the foot, observations are limited largely

TABLE 19-1. Frequency (%) of Pattern Types on the Fingers*

	Digit					
Pattern	1	2	3	4	5	Total
A	3	10	8	2	1	5
U	65	36	72	58	86	63
R	0	23	4	1	0	6
W	32	31	16	39	13	26

*The values for left and right and male and female do not differ appreciably and have been combined for simplicity. (Adapted from Holt, S. B.: The Genetics of Dermal Ridges. Springfield, Ill., Charles C Thomas, 1968.)

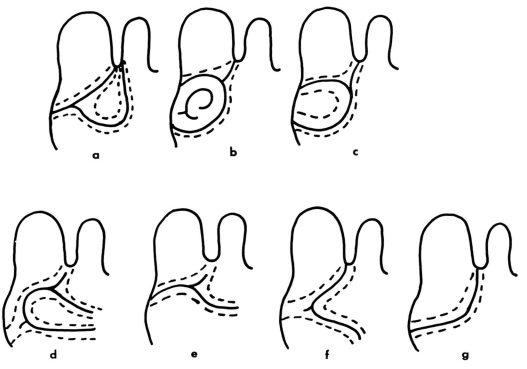

Figure 19-3. Hallucal patterns in order of frequency: (a) distal loop; (b) whorl; (c) tibial loop; (d) fibular loop; (e) proximal arch; (f) fibular arch; (g) tibial arch (no triradius).

to the hallucal area, although other areas can also give valuable information. The patterns in the hallucal area are shown in Figure 19-3. The most frequent patterns in normal individuals are the whorl and the large distal loop ($<$ 21 ridges).

Flexion Creases. Strictly speaking, the flexion creases are not dermatoglyphics but have come to be included in dermatoglyphic analysis. They represent places of attachment of the skin to underlying structures and are formed between the seventh and 14th week of development.[7]

The palmar creases generally consist of a distal and proximal transverse crease and a thenar crease (Fig. 19-4). About 6% of normal individuals have at least one **simian crease**—a single crease extending across the entire palm—or a **transitional** simian crease

—two transverse creases joined by an equally deep, short crease (type 1) or a single crease with a branch above and below the main crease (type 2). Considerable variations in reported frequencies result from whether transitional forms are counted as simian creases. About 11% of normal individuals have a **Sydney line**, in which the proximal transverse crease extends across the entire palm, rather than stopping short of the ulnar border.

METHODS OF OBSERVATION AND PRINTING

If the dermal ridges are too small or poorly developed to observe directly, as in the newborn, an ordinary otoscope provides a satisfactory light and magnification for observation. The position of the hand or foot is adjusted to get the best interplay of

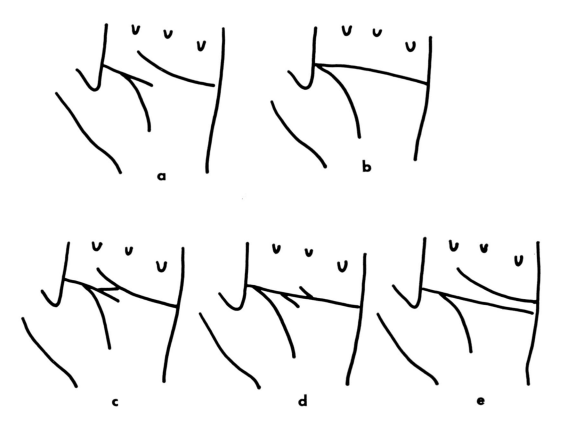

Figure 19-4. Palmar creases: (a) normal; (b) simian; (c) transitional type 1; (d) transitional type 2; (e) Sydney.

available and direct light. Depending on the interests of the observer and the nature of the patient's defect, the patterns may be recorded directly or printed for a permanent record.

For printing of infants, Hollister* ink pads and paper are useful. The area to be printed should be clean, dry and warm; after being "inked" with the pad, the area is placed lightly on the paper. Too much pressure will blur the print. For children over four years and for adults the Faurot† inkless method works well. Placing the paper over a sponge rubber pad helps one to get a complete print when the hand is too large to manipulate easily. Care must be taken not to use too much ink or pressure. A detailed description of the inkless method by Walker[11] is useful to anyone using either method of printing.

USES AND LIMITATIONS OF DERMATOGLYPHIC ANALYSIS

The strong resemblance of dermatoglyphic patterns in pairs of monozygotic twins suggests that their determination has a major genetic component. One would therefore expect that when a large number of genes were missing or present in excess the dermatoglyphics would be altered. This appears to be so. In several chromosomal syndromes these alterations are consistent enough to be of diagnostic value.

Intuitively, one might expect that the dermal ridge patterns reflect the conformation of the fetal hand at the time of ridge development, as first suggested by Cummins (1926). If so, we would expect the dermal ridges to be altered when the limbs are deformed, and they are.[4] We would therefore not expect the dermatoglyphic patterns to be diagnostically useful if the patient has gross malformations of the limbs, as in Apert syndrome; the patterns reflect the obvious anatomic defect. They may be useful, however, as a reflection of more subtle morphologic changes in the embryo. Cu-

*Hollister, Inc., 833 New Orleans St., Chicago, Ill.
†Faurot Inc., 299 Broadway, New York, N.Y.

taneous syndactyly, for instance, is a feature of a number of syndromes but it is sometimes difficult to decide on gross examination whether it is present in a minor degree. Fusion of the triradii at the base of the digits is good evidence that the basic defect resulting in syndactyly was present when the ridges formed, even if the syndactyly is not obvious at birth.

Another example is the de Lange syndrome. Patients generally have short fingers, syndactyly, low-set thumbs and characteristic dermal patterns. We are not surprised that the few de Lange patients we have seen who do not have the "typical" hand shape also do not have the "typical" dermatoglyphics.

Examination of dermatoglyphics may help to decide whether a causative agent was acting early or late. For example, the unusual longitudinal mainline configurations in a number of patients with arthrogryposis[1] suggest that the defect was present in these patients at least as early as the 13th to 19th week. When there is no early anatomic effect, as in the simple biochemical disorders, there is also no change in the dermatoglyphics.

BIASES AND PITFALLS

It is often assumed that a pattern on one finger has no relation to the patterns on other fingers of the same individual, but in fact there is a tendency for them to be alike more often than expected if they were independent of one another. This has been shown in both normal individuals and those with Down syndrome. Chi square tests on differences in pattern frequency between groups assume independence of observations and are therefore unreliable indicators of statistical significance. Furthermore, dermal patterns are largely inherited and inclusion of several members of a single sibship will bias the sample. Neglect of these points, use of too small a sample, failure to match control populations for race and sex, and inappropriate use (or nonuse) of statistical tests can lead to much confusion, as has been pointed out for the dermatoglyphics of patients with congenital heart disease,[8] leukemia and schizophrenia.

Another bias in establishing the dermatoglyphic features of a syndrome may arise if the etiology is unknown. Since syndromes are identified by a characteristic association of features, each of which may sometimes be absent, cases with relatively few features or lacking the supposedly "cardinal" features may not be accepted as "true" cases of the syndrome. This creates a bias in assessing the frequency of the various features of the syndrome.[6] If a dermatoglyphic pattern is a feature of the syndrome or related to it, it is subject to this bias. For example, one of the criteria for the diagnosis of the de Lange syndrome has been micromelia, with low-set thumbs and syndactyly, and an invariable criterion for the diagnosis of Rubinstein-Taybi syndrome has been broad thumbs and great toes. If the shape of the hand influences the dermal configurations, then omission of cases without these anatomic features will bias the estimate of the frequency of the associated dermatoglyphic features.

In the following sections the dermatoglyphic features of a number of syndromes are reviewed, with emphasis on the features that are sufficiently frequent in the patient and rare in the general population to be diagnostically useful per se.

ZYGOSITY DIAGNOSIS IN TWINS

If dermatoglyphic patterns are in large part genetically determined, then the hands of monozygotic twins should resemble one another as closely as do the two hands of a single individual, which are also genetically identical. This appears to be true, and the argument can be used in reverse to develop an aid to the diagnosis of zygosity. That is, the more closely do the hands of twins resemble one another, the more likely it is that the twins are monozygotic. Several methods have been developed to estimate the probability of monozygosity.[2]

DERMATOGLYPHIC FEATURES OF SYNDROMES

Chromosomal Syndromes. *21 Trisomy (Down) Syndrome.* The dermatoglyphic features of Down syndrome are summarized in Table 19-2. The most useful is the hallucal tibial arch, which is so rare in normal individuals that its presence in a child suspected of having Down syndrome is strong evidence in favor of the diagnosis.

Long before the chromosomal basis of Down syndrome was established, Cummins demonstrated characteristic differences in dermal configurations between affected and normal children. In 1957, Walker used these differences in frequency to derive an estimate of the probability that a child has Down syndrome on the basis of the der-

TABLE 19-2. Dermatoglyphic Features of 21 Trisomy (Down) Syndrome

	Down syndrome %	Control %	Ratio %
hallucal tibial arch	72	ca .5	144.0
small distal loop (< 21 ridges)	32	11	2.9
single crease on digit 5	17	.5	34.0
bilateral t″	82	3	27.3
bilateral simian crease	31	2	15.5
10 ulnar loops on fingers	31	7	4.6
radial loop on digit 4 or 5	13	4	3.3
bilateral I₃ pattern	46	26	1.8
thenar pattern	4	11	0.4

matoglyphics alone. The principle is that for any particular pattern present, the probability that the individual has Down syndrome varies directly with the ratio of that pattern's frequency in patients with Down syndrome to that in normal individuals. A probability index may be derived by multiplying the probabilities for each pattern or, after conversion to logarithms, by adding them. The more differences, and the greater their magnitude, the better the discrimination. The frequency distributions of the index for a group of patients with Down syndrome and controls overlap somewhat, but scores in the nonoverlapping range are strong evidence for or against the diagnosis of Down syndrome. It is assumed that the patterns in the various areas are independent of one another, and although this is not strictly so, the method allows discrimination of about 70% of affected individuals from controls and 76% of controls from affected individuals. The remainder fall into the overlap zone. As Walker suggested, this index could be improved by including other characteristics. Indeed, over 90% of patients with Down syndrome and over 80% of controls can be separated by including such stigmata as Brushfield spots, simian crease, high palate and other features.

Another method using predictive discrimination has been simplified by Reed et al.,[10]

who constructed a nomogram using only four dermatoglyphic traits chosen for their high discriminant value. By this method 81% of patients with Down syndrome and 67% of controls can be discriminated, but more individuals, either normal or affected, fall in the overlap zone than for either of the previous methods. This method has the advantage of simplicity, but occasionally gives false positive results—a more serious error than false negatives.

Another approach was taken by Lu,[3] who has listed all possible combinations of finger patterns and their frequencies in a group of patients with Down syndrome and controls. This will discriminate 89% of those with Down syndrome from those without. With the addition of other dermatoglyphic and clinical information, his method may be very useful.

Finally, Penrose and Loesch[5] have recently developed a dermatoglyphic discriminant for trisomy 21 using a new system of classification and more emphasis on sole patterns. Using this method only 4.6% of cases are misclassified. However, the computations are time-consuming.

13 Trisomy (D_1). Table 19-3 presents the dermatoglyphic features of trisomy D_1. A dermatoglyphic discriminant developed by Penrose and Loesch misclassifies only 5.2% of cases.

TABLE 19-3. Dermatoglyphic Features of 13 Trisomy Syndrome

	Trisomy D_1 %	Control %	Ratio %
bilateral t″	81	3	27.0
bilateral simian crease*	62	2	31.0
4 or more arches	24	3	8.0
radial loop on other than digit 2	55	7	7.9
thenar exit of A-line	81	11	7.5
hallucal tibial loop	42	9	4.7
fibular loop or arch	38	9	4.2
thenar/I_1 pattern	45	11	4.1
bilateral I_3 pattern	58	26	2.2

*Among those who did not have simian creases, several had other types of unusual crease.

TABLE 19-4.   Dermatoglyphic Features of 18 Trisomy (E) Syndrome

	Trisomy E %	Control %	Ratio %
7 or more arches	80	1	80.0
single crease on digit 5	40	.5	80.0
radial loop on digit 1	16	.5	32.0
bilateral simian crease	25	2	12.5
bilateral t″	25	3	8.3

TABLE 19-5.   Dermatoglyphic Features of 5p— Syndrome

	5p— %	Control %	Ratio %
bilateral simian crease	35	2	17.5
8 or more whorls	32	8	4.0
thenar/I_1 pattern	45	11	4.1
bilateral t′	80	35	2.3
I_4 loop left	77	60	1.3
right	86	47	1.8

There is a marked increase in frequency of bilateral high triradii and of bilateral simian creases, but the other differences are not sufficiently striking to carry much weight by themselves.

18 Trisomy (E). Table 19-4 presents the dermatoglyphic features of trisomy E. The high frequency of arches is so striking that less than six arches or more than two whorls would argue strongly against the diagnosis of trisomy E.

4p— Syndrome. There is said to be an increased frequency of low arch patterns on the digits. Of 12 patients in the literature with dermal patterns reported, four had at least four arches on the digits (control 7%). Four out of 20 had bilateral simian creases and 12 out of 16 had hypoplastic ridges.

5p— Syndrome. The dermatoglyphic features of the 5p— syndrome are presented in Table 19-5. All these patients sometimes have partial syndactyly of the hands and feet and fusion of the b and c triradius with or without obvious syndac-tyly. There is some confusion as to the frequency of simian creases in this syndrome because of differences in terminology and definition; however, about one-third of these patients probably have a simian crease bilaterally, which is a striking increase. None of the other differences is striking enough individually to have much diagnostic significance at the level of clinical screening. The triradius is most often in the t′ position and usually does not have an associated hypothenar pattern. The frequency of I_4 loops is increased and in patients with 5p— syndrome, the loop more frequently results from the d rather than the c mainline exiting in I_4. The difference in dermal patterns between 5p— individuals and controls can be used to discriminate the two with 10.5% misclassification.[5]

18p— Syndrome. In this syndrome the finger patterns are not striking. There may be a high axial triradius or simian crease in a few patients. Both of the patients reported by Penrose have a missing c triradius.

18q— Syndrome. Of 25 patients with this syndrome for whom there is some dermatoglyphic information, six have eight or more whorls (control 8%); five have bilateral simian creases (control 2%); four out of 11 have a missing or misplaced triradius at the base of the digits, and three out of five have a fibular arch in the hallucal area (control 4%). Further studies would be of interest to confirm these findings.

45 XO (Turner) Syndrome. In individuals with XO Turner syndrome the A-line exits in the thenar area more frequently than in normal individuals. Unilateral or bridged simian creases and absence of the triradius may be somewhat more common than in normal individuals. Patterns in I_4 are probably less common in Turner syndrome. The total ridge count (TRC), atd angle and ab ridge count are all significantly higher in Turner syndrome than in normal individuals, but there is so much overlap in the distributions that they are not individually useful as diagnostic aids. In Table 19-6 we have chosen cut-off points to provide the best separation, but the degree of discrimination is not impressive.

47 XXY (Klinefelter) Syndrome. Of patients with Klinefelter syndrome, 15% have three or more arches compared to 4% of male controls. There is a slight increase in mean height of the axial triradius and in frequency of hypothenar patterns, and a decrease in frequency of thenar patterns. Although there are some statistically significant differences between Klinefelter patients and normal males, they are not frequent enough or great enough to be of diagnostic value in the individual case.

Gene-determined Syndromes. *Cerebrohepato-renal Syndrome.* A few of these patients initially have been suspected of having Down syndrome, so their dermatoglyphic patterns are of some interest. Of 15 patients from the literature plus one unpublished case, eight had bilateral simian creases or bridged creases, three had hypoplastic ridges, two had a wide-spaced first toe and one had a single crease on the fifth digit, all features in common with Down syndrome. In contrast to Down syndrome, camptodactyly was frequent and a few had long fingers with narrow fingernails. Unfortunately, finger and palm prints are

TABLE 19-6. Dermatoglyphic Features of XO (Turner) Syndrome

	XO %	Control %	Ratio %
ab ridge count, 105	13	2	6.5
atd angle, 120	23	4	5.8
TRC ≧ 200	28	6	4.7
thenar exit to A-line	57	14	4.1
bilateral hypothenar patterns	48	18	2.7

TABLE 19-7. Dermatoglyphic Features of Smith-Lemli-Opitz Syndrome

	S.L.O. %	Control %	Ratio %
hallucal tibial arch	(6/19)	.5	64.0
bilateral simian creases	55	2	27.5
bilateral t″	12	3	4.0
8 or more whorls	33	8	4.1

available on only two patients. One of these had ten ulnar loops and one has nine whorls. Both have low axial triradii bilaterally. More information on the dermatoglyphic patterns would be of interest.

Smith-Lemli-Opitz Syndrome. The dermatoglyphic features of this syndrome are presented in Table 19-7. Apart from the tibial arch, none of the differences appears sufficiently distinctive to be of much diagnostic aid individually.

Syndromes of Undetermined Etiology. *Arthrogryposis Multiplex Congenita.* Brehme and Baitsch[1] have described the dermatoglyphics of 14 patients with this syndrome. Half of them had marked longitudinal orientation of the mainlines. Six of the remaining patients have a less striking longitudinal orientation. Some show extension of finger patterns to the skin over the middle phalanges. Analysis of dermal ridges in patients with this disorder may be helpful in determining the time at which the causative agent was acting. Correlations of dermatoglyphic findings with the various types of arthrogryposis would also be of interest.

de Lange Syndrome. The dermatoglyphic features of the de Lange syndrome are shown in Table 19-8. There is an overall increase in arch patterns and a decrease in whorls in this series, but only one patient

TABLE 19-8. Dermatoglyphic Features of de Lange Syndrome

	de Lange %	Control %	Ratio %
single crease on digit 5	78	> .5	156.0
bilateral simian crease	34	2	17.0
absence of a, b, c, or d triradius	48	5	9.6
bilateral t″	22	3	7.3
radial loop on other than digit 2	49	7	7.0
0 whorls on digits	77	24	3.2
thenar/I₁ pattern	22	11	2.0
Hallucal tibial arch	9	.5	18.0
tibial loop	31	9	3.2
bilateral whorl	9	27	.3

TABLE 19-9. Dermatoglyphic Features of Rubinstein-Taybi Syndrome

	Rubinstein-Taybi %	Control %	Ratio %
bilateral I₂ pattern	13	1	13.0
4 or more arches	19	3	6.3
thenar/I₁ pattern	60	11	5.5
bilateral t″	16	3	5.3
bilateral ulnar loop in hypothenar	24	5	4.8
radial loop on other than digit 2	19	7	2.7
bilateral I₃ pattern	47	26	1.8
hallucal distal loop	76	57	1.3
triradius at tip of digit 1	28	?	—

TABLE 19-10. Summary of Unusual Dermatoglyphic Findings in Various Syndromes*

Feature	Control %	Trisomy 21	Trisomy D	Trisomy E	5p−	4p−	18q−	XO Turner	Smith-Lemli-Opitz	Cerebro-hepato-renal	Arthrogryposis multiplex	Rubinstein-Taybi	de Lange	Rubella
8 or more whorls	8	—	—	—	4	—	3	4	4			—	—	4
0 whorls	24	2	2	4	9	+	—	—	—		+	9	3	—
7 or more arches	1	2	12	80								3	7	
radial loop on other than digit 2	7		8	3							+			
radial loop on digit 1	.5	3	24	32									4	
radial loop on digit 4 or 5	4	4	10	2	2									
10 ulnar loops	7		—	—										
triradius at tip of digit 1	?	27	27	8			—	4	4		+	+	7	
bilateral t″	3	—	—	—	2			+			+	5		
bilateral t′	35	3	4	—									2	
bilateral hypothenar pattern	18	—		—	4		+	3			+	2		
thenar/I₁ pattern	11											5		
bilateral I₂ pattern	1	2	2	2			+					13		
bilateral I₃ pattern	26	—	2	4			—					2		
bilateral I₄ pattern	34		—	—	2		++							
thenar exit of A-line	11	—	8	+			+	4			+	—		
ab count of 105 or more	2			+			+	7				+	10	
absent a, b, c, or d triradius	5	72		++							+		9	
hallucal tibial arch	1	—		10					32		+		3	
tibial loop	9		5				+					2	2	
fibular loop or arch	9	3	4	3										
small distal loop	11	—	—	—				+	—			—		
large distal loop	48	8	5	4	17	10	11						6	5
arch (any type)	9	16		13							+	+	18	
bilateral simian crease	2	17	31	40					28	++	+		80	
single crease on digit 5	1	++			+				+					
deep plantar crease	.1		+		+	+			++	+		+		
hypoplastic ridges	?			++								+		
overlapping fingers	?												+	

*The numbers below the syndromes represent the magnitude of increase in frequency of a feature above that of controls: + indicates an increase where accurate figures are not available; − indicates a decrease. A blank space indicates that there is no known change in frequency.

has more than three arches. Radial loops are more frequent than in controls and are often present on digits other than the second. A variety of patterns found in the hallucal area of the feet have frequencies differing from normal. The single crease on the fifth digit is very rare in normal individuals and very common in patients with the de Lange syndrome, and its presence has strong diagnostic value. Bilateral simian creases and hallucal tibial arches are less discriminating, but nevertheless carry some weight. The other differences are not large enough to be individually useful.

Rubinstein-Taybi Syndrome. The dermatoglyphic features of this syndrome are presented in Table 19-9. The individual differences are not likely to be useful in discrimination. Distorted and unusually long distal loops in the hallucal area have been reported in several patients. A more detailed documentation and classification of patterns in this area may be of interest. More information is needed on the correlation of the dermatoglyphic findings with the shape of the hand. However, this requires acceptance of patients without broad thumbs as examples of the syndrome.

Teratologic Syndromes. *Rubella Syndrome.* The evidence that prenatal rubella may cause disturbances of the dermatoglyphic patterns is conflicting. There is probably some increase in frequency of bilateral simian creases, although not enough to be diagnostically helpful,[8] and a statistically significant increase in whorls (28% as compared to 7% of controls). Data on axial triradii are confused by the use of the atd angle, which is age-dependent, and failure to match controls for age. Thus dermatoglyphics do not appear to have any diagnostic value in the rubella syndrome since the differences are neither large nor numerous nor consistent.

DERMATOGLYPHICS AS A DIAGNOSTIC AID

The clinician may be presented with a patient who has certain dermatoglyphic patterns, and he must decide whether they suggest a syndrome. Table 19-10 is therefore presented as an aid to the clinician. Herein he may look up the dermatoglyphic features of his patient and the syndromes in which these features are frequent, whereas the preceding tables have presented syndromes and the frequencies of their dermatoglyphic patterns. In this way he may find support for the diagnosis of a particular syndrome which, though not conclusive, may provide a guide as to whether a karyotype should be performed and a suggestion as to which syndrome to consider.

For example, an infant was recently referred to us as a suspected case of E trisomy on the basis of his physical appearance. He had ten digital whorls, bilateral simian creases, overlapping digits, hypoplastic palmar ridges, bilateral hallucal tibial arches and a single crease on digit 5. From Table 19-10 one can list the syndromes in which each of these features has an increased frequency. Thus the Smith-Lemli-Opitz syndrome appears six times, E trisomy five times, and de Lange and trisomy 21 four times. The facts that 80% of E trisomy patients ($80 \times 1\%$) have seven or more arches (whereas our patient has 10 whorls) and that 0 whorls is a common finding in the de Lange and trisomy 21 syndromes argue against these diagnoses. This evidence in favor of the Smith-Lemli-Opitz syndrome was borne out by the other physical features and a normal karyotype. By summing the figures in the body of the table one can get a more quantitative rough evaluation.

The important point is that the table may suggest a diagnosis that, once thought of, can be confirmed by other means. It must be realized, of course, that for the table to be useful, the patient must have one of the syndromes listed therein.

Much of the material in this chapter has been borrowed or adapted from Preus, M., and Fraser, F. C.: Dermatoglyphics and

Syndromes. Amer. J. Dis. Child., 124:933, 1972. Copyright 1972, American Medical Association.

REFERENCES

1. Brehme, H., and Baitsch, H.: Hautleistenbe-funde bei 15 Patienten mit Arthrogryposis multiplex congenita. Humangenetik, 2(2): 344-354, 1966.
2. Holt, S. B.: The Genetics of Dermal Ridges. Springfield, Ill., Charles C Thomas, 1968.
3. Lu, K. H.: An information and discriminant analysis of fingerprint patterns pertaining to identification of mongolism and mental re-tardation. Amer. J. Hum. Genet., 20(1):24-43, 1968.
4. Mulvihill, J. J., and Smith, D. W.: The gene-sis of dermatoglyphics. J. Pediat., 75:579-589, 1969.
5. Penrose, L. S., and Loesch, D.: Diagnosis with dermatoglyphic discriminants. J. Ment. Defic. Res., 15:185-195, 1971.
6. Pinsky, L., and Fraser, F. C.: Atypical mal-formation syndromes. J. Pediat., 80:141-144, 1972.
7. Popich, G. A., and Smith, D. W.: The gene-sis and significance of digital and palmar hand creases: Preliminary report. J. Pediat., 77: 1017-1023, 1970.
8. Preus, M., Fraser, F. C., and Levy, E. P.: Dermatoglyphics in congenital heart malfor-mations. Hum. Hered., 20:388-402, 1970.
9. Preus, M., and Fraser, F. C.: Dermatoglyph-ics and syndromes. Amer. J. Dis. Child., 124:933-943, 1972.
10. Reed, T. E., et al.: Dermatoglyphic nomo-gram for the diagnosis of Down's syndrome. J. Pediat., 77(6):1024-1032, 1970.
11. Walker, N. F.: Inkless methods of finger, palm and sole printing. J. Pediat., 50:27-29, 1957.

Chapter 20

IMMUNOGENETICS AND IMMUNOLOGIC DISORDERS

The subject matter of modern immunology has its roots in clinical medicine, but it spreads its branches to shade a wide area of biology.[5] In this chapter several topics are presented: the development of immunity; histocompatibility; transplantation; maternal-fetal interaction; autoimmune diseases; and immunologic deficiency diseases. Immunogenetics as it pertains to blood groups is discussed in Chapter 21.

DEVELOPMENT OF IMMUNITY

The basis of immunity is the capacity within each individual to recognize what is "self" and what is "nonself."[2] This capacity is vital for survival so that when bacteria or viruses or cancer cells appear, the body can recognize the invaders as being nonself and destroy them before being destroyed by the invading cells. The appearance of lymphoid tissue (in man at about 12 weeks in utero) coincides with and is directly related to the beginning of immune defense capability. However, there is some evidence that immunity may be induced in sheep and man before the appearance of lymphoid tissue.

At present, it is widely accepted that there are two major immune systems—the bursa system and the thymus system—which originate and differentiate from the same stem cells.[3] The **bursa system** is responsible for humoral immunity; i.e., immunity carried by circulating **antibodies,** small globulin molecules that arise in response to stimulation from an antigen. An **antigen** is a substance (a protein or related material) that stimulates the formation of an antibody.

To illustrate how the bursa system works in the development of immunity, let us hypothesize that the body is invaded by bacteria, in this case beta hemolytic streptococci group A, type 3. The first cells that try to halt this invasion are macrophages, which engulf the bacteria. Following this initial contact, a series of transformations takes place in which antigens (parts of bacteria or products of bacteria) processed by the macrophage are taken up by small lymphocytes, which become transformed to lymphoblasts and then to plasma cells. It is in the **plasma cells** that the immunoglobulins, which constitute the antibodies, are manufactured. There are five types of immunoglobulins, designated IgG, IgM, IgA, IgD, and IgE. Each is called upon for certain functions.

These immunoglobulins are then released

into the circulation as antibodies capable of combining specifically with the corresponding antigens. In the case of the invasion of bacteria, the antibodies inactivate the antigens in collaboration with other constituents of the blood, such as complement and polymorphonuclear cells. In the example of the beta hemolytic streptococcus group A, among the antigens that stimulate antibody production are: erythrogenic toxin; streptolysin O; and M substance, a protein fraction of the cell.

It is not clearly understood how an antibody is made to be specific for an antigen. Among the theories advanced are:

1. **clonal selection theory**—the antigen selects from a library of pre-existing antibody patterns a unit that will combine with itself;

2. **direct template theory**—the antigen becomes part of the immunoglobulin manufacturing unit;

3. **indirect template theory**—the antigen alters an existing manufacturing unit to fit itself.

Some of the functions of the specific immunoglobulins have been defined. IgG accounts for the major portion of the immunoglobulins and takes part in reactions against a variety of bacteria, viruses and toxins. It plays the central role in fighting the streptococcal invasion and is the immunoglobulin best suited to neutralize toxins such as erythrogenic toxin. IgM, on the other hand, may be adapted to deal with particulate antigens, such as bacterial cells, and may combine with cell-membrane antigens, activate complement and provoke immune lysis of the cell. IgA has the remarkable property of being secreted locally into saliva, respiratory secretions (where it protects mucous membranes), intestinal juice and colostrum. It is now known that IgE is involved in allergy such as hay fever, but a role for IgD has not been elucidated at the time of this writing.

Since this example represents a first exposure to this type of streptococcus, the patient would become clinically ill while developing antibodies to fight the infection. The response to the streptolysin O antigen is a rising antistreptolysin O (ASO) titer, which assists in the diagnosis of the streptococcal etiology. The development of antibodies against the M substance confers a permanent immunity against the specific type 3, group A beta hemolytic streptococcus that was the infecting agent in our hypothetic case. However, the patient is still vulnerable to any of the other types of group A streptococci.

What would happen should the patient be exposed to another invasion of type 3, group A streptococci? There would be a prompt and vigorous response that would eradicate the invader without allowing it a sufficient foothold to produce clinical illness. The patient is said to be "immune" and this is a manifestation of "immunologic memory." The weight of current evidence favors the small lymphocyte as the "memory cell."[4] On antigenic stimulation, "memory" is rapidly translated into the activity of antibody production in plasmoblasts. The memory cell immediately recognizes the M substance of the type 3 organism. Memory cells may live in the circulation for ten years.

The second system of immunity, the **thymus system,** is mediated by entire cells, small lymphocytes that have been derived from the thymus gland. This system of cellular immunity plays a key role in the rejection of allografts, delayed hypersensitivity and graft-versus-host reactions. It may be a major factor in the body's natural defense against cancer as well as against many viral, bacterial, fungal and protozoal diseases. The sequence of events following the introduction of foreign cells such as a kidney allograft is similar to that found in the invasion of bacteria discussed previously. The antigens present in the cells of the kidney allograft are detected as being nonself by small thymus-dependent lymphocytes, probably after the antigen has been processed by the macrophages. These lymphocytes are now sensitized. They are transformed to lymphoblasts that divide into many new lymphocytes, each one sensitized to the grafted kidney and each one bearing antibodies against the foreign kidney cells. Unlike humoral antibodies which circulate freely in the blood, the antibodies in cellular immunity remain fixed to the lymphocytes. What happens next is not precisely understood, but the sensitized lymphocytes return to the kidney allograft and initiate a rejection of the graft, possibly by enlisting the aid of macrophages.

The defense mounted against the invasion of streptococci in our earlier example may not always result in an unqualified victory. The immune response may turn against some patients and produce damage. Such is the case with rheumatic fever and glomerulonephritis, which will be discussed later in this chapter. It is also true that the body may not respond to a foreign antigen by developing immunity. It may, instead, develop tolerance—accept the antigen as self. This has been demonstrated to occur in the immunologically immature (or deficient) individual. The concept of tolerance is particularly relevant to organ transplantation.

HISTOCOMPATIBILITY—THE GENETIC BASIS OF TRANSPLANTATION

That every human being differs genetically from every other human being (except for monozygotic twins) does not require elaboration. Knowing that "nonself" is open to immunologic attack whether it is a virus, bacterium, cancer cell or transplanted organ would appear to present a formidable barrier to transplantation. How, then, can one even consider transplanting an organ, which cannot avoid being genetically dissimilar, into a recipient? Fortunately, in the totality of genetic differences between the donor and recipient, only certain genetic differences play significant roles in whether a transplanted organ will be accepted as self or rejected as nonself. The ABO blood groups and the histocompatibility antigens are of major importance.

Great progress has been made in elucidating the genetic basis of the histocompatibility (HL-A) antigens. The situation appears complicated, as there are now more than 40 histocompatibility antigens. It now appears that they are all controlled by alleles at two closely linked loci, with less than 1% crossing-over between them. Thus there are several thousand possible phenotypes, which is why it is rather unlikely to find an unrelated donor who is histocompatible with a would-be recipient. However, siblings have a much higher chance of being histocompatible, specifically one chance in four, as demonstrated in Figure 20-1.

This one-in-four chance of histocompatibility among siblings may be exploited to obtain a kidney that will not undergo rejection. The mixed leucocyte culture test consists of culturing leucocytes together from donor and recipient and adding mito-

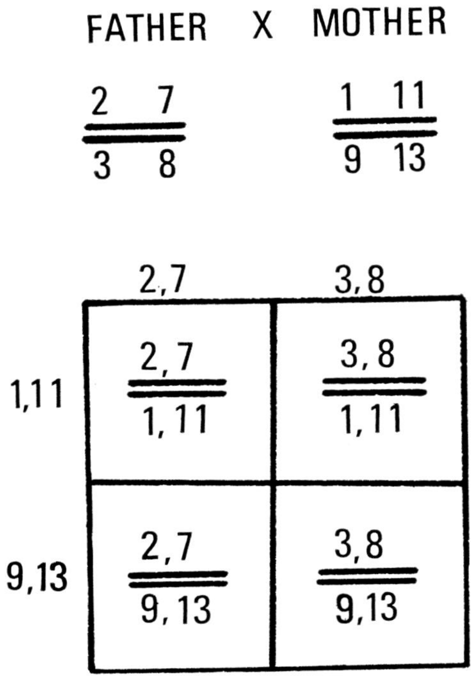

Figure 20-1. HL-A maternal and paternal specificities derived from each of the two loci yield four different genotypes, each with a one-in-four chance to recur.

mycin C after seven days to stimulate division. If stimulation occurs incompatibility is recognized. The basis of the test is that lymphocytes exposed to materials that are antigenically incompatible (including other lymphocytes) undergo a lymphoblastic transformation. This test may be used in any elective situation in which there is a living donor and at least one week to complete the study. Obviously this approach cannot be applied to cadaver donors for heart and liver transplants, when there are only several hours to prepare for the procedure.

Perhaps the clearest way to illustrate histocompatibility in man is to begin with a clinical situation. A patient who has been in an automobile accident has sustained massive and irreparable brain injury and is about to die in the emergency room of a university hospital that has an active transplantation service. The relatives of the patient wish to see something salvaged from this senseless waste of a human life, so they make known their wishes to donate the dying patient's organs to the transplantation service. What steps are now followed to prepare for organ transplantation and reduce the risk of incompatibility and rejection? To heighten the urgency of the situation, we will specify that heart transplantation is the procedure being considered.

1. ABO Incompatibility. This is the first and strongest barrier to transplantation, so the donor's blood groups must be compared with the blood groups of potential recipients in the same way that blood groups are matched for transfusion. If the donor is type A, the only suitable recipients would be types A or AB. However, if the donor is type O, he may be considered a universal donor; that is, he would be compatible in this first step of matching with recipients of groups O, A, B and AB.

2. Lymphocyte Crossmatch. The lymphocytes of the donor are presumed to carry the antigens present in other tissues and hopefully to reflect the antigen content of the donor organs. These donor lymphocytes

are crossmatched with the blood serum of the recipient in an effort to detect in the recipient the presence of antibodies already formed against the donor antigens. Such preformed antibodies could be responsible for hyperacute rejection of the donor organ. Of course, the decision whether or not to proceed with transplantation cannot be made until some potential recipients are selected for crossmatching on the basis of the information obtained in steps 1 and 3.

3. Histocompatibility Antigen Matching. The specific antigens possessed by the donor are determined by a serologic means using the lymphocytes as the source of antigen.[10] Let us assume that the donor turns out to have the antigens HL-A2, HL-A9 and HL-A12. The antigen profile of available recipients who have already been typed is now studied. First, the potential recipients are selected on the basis of ABO compatibility. The donor is blood type A_1, so only type A_1 recipients will be considered initially. Three critically ill cardiac patients are found who are type A_1 and for whom no treatment less drastic than heart transplantation remain. (See Table 20-1.) Recipient 3 has no HL-A2 or HL-A9 antigens. This is a two-group mismatch of specificities for which the laboratory is currently able to test (not to mention potential mismatches for which no test was performed due to the limits of the current state of the art). Patient 2 has no HL-A12; this is a one-group mismatch of known specificities. Recipient 1 has all three antigens that the donor has: HL-A2, HL-A9 and HL-A12. However, like recipients 2 and 3, recipient 1 also has additional antigens not present in the donor (HL-A1, HL-A7). The match between the donor and recipient 1 discloses no mismatch of an antigen present in the donor and not in the recipient. A completely compatible match, which would be judged confidently only in identical twins, would require not only that there be no antigen in the donor that the recipient does have, but also that there not be an antigen in the recipient that the do-

TABLE 20-1. Histocompatibility Typing in Clinical Example of Cardiac Transplantation

	ABO	HL-A1	HL-A2	HL-A3	HL-A9	HL-A10	HL-A11	HL-A5	HL-A7	HL-A8	HL-A12	HL-A13	Cross-match
Donor	A	−	+	−	+	−	−	−	−	−	+	−	Negative
Rec. 1	A	+	+	−	+	−	−	−	+	−	+	−	
Donor	A	−	+	−	+	−	−	−	−	−	+	−	Negative
Rec. 2	A	+	+	+	+	−	−	+	−	−	−	−	
Donor	A	−	+	−	+	−	−	−	−	−	+	−	Negative
Rec. 3	A	−	−	+	−	−	+	+	−	−	+	−	

nor lacks. That is, every group must be identical.

It has been calculated from data on ABO and HL-A antigen compatibility between donors and recipients that a minimum of 500 prospective recipients may be required to give a cadaver organ donor a 95% chance of being transplanted into a compatible recipient.

In this clinical example, the least incompatible match would be accepted (at some of the few institutions still interested in performing cardiac transplants in humans) as a satisfactory basis for proceeding with transplantation after determining that the lymphocyte crossmatch was also negative. This would be recipient 1. It should be noted that some active transplantation groups believe that histocompatibility matching is unrelated to survival of transplant patients and that only ABO compatibility is required. Most have abandoned the Terasaki grading system. What is really being criticized here is the failure of present-day histocompatibility matching techniques to discriminate between poor matches and poorer matches by methods that are yet weak and imperfect. The basic biologic law of incompatibility between self and nonself has not been abrogated. The issue is a philosophic one as to whether one wishes to perform transplantations without making every effort to refine progressively the immunologic raw material underlying the procedures.

If the clinical situation were less urgent and involved kidney transplantation, a careful search for the best possible cadaver donor should be made. Even better, a relative could be sought and in this case not only could the histocompatibility antigen matching be done, but a special mixed leucocyte culture test could be performed. As has been stated earlier, the latter test requires one week, but if the clinical urgency is not great it should provide the means for selecting the most compatible relative who is willing to donate one of his kidneys.

TABLE 20-2. Human HL-A Leucocyte Antigen Groups

Locus 1	Locus 2
HL-A1 (LA1)	HL-A5 (Da5, Te11)
HL-A2 (Mac, LA2)	HL-A7 (Da10, 4d)
HL-A3 (LA3)	HL-A8 (Da8)
HL-A9	HL-A12 (Da4, Te9)
HL-A10 (Da17, Te12)	?HL-A13 (HN)
HL-A11 (Da21, Te13)	?Da6
?Da15 (Te40)	?Da9

Human Leucocyte Antigen Groups. As was stated earlier, the assumption has been made that the leucocytes reflect the antigen content of other tissues, although it is appreciated that there are some organ-specific antigens. There appear to be two series of segregating leucocyte antigen groups. The convention has been followed in Table 20-2 that there are two loci. WHO committee nomenclature has been used. There is agreement as to some of the antigens that belong to each locus and question about others. How many antigen specificities will eventually be determined for these loci probably depends on the amount of effort expended in searching for them.

Thus, the major deficiency to present serologic histocompatibility typing remains the acknowledged fact that many antigens relevant to compatibility and organ transplant survival have not yet been detected and defined. It is easy to visualize how a laboratory could assign a satisfactory match to a donor-recipient pair on the basis of nine antigens tested, when two or three of the next six antigens tested could be mismatched—if only those next antigens were known. With these deficiencies, however, remarkable advances have been made in serologic typing in just the past five years.

Transplantation. The central problem in transplantation is how to violate a basic biologic law—the recognition and rejection of nonself—and get away with it. As was pointed out in the previous section, grafts between identical twins and grafts between individuals completely compatible in ABO and histocompatibility specificities will not

be recognized as nonself. However, in the clinical setting, the occasion rarely arises for an identical twin to be a donor, and the limitations in present techniques of histocompatibility matching and donor availability do not permit ideal matching.

A brief historical review can only mention that transplantation was described in Greek mythology and early Christian legends. Tagliacozzi, in the sixteenth century, gained a reputation for being able to reconstruct noses lost in duels and to syphilis. He appreciated (empirically?) that one could not transplant the nose from one person to another, and thus devised the operation, used to this day, of utilizing a flap from the patient's own upper arm (autograft). (The terminology of transplantation is provided in Table 20-3.)

A number of workers have been responsible for the accelerated advancement in knowledge in transplantation in our own century, among them Jensen, Carrel, Murphy and Medawar. It was the series of classic experiments conducted by Medawar in the 1940's that provided the basis for contemporary transplantation research.[7] Certain principles have emerged from the work of Medawar and other investigators:

1. Allograft immunity is cell-mediated (although humoral mechanisms probably play a role).

2. Grafts between genetically dissimilar individuals may first appear to be accepted, but are then rejected within a period of about ten days, depending on the strength of the genetic difference (first-set rejection). If another

TABLE 20-3.   Terminology of Tissue Transplantation

New Terminology	New Adjective	Old Terminology	Definition	Result
Autograft	Autologous	Autograft	Graft in which donor and recipient are the same individual	Acceptance
Isograft	Isogeneic	Isograft	Graft between individuals with identical histocompatibility antigens (e.g., MZ twins)	Acceptance
Allograft	Allogeneic	Homograft	Graft between genetically dissimilar members of same species (e.g., man to man)	Rejection
Xenograft	Xenogeneic	Heterograft	Graft between species (e.g., ape to man)	Rejection

transplant from the same donor (or donor of the same genotype) is attempted, rejection is accelerated (second-set rejection). The process may require only three to six days. The recipient has been sensitized (has immunologic memory) and quickly attacks the graft.

3. Tolerance to a graft is an alternative to rejection. The foreign cells may be accepted as self, especially in the immunologically immature (or deficient) individual, rather than rejected as nonself. Methods that take advantage of this weakness in the immunologic armor may provide the answer to long-term survival of all allografts without resorting to drastic immunosuppression.

Rejection. The mechanism of rejection has been introduced in the section on development of immunity. Certainly the cell-mediated immunity of the thymus system plays the major role. Small lymphocytes are transformed to lymphoblasts after detecting the foreign antigen and return to the graft as "sensitized" cells capable of participating in the graft rejection. Figure 20-2 illustrates rejection of a skin allograft between

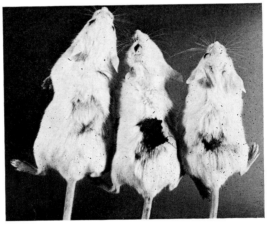

Figure 20-2. From left to right: A/J mouse receiving transplant of A/J skin without rejection; A/J mouse receiving C57 skin without early rejection because of cyclophosphamide immunosuppression; A/J mouse without immunosuppression showing active rejection of C57 skin.

genetically dissimilar strains of mice; acceptance of an isograft between mice of the same genetic constitution; and temporary acceptance (overriding of rejection) of an allograft between genetically dissimilar mice under the influence of immunosuppressive medications.

The use of immunosuppressive agents is the primary tool of physicians to cope with rejection, which is bound to occur if the histocompatibility match is not ideal. Adrenocorticosteroids such as prednisone are administered in large doses before transplantation and during the critical first two weeks, then the dosage is decreased gradually depending on the response of the patient. Rapidly acting steroids such as intravenous hydrocortisone are used at the time of transplantation and as a supplement during periods of rejection. Azathioprine, administered before transplantation and at high doses for two weeks after surgery before decreasing gradually, is the mainstay of immunosuppressive therapy. However, cyclophosphamide has proved to be a highly effective immunosuppressant that elicits a more rapid response in the human subject than azathioprine.

Antilymphocyte globulin (ALG), a biologic product prepared by immunizing horses with human lymphocytes or preferably thymus cells, was considered from animal studies to be the most potent and true immunosuppressant. Its effectiveness in the human has been variable. Some preparations appear to have high biologic activity and others essentially no activity. In some preparations, the ALG is more "antihuman" than antilymphocytic. Immune clearance of this agent is also a problem; the patient raises antibodies against ALG. This problem may be lessened by pretreating the patient with the other immunosuppressants and administering disaggregated horse IgG before giving ALG. The potential benefits of ALG in human transplantation are as yet largely unrealized.

The clinical picture of rejection has been elucidated for the commonly transplanted organs.

Rejection of the Kidney. The kidney may be rejected immediately after transplantation (hyperacute rejection). This is likely to occur if there are pre-existing humoral antibodies in the recipient or in some instances of ABO incompatibility. The kidney may secrete urine for two to ten minutes and then gradually cease. In appearance, the kidney becomes cyanotic, mottled and flabby. Complete anuria persists postoperatively and the kidney must be removed.

The function of the kidney that has been successfully transplanted is the guide to the presence or absence of rejection.[6] Anuria, of course, is the ultimate in lack of function. However, the usual tests of renal function serve to monitor rejection: urinalysis; creatinine, inulin and urea clearance; blood urea nitrogen, serum creatinine; sodium, potassium, PSP and protein excretion; and pH. Fever, palpably enlarging kidney and hypertension are among the clinical manifestations of rejection.

Morphologic findings of rejection in the kidney depend on the age of the graft and the vigor of the process. Small lymphocytes dominate a pleomorphic interstitial cell population. Tubular atrophy and arterial narrowing secondary to intimal thickening are characteristic findings.

Rejection of the Heart. The heart is also subject to hyperacute rejection. In human transplants this has been seen in the attempt to implant a cardiac xenograft. It has also been witnessed in a milder form in a second cardiac transplant in a man who rejected a heart implanted seven months earlier. The hyperacutely rejected heart contracts tightly into a ball and does not beat. In the case of the second cardiac allograft in the same man, the hyperacute rejection was temporarily overridden at the surgical table by the administration of adrenocorticosteroids.

Acute first-set rejection of the heart has its onset between the fifth and eighth postoperative day and is characterized by: electrocardiographic changes (loss of QRS voltage, S-T segment and T wave abnormalities); congestive heart failure; malaise; pericardial friction rub; and elevated LDH-1 (cardiac isozyme of lactate dehydrogenase).[8] The histopathology of acute rejection reveals an interstitial infiltrate of lymphocytes, histiocytes and polymorphonu-clear leucocytes.

Chronic (or late) rejection is more insidious. There is gradual loss of electrocardiographic QRS voltage with progressive malaise and congestive heart failure. The morbid findings of chronic rejection include striking vascular changes with intimal thickening and fibrosis of the coronary arteries, focal areas of myocardial necrosis and interstitial infiltrates of lymphocytes, plasma cells and histiocytes.

Other organs have been transplanted less commonly than the kidney and the heart, most notably the liver and the lung. Rejection of these organs is signaled by diminished function (e.g., jaundice and abnormal liver function studies in liver transplants and pulmonary insufficiency in lung transplants). However, infection more often supervenes in these patients.

Infection highlights the problem faced by the physician managing a patient with an organ transplant. Because the patient is at risk from rejection, he must have his immunologic mechanisms of nonself suppressed. However, immunosuppression is not yet sufficiently specific, so the patient's immune system is suppressed not only with respect to the transplant, but also to bacterial and viral infections and to cancer. He walks a tightrope between rejection and infection.

It has already been pointed out that if there were complete histocompatibility, as in identical twins, immunosuppressants would be unnecessary. Since this situation rarely occurs in kidney transplants and is not applicable in heart transplants, the need is for techniques that will more accurately define and test the histocompatibility of donor and recipient. Serologic tests are the most popular and are becoming more definitive. Mixed leucocyte cultures add a new dimension to histocompatibility, but are too time-consuming (one week) to be applicable to cadaver donors when only hours are available, unless there is an important advance in long-term organ preservation.

What is needed to make organ transplantation an unqualified therapeutic success is an authentic breakthrough in immunology. It is true that five-year survivors of kidney transplants are becoming more common. However, kidney recipients have advantages over heart recipients in that there is more time to get a good tissue match (including the opportunity to use relatives as donors) and the recipient is initially immunosuppressed by his uremic condition. If heart transplantation is to become a genuine therapeutic alternative, ways to utilize poor histocompatibility matches and even xenografts will be necessary to meet the potentially enormous demands for heart replacement.

It is here that the concept of tolerance and methods of inducing tolerance might be relevant.[9] The need is for immunologic specificity. The recipient should not have his ability to fight infection and cancer disastrously compromised. The ideal would be to leave the recipient with only one immunologic blind spot, i.e., the inability to recognize the transplanted organ as being nonself.

Graft-versus-host Reactions. Not only does the recipient recognize the transplant as being nonself, but the transplant may recognize the recipient as being nonself and attempt to attack it. This can occur if the donor cells are immunologically competent, such as lymphoid tissue. In the mouse, a form of this reaction has been called "runt disease." The growth of the host is strikingly impaired, for example, if spleen cells are injected into the newborn animal. If a transplant of hematopoietic tissue is introduced into a subject following total body irradiation and destruction of host immunity, the transplanted immunologically competent cells raise antibodies against the host leading to wasting and death. A rapidly fatal graft-versus-host reaction may follow a blood transfusion that contains incompatible, immunologically competent lymphocytes in patients with Swiss-type agammaglobulinemia.

Maternal-Fetal Interaction. In Chapter 1, we stated that the three major categories of genetically determined diseases were: (1) single mutant gene, (2) chromosomal, and (3) multifactorial. To these could be added a fourth category: diseases of maternal-fetal interaction. Some examples are hemolytic disease of the newborn (discussed in Chapter 21) and maternal antithyroid antibodies.

Maternal Antithyroid Antibodies. Familial nongoitrous cretinism has been attributed to maternal antithyroid antibodies crossing the placenta and attacking the thyroid gland of the fetus. Of great interest are the data of Fialkow and others demonstrating the presence of antithyroid antibodies in children with Down syndrome and in their mothers more frequently than in their fathers or in control populations. Similar findings have been reported for Turner syndrome. Thyroid disease is also increased in mothers and maternal relatives of children with Down syndrome. This suggests that there is a genetic predisposition to the formation of antithyroid antibodies that is related in some way to the predisposition to nondisjunction. It remains to be seen whether the presence of antibody predisposes to nondisjunction or whether the genetic difference predisposes both to antibody formation and nondisjunction.

AUTOIMMUNE DISEASES

The autoimmune nature of the diseases of connective tissue such as rheumatoid arthritis and systemic lupus erythematosus is well recognized. A variety of other systemic and organ-specific diseases have been attributed to autoimmune mechanisms (Table 20-4). A definitive discussion of these diseases exceeds the scope of this presentation. In fact, the underlying mechanism of an autoimmune disease remains unclear. It has been frequently conceded that an autoimmune disease represents immunologic hyperactivity although the mechanism may turn out to be selective or generalized immunologic deficiency.

Only a single disease, rheumatic fever (the autoimmune basis of which is becoming more apparent) will be discussed briefly. Although there are still some reservations about the immunologic aspects of this disorder, it makes an interesting sequel to our introductory example of the development of immunity to a group A beta hemolytic streptococcal infection. The vast majority of patients who have a streptococcal infection respond as in the example in the first section of this chapter. They develop immunity to the specific type of streptococcus that infected them. Some patients, however, develop the systemic disease that is particularly damaging to the heart, rheumatic fever.

In patients with active rheumatic fever, there is evidence of circulating antiheart antibodies. The group A streptococcus appears to share a common antigen (cross-reactive antigen) with human myocardium. Kaplan first recognized the cross-reactive antigen and showed by immunofluorescent techniques that the sera of patients with active rheumatic fever frequently contain antibodies to this shared antigen. One can thus visualize that in raising antibodies to

TABLE 20-4. Examples of Diseases Considered Autoimmune

Systemic lupus erythematosus	Stevens-Johnson syndrome
Rheumatoid arthritis	Goodpasture syndrome
Ankylosing spondylitis	Sjögren syndrome
Dermatomyositis	Rheumatic fever
Scleroderma	Glomerulonephritis
Polyarteritis nodosa	Hashimoto thyroiditis
Henoch-Schönlein purpura	Acquired hemolytic anemia
Takayusu arteritis	

TABLE 20-5. Selected Immunologic Deficiency Diseases

Disease	Inheritance	Deficiency	Manifestations
Agammaglobulinemia (Bruton disease)	X-linked recessive	IgG and IgM markedly decreased; IgA absent. Plasma cells virtually absent but lymphocytes are present. Normal thymus structure.	Excessively prone to pyogenic bacterial infections but not viral. "Arthritis." Able to reject grafts.
Swiss-type (alymphocytic) agammaglobulinemia	Autosomal recessive (there is also an X-linked form)	IgG, IgM and IgA absent or markedly decreased. Absence or gross deficiency of plasma cells *and* lymphocytes. Dysplastic or vestigial thymus.	Excessively prone to bacterial, viral and fungal infections. Unable to reject allograft or resist graft-versus-host reactions.
Ataxia-telangiectasia	Autosomal recessive	Hypoplasia of thymus; IgA absent or markedly decreased.	Ataxia, telangiectases; sinus and pulmonary infections; broken chromosomes.
Wiskott-Aldrich syndrome	X-linked recessive	Variable cellular and humoral immune deficiency.	Thrombocytopenia; eczema, bloody diarrhea, prone to infections.
Congenital thymic aplasia (DiGeorge syndrome)	No genetic basis	Complete absence of thymus and thymus-dependent lymphocytes. Normal immunoglobulins and plasma cells.	Excessively prone to infections, especially viral and fungal. Hypoparathyroidism with neonatal tetany. Anomalies of mouth, neck and great vessels.

fight a streptococcal infection the patient may also raise antibodies capable of attacking the heart. Why this occurs in some patients and not in others appears to be related to a polygenic hereditary predisposition mediated at levels as yet undefined. The genetic background of rheumatic fever is briefly described in Chapter 24.

IMMUNOLOGIC DEFICIENCY DISEASES

In 1952, Bruton[1] reported the first patient with agammaglobulinemia after Glanzmann and Riniker had described the alymphocytic disorder that has been further elucidated by several Swiss investigators and termed Swiss-type agammaglobulinemia. Since then, Good estimates that more than 1000 patients with immunologic deficiency diseases have been studied throughout the world. These patients provide the Baconian opportunity to study the exceptions in Nature in order to reach an understanding of normal immunologic development.

At least 20 distinct and separable disorders of immunologic deficiency have been defined. Agammaglobulinemia (Bruton disease) and Swiss-type (alymphocytic) agammaglobulinemia, ataxia-telangiectasia, Wiskott-Aldrich syndrome and DiGeorge syndrome are among these disorders and are considered in other chapters and in Table 20-5.

REFERENCES

1. Bruton, O. C.: Agammaglobulinemia. Pediatrics, 9:722, 1952.
2. Burnet, F. M., and Fenner, F.: The Production of Antibodies. London, Macmillan and Co., 1948.
3. Cooper, M. D., Peterson, R. D. A., and Good, R. A.: Delineation of the thymic and bursal lymphoid systems in the chicken. Nature, 205:143, 1965.

4. Gowans, J. L., Gesner, B. M., and McGregor, D. D.: Biological Activity of the Leucocyte. Wolstenholme, G. E. W., and O'Connor, M., eds. London, Churchill, 1961. p. 32.

5. Holborow, E. J.: An ABC of Modern Immunology. London, The Lancet Ltd., 1968.

6. Hume, D. M., et al.: Experiences with renal homotransplantation in human: report of 9 cases. J. Clin. Invest., 34:327, 1955.

7. Medawar, P. B.: Behavior and fate of skin autographs and skin homografts in rabbits (report to War Wounds Committee of Medical Research Council). J. Anat., 78:176, 1944.

8. Nora, J. J., et al.: Rejection of the transplanted human heart: Indexes of recognition and problems in preventing. New Eng. J. Med., 280:1079, 1969.

9. Nossal, G. J. V.: Immunological tolerance in organ transplantation. Fair prospect or fanciful folly? Circulation, 39:5, 1969.

10. Van Rood, J. J., and van Leeuwen, A.: Leukocyte grouping: method and its application. J. Clin. Invest., 42:1382, 1963.

Chapter 21

BLOOD GROUPS AND SERUM PROTEINS

In the discipline of human genetics, few areas of investigation have been more informative than blood groups and, more recently, serum proteins.

The ABO blood groups were discovered by Landsteiner in 1900. This important contribution received ultimate recognition in the award of a Nobel Prize 30 years later. During the first 25 years after their discovery, the mendelian inheritance of blood groups was intensively studied and firmly established. Now blood groups have broad application in population and family studies, in linkage analysis and chromosome mapping, and in forensic medicine. Safe blood transfusion, which represents one of the few indispensable therapeutic options of modern medicine, could not exist without blood-typing, which depends on the accurate identification of blood groups.

Serum proteins, as a polymorphism, were found to provide the same sort of genetic information as blood groups when methods for their identification were developed in 1955. Starch gel electrophoresis and subsequently a number of other media have been used in the methodology.

The advantages to genetic investigation offered by blood groups and serum proteins include the relative simplicity of their identification and inheritance. Codominance is the rule (making heterozygotes as readily detectable as homozygotes), although there are notable exceptions, including the O and I alleles, which are recessive.

BLOOD GROUPS

ABO Blood Groups. On the basis of agglutination reactions Landsteiner was able to divide humans into four distinct phenotypes. Only two antigens were required to explain the four groups. Landsteiner also recognized that an individual's serum does not contain the antibody against the antigen present in his own red cells. The four major phenotypes are A, B, AB and O, produced by alleles A, B and O. Groups A and AB can be further subdivided by subgroups A_1 and A_2 to increase the phenotypes to six: A_1; A_2; A_1B; A_2B; B and O. Group A_1 accounts for about 85% of individuals with type A blood.

ABO blood groups are inherited by mendelian laws, with the above three alleles producing the genotypes as listed in Table 21-1. With respect to the ABO system there is a reciprocal relation between the antigens and the antibodies of an individual.

TABLE 21-1.　ABO Blood Groups

Genotype	Phenotype	Red Cell Antigen	Serum Antibody
AA AO	A	A	anti-B
BB BO	B	B	anti-A
AB	AB	AB	none
OO	O	none	anti-A, anti-B

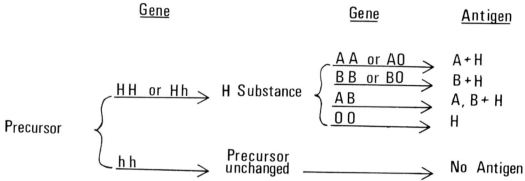

Figure 21-1.　Possible pathway for biosynthesis of blood groups.

Group A individuals possess A antigen on their cells and anti-B antibodies in their serum. Group B people have B antigen and anti-A antibody. Both A and B antigens, but not antibodies, are possessed by group AB individuals. Finally, group O persons possess no antigens but their serum contains both anti-A and anti-B antibodies. Incompatible donor cells are agglutinated by recipient antibodies.

Any anti-A or anti-B antibodies possessed by the newborn are passively transferred from the mother. Passive antibodies remain for three to six months while the infant gradually acquires these antibodies—possibly through an inherited immunologic mechanism that requires an interaction with bacterial flora of the host.

Exact genotypes of A_1, A_2 and B people are often revealed when other family members are blood-typed. The blood of A_1B, A_2B and O people can be accurately genotyped by the use of anti-A_1, anti-A_2 and anti-B.

The gene frequency of the ABO groups varies widely in different populations. In England group O occurs in about 46% of the population. Group A is almost as common with 42%. Group B is 9% and group AB, 3%. The gene frequency can be calculated from the population frequency using the Hardy-Weinberg law. Group B is more common in eastern countries than in northern Europe.

The actual immunologic specificities of the ABO blood groups are carbohydrate in nature and therefore not primary gene products. It is postulated that the primary gene products may be enzymes specified by the A, B and H genes, which participate in the biosynthesis of the blood group product as illustrated in Figure 21-1. A glycoprotein precursor is acted upon by the enzyme specified by a gene (H), leading to the production of H substance. The H substance in turn is acted upon by the enzymes specified by genes A or B to produce the antigens A or B. In the absence of A or B genes the H substance is not modified and only H antigen results. Apparently the O gene does not specify an active product.

Almost all individuals have H genes (HH or Hh). The rare individual who does not possess this gene (hh homozygous) is incapable of modifying the precursor to H substance, and thus the biosynthetic pathway is interrupted. The red cells are not agglutinated by anti-A, anti-B or anti-H; and the serum contains anti-A, anti-B and anti-H. Such persons are said to possess the **Bombay phenotype.**

The immunodominant sugars for the blood group substances have been identified as L-fucose for group H, N-acetyl-D-galactosamine for group A and D-galactose for group B. The enzymes thought to be specified by genes H, A and B and the biosynthetic pathways for the formation of the blood substances have been proposed although not definitively demonstrated. However, available evidence supports the concept that the blood groups are built by the sequential addition of sugar units to the precursor glycoprotein.

ABO variants may occur as a result of three possible causes:

1. influence of other genes on biosynthesis of A and B antigens (see Bombay phenotype);
2. rare alleles of ABO (e.g., A_3, Ax, Am);
3. environmental action on normal ABO genes (leukemia, blood mixtures).

Rare alleles of ABO are *weak* antigens, although usually dominant genes, which are masked by the presence of normal A or B antigen. B variants are more uncommon than A variants but both have been described and studied in different pedigrees.

The action of environment on genes occurs on rare occasions and is evidenced by the effect of leukemia on the A antigen. Reports of changes from A to weak A antigen following the onset of leukemia were among the first hints that environment could alter the action of genes. One group of investigators reported a patient diagnosed as having acute monoblastic leukemia whose red cells produced only 2% agglutination with anti-A. During remission of his disease, 35% of his cells produced agglutination with anti-A. With leukemia relapse, the agglutinable cells dropped to 8%.

Reports of changes in H, B, I and D antigens, as well as in A, appear in the literature. An acquired, weak anti-B has been reported in a group of persons who had carcinoma of the rectum or colon. Bacterial filtrates will produce similar changes in vitro. Mixtures of blood either through transfusion or fetomaternal bleeding could produce the appearance of a weak antigen.

ABO antigens are not limited to red cells but are distributed throughout many tissues. In 1926, ABO antigens were noted to be present in saliva and four years later it was discovered there were **nonsecretors** as well as **secretors.** The ability to secrete ABO antigens in the saliva is inherited as a mendelian dominant character (secretor gene) not linked to the ABO genes, but closely linked to the Lutheran gene on the same chromosome (recombination frequency 0.15). It provides the first example of autosomal linkage in man. Attempts have been made to separate the homozygote secretor (Se Se) from the heterozygote (Se se) serologically, but the results have not been totally successful.

Rh Blood Groups. The Rh blood groups have, since their discovery in 1940, turned out to be an important example of maternal-fetal interaction. They received the designation Rh because antibodies obtained from immunizing rabbits and guinea pigs with blood from the *rhesus* monkey (*Macacus rhesus*) agglutinated the red cells of about 85% of a white population in New York City. Landsteiner and Wiener designated these people as Rh-positive while the remaining 15% were called Rh-negative. Later it was discovered that the human anti-Rh and the rabbit antirhesus antibodies were not the same, although cross-reacting. Rapidly other blood group differ-

from plasma antigens. There is an abundance of theories about the Lewis blood groups that cannot be amplified within the limited scope of this presentation.

Duffy Blood Groups. The antibody leading to the discovery of the Duffy group was found in the serum of a patient of that name who had hemophilia and who had received multiple transfusions. The gene was designated Fy^a and its allele Fy^b. Later it was discovered that the phenotype $Fy(a-b-)$ was present in 85% of New York blacks. This blood group provides the greatest distinction between blacks and whites.

Kidd Blood Groups. Jk^a and Jk^b are the alleles in Kidd blood group system. The phenotype $Jk(a-b-)$ may be due to an inhibitory gene or another allele at the Kidd locus. This system is of anthropologic interest. $Jk(a+)$ is present in about 95% of West Africans, about 93% of American Negroes, about 77% of Europeans and about 50% of Chinese. Both anti-Jk^a and anti-Jk^b have been known to cause HDN and anti-Jk^a has produced transfusion reactions.

Diego Blood Group. This blood group system was discovered in Venezuela when it produced hemolytic disease of the newborn in a family possessing some physical characteristics of the native Indians. The antigens are called Di^a and Di^b and their respective antibodies are anti-Di^a and anti-Di^b. This antigen is reported in Chinese, Japanese, South American Indians, the Chippewa Indians and other phenotypically similar populations with the notable exception of the Eskimos.

I Blood Groups. This antigen has been studied in patients with acquired hemolytic anemia of the "cold antibody" type. The antigen I differs in certain respects from other blood group antigens. Almost everyone has some trace of the antigen and the amount of I antigen on the red cells increases from birth until adult levels are reached at about 18 months of age. The corresponding levels of i decrease as I increases. The i antigen appears to be inherited in a recessive manner, but there seems to be a disturbing excess of i siblings. There are two types of anti-I: autoanti-I, which occurs in people who have acquired hemolytic anemia with cold antibodies; and natural anti-I, which appears in i phenotype adults. Natural anti-I does not cross the placenta. Examples of anti-i have been found in persons with some types of reticulosis. Transient anti-i is often present in patients with infectious mononucleosis.

Xg Blood Group. The Xg blood group differs from previous groups in that it is X-linked and dominantly inherited. The discovery of this X-linked blood group offers more hope for mapping of the X chromosome than has yet been realized. A large number of X-linked conditions have been studied and found not to be measurably linked to the Xg locus. X-linked ichthyosis and ocular albinism have thus far been reasonably well established as linked with the Xg locus, but precisely where the Xg locus is on the X chromosome is still a matter of conjecture. An attractive theory, based on modest data, is that it may be located at the distal end of the short arm. Although there is conflicting evidence on Lyonization of the Xg blood group, evidence against Lyonization could support the concept of lack of inactivation of the Xg locus and adjacent segments of the short arm of the X chromosome, which would account nicely for the phenotypic abnormality in XO Turner syndrome.

$Xg(a+)$ hemizygous males react as strongly as homozygous females. The heterozygote female may or may not produce a weaker reaction. How this evidence can be made to agree with the speculation in the preceding paragraph remains an open question.

Other Blood Groups, Public and Private. The Y+ blood groups discovered in 1956, the Auberger in 1961 and the Dombrock in 1965 have been the subjects of considerable investigation. A number of other "public" antigens have been described, including August, Colton, Gerbich, Gregory, Lan and

Vel. The term "public" antigen is used to describe antigens that are encountered frequently, as opposed to a "private" antigen that is limited to a single kindred.

SERUM PROTEINS

A number of genetically informative serum protein polymorphisms have been determined by electrophoresis, including haptoglobins, immunoglobulins, complement, transferrins and the X-linked Xm system. Figure 21-2 is an illustration of a simple electrophoretic separation of serum proteins into albumin and globulin fractions. Further separation of these fractions is achieved by special methods. For example, gamma globulin is separated into IgA, IgD, IgE, IgG and IgM. These **immunoglobulins** are discussed in Chapter 20. **Transferrins** are beta globulins that bind iron. The **Xm serum system** has the potential to be another useful marker in mapping the X chromosome. Recent findings suggest linkage between the Hunter and Xm loci.

The **haptoglobins** are the earliest and most extensively studied of serum protein polymorphisms. These proteins are alpha-2-globulins and have the property of binding hemoglobin. Two allelic genes, Hp^1 and Hp^2, determine three main phenotypes: Hp1-1 (genotype Hp^1Hp^1); Hp2-1 (genotype Hp^1Hp^2); and Hp2-2 (genotype Hp^2Hp^2). In addition to these three common types of haptoglobin, which form characteristic patterns through electrophoresis on starch gel and certain other media, a number of other variants have been described. Two loci appear to be involved in haptoglobin synthesis, one for alpha and one for beta chains, each chain susceptible to point mutations as are the hemoglobin chains. There is evidence that some of the alleles at the haptoglobin locus have arisen through duplication by nonhomologous crossing-over. Haptoglobins may prove to be useful in linkage studies. The alpha locus has been proposed by one group of investigators to be on chromosome 13 and by

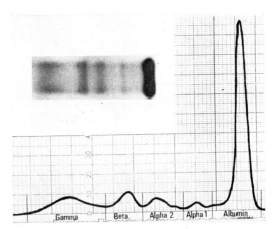

Figure 21-2. Serum proteins separated by electrophoresis on agar gel with densitometric display.

another group to be on chromosome 16. The common evolutionary origin for the alpha chain of haptoglobin and the light chain of gamma globulin has been postulated and would represent a step toward a unifying concept in the development of serum proteins.

The existence of **complement** has been recognized for almost a century and its participation in antigen-antibody reactions for decades, but it has only been within the last five years that polymorphism in the various components of complement has been investigated. Currently there are nine components of complement, designated C1 through C9 in conformity with a standardized nomenclature for variants of complement recommended by the World Health Organization. Deficiencies of identifiable components of complement have been identified in kindreds and associated with immunologic abnormalities.

REFERENCES

1. Race, R. R., and Sanger, R.: Blood Groups in Man. 5th ed. Philadelphia, F. A. Davis, 1968.
2. Ruddy, S., and Austen, K. F.: Inherited abnormalities of the complement system in man. *In* Steinberg, A. G., and Bearn, A. G. (eds.):

Progress in Medical Genetics. vol. 7, p. 69. New York, Grune & Stratton, 1970.

3. Sutton, H. E.: The haptoglobins. *In* Steinberg, A. G., and Bearn, A. G. (eds.): Progress in Medical Genetics. vol. 7, p. 163. New York, Grune & Stratton, 1970.

4. Watkins, W. M.: The possible enzymic basis of the biosynthesis of blood group substances. *In* Crow J. F., and Neel, J. V. (eds.): Proceedings Third International Congress of Human Genetics. Baltimore, Johns Hopkins Press, 1967. p. 171.

Chapter 22

SOMATIC CELL GENETICS

Techniques for the study of mammalian cells in tissue culture have been available for many years, but recent developments have opened up exciting possibilities for their application in human genetics. Human fibroblasts provided the material from which the correct human chromosome number was demonstrated, as well as the first cases of human chromosomal disease. Later it was discovered that lymphocytes could be cultured from peripheral blood following stimulation by phytohemagglutinin, and this is now the technique most widely used for diagnostic cytogenetics, supplemented where necessary by preparations from fibroblasts or bone marrow (Chapter 2).

The great advantage of somatic cell lines grown in culture are: (1) one can perform therapeutic trials and other procedures on cell cultures that are inappropriate on patients; (2) the cell environment can be much more accurately defined and controlled than that of the cell *in vivo*; and (3) cell lines from patients with rare genotypes can be maintained for study long after the patient is unavailable. For these reasons fibroblast and blood cell cultures have become useful in the antenatal diagnosis (Chapter 16) and investigation of inborn errors of metabolism.[1]

Most cultures of normal human fibroblasts become senescent after a certain number of generations (usually about 50), whereas lines developed from malignant tissues may have an indefinite life span. However, the latter lines are aneuploid and therefore not representative of the normal cell. It has recently been discovered that leucocyte cultures may be induced to become permanent euploid lines, which will be a boon to further studies.

Differentiated cells usually do not grow in culture or, if they do, usually lose their differentiated properties, although in some cases (retinal pigment cells, cartilage cells) they can be coaxed to redifferentiate under special culture conditions. Furthermore, cultures from some endocrine gland tumors (adrenal, pituitary, thyroid) will continue to produce hormones, presenting the possibility of commercial hormone production from such sources.

The ability to "clone" cells, i.e., to grow colonies all descended from a single progenitor, provided critical proof of the Lyon hypothesis (Chapter 4). It has also been used to demonstrate the somatic mutation theory of neoplasia. Leiomyomas of the uterus were taken from women who were heterozygous for G6PD types A and B, and who would therefore be a mosaic of cells with either the A or B allele active. Any particular leiomyoma typed either A or B, showing that all the cells from one tumor arose from one progenitor cell. On the other hand, the same experiment with trichoepitheliomas (dominantly inherited) showed that the tumors had both G6PD types, suggesting that they arose from multiple foci.

Cultured human cells have also been extensively utilized in the study of those inborn errors of metabolism in which the error is manifest in culture. Intensive biochemical studies on such diseases as the Lesch-Nyhan syndrome and orotic aciduria are beyond the scope of this book, but are throwing new light on the important question of gene regulation.[1]

Another use of somatic cell genetics has been in the detection of heterogeneity through complementation. In Chapter 8 we mentioned the demonstration that cells from patients with the Hurler type of mucopolysaccharidosis would prevent storage of mucopolysaccharides in cells from patients with the Hunter type and vice versa, thus showing that each provided something the other lacked and they were therefore nonallelic. Cells from patients with Hurler type did not complement cells from patients with Scheie type, suggesting that they are allelic.

The most dramatic development in somatic cell genetics has been the discovery that fibroblasts may fuse with one another to form a heterokaryon (with two individual nuclei), which may be followed by nuclear fusion. The cell fusion may occur spontaneously at a low frequency, and the rate is markedly increased by the use of inactivated Sendai virus. Fusion may occur between cells of quite different species (for instance, man and mosquito!). Following nuclear fusion the chromosomes of one parental type tend to get lost, a fact that has ingeniously been used for chromosome mapping.

For example, a line of mouse cells was developed by selection that lacked the enzyme thymidine kinase (TK). These were mixed with cells from a human line lacking the enzyme hypoxanthine-guanine-phosphoribosyl transferase (HGPRT). Both of these lines will grow on normal medium since the enzymes are not involved in the major biosynthetic pathways for thymidylic acid and purines respectively. However, the mutants do not utilize exogenous thymidine and hypoxanthine, respectively. Neither mutant will grow in the presence of aminopterin. Cells derived from fusion of these two lines can grow in the presence of aminopterin if thymidine and hypoxanthine are provided in the medium. The mixture of cells from the two lines is therefore grown in the "HAT" medium, containing hypoxanthine (H), aminopterin (A) and thymidine (T). Only hybrid cells between the two lines would be able to grow on the medium, since they and only they would have both TK and HGPRT, and thus we have a rapid and efficient way of selecting hybrid cell lines. Sublines are then maintained, in which progressive loss of human chromosomes occurs. Only lines that retain the human chromosome with the gene for TK will grow in the HAT medium. It was soon apparent that only lines retaining chromosome 17 grew on the HAT medium, and it was thus demonstrated that the gene for thymidine kinase is on chromosome 17.[3]

A recent paper by Ruddle and associates[4] shows how rapidly chromosome mapping is progressing. They report evidence from cell hybridization experiments that the locus for peptidase C is on chromosome 1. Similar studies have shown that the genes for phosphoglucomutase-1 (PGM1) and for 6-phosphoglucomutase (6PDG) are also on chromosome 1. Classic linkage studies have shown that the PGM1 locus is linked to the Duffy (Fy) blood group locus, which in turn is linked to the salivary and pancreatic amylase loci Amy-1 and Amy-2, and to the locus for nuclear cataract, Cae, and further that the 6PDG locus is linked to the Rh locus which in turn is linked to the elliptocytosis locus. Thus chromosome 1 is the best mapped autosome, to which at least nine genes have now been assigned. Progress in human chromosome mapping should be rapid in the next few years. Table 22-1 illustrates the rapid progress being made in the field of chromosome mapping by the cell hybridization technique.

Cell hybridization is also throwing new light on the question of differentiation and gene regulation. For instance, when cells from a heteroploid mouse strain that are rapidly synthesizing DNA and RNA form heterokaryons with nucleated erythrocytes of the chicken that are synthesizing virtually no nucleic acids, the hen nuclei immediately begin synthesizing nucleic acids and after about a week develop nucleoli, at which time hen-specific proteins begin to be synthesized. This suggests that the cyto-

TABLE 22-1. Autosomal Linkages in Man[2]

---

1. Linkage groups assigned to specific chromosomes:

Chromosome 1   centromere
    uncoiler
    zonular pulverent cataract
    Duffy blood group
    auriculo-osteodysplasia
    salivary amylase
    pancreatic amylase
    *phosphoglucomutase$_1$
    elliptocytosis 1
    Rh blood group
    *peptidase C
    *6-phosphogluconate dehydrogenase

Chromosome 6   *malate dehydrogenase
    *indophenoloxidase A

Chromosome 7   *mannose phosphate isomerase
    *pyruvate kinase

Chromosome 10   *regulator for esterase Es$_2$
    *glutamic oxaloacetic transaminase, soluble

Chromosome 11   *lactic dehydrogenase A
    *esterase A$_4$

Chromosome 12   *lactic dehydrogenase B
    *peptidase B

Chromosome 14   *nucleoside phosphorylase

Chromosome 16   alpha-haptoglobin
    *adenine phosphoribosyl transferase

Chromosome 17   *thymidine kinase

Chromosome 18   *peptidase A

Chromosome 19   *glucosephosphate isomerase

Chromosome 21   *indophenoloxidase B

2. Linkage groups unassigned to specific chromosomes:
   a. Lutheran blood group, secretor, myotonic dystrophy
   b. ABO blood group, nail-patella, adenylate kinase
   c. beta hemoglobin, delta hemoglobin
   d. Am$_2$ immunoglobin, Gm immunoglobulin, alpha 1-antitrypsin
   e. transferrin, pseudocholinesterase$_1$
   f. albumin, group-specific component
   g. MNS blood group, sclerotylosis
   h. HL-A, phosphoglucomutase$_3$, adenosine deaminase, P blood group
   i. isocitrate dehydrogenase, malate dehydrogenase

---

*Linkages established or continued by cell hybridization

plasm regulates nuclear activity and that the nucleolus plays an important role in transferring genetic information from nucleus to cytoplasm.

A final example of the use of cultured cells in somatic cell genetics relates to the question of genetic engineering, or directed genetic change. This has been demonstrated in the case of galactosemia, in which a virus was used to transfer DNA from a normal cell line to a strain from a galactosemic patient, following which cells from the galactosemic line were shown to be producing the missing enzyme. This approach opens exciting therapeutic possibilities and also presents some difficult questions to those concerned about the possible dangers of tampering with the human germ plasm.

REFERENCES

1. Davidson, R. G.: Application of cell culture techniques to human genetics. *In* Emery, A. E. H. (ed.): Modern Trends in Human Genetics. vol. I, p. 143. London, Butterworths, 1970.
2. McKusick, V.: Personal communication.
3. Migeon, B. R., and Childs, B.: Hybridization of mammalian somatic cells. *In* Steinberg, A. G., and Bearn, A. G. (eds.): Progress in Medical Genetics. vol. 7, p. 1. New York, Grune & Stratton, 1970.
4. Ruddle, F., *et al.*: Somatic cell genetic assignment of peptidase C and Rh linkage group to chromosome A-1 in man. Science, 176:1429, 1972.

Chapter 23

GENETICS AND CANCER

Over the past several decades the familial nature of neoplasia has been more and more widely recognized. Clearly, there are families with strong predispositions to develop neoplasms. Just as clearly, there is evidence for the existence of a number of oncogenic (cancer-producing) agents, viruses, chemicals and radiation. Many of these categories of agents have been encountered elsewhere in this text as teratogens implicated in the production of malformations. In fact, families displaying an unusually high frequency of cancer often have a high frequency of birth defects.[4]

In the minds of some investigators, it has been as difficult to reconcile the roles of genetic predisposition and oncogenic agents in cancer as it has been to appreciate the interaction of heredity and environment in the production of common diseases and malformations. There are equally strong temptations to say that nothing is known about the genetics of cancer or that bacterial models have unequivocally demonstrated the aberrancies of cell regulation that could lead to malignant transformation. Both temptations should be resisted. A great deal is known about the genetics of cancer, but one must be cautious about simplistic explanations, however appealing, derived solely from unicellular models.

It does not seem unreasonable to approach the genetics of cancer as one would approach the genetics of other common diseases and be prepared to accept that, although some cancers may be associated with chromosomal anomalies (e.g., 21 trisomy) and others with single mutant genes (e.g., hereditary adenocarcinomatosis), the majority of cases might best be explained by a genetic-environmental interaction.

There is compelling evidence for an important viral role in many malignancies, such as leukemia. How could this be reconciled with the familial cases of leukemia in successive generations with no direct personal contact between affected individuals? To the traditional concept of horizontal transmission must be added the concept of vertical transmission of viruses. As for other oncogenic agents, they may eventually be demonstrated to act as environmental triggers on individuals with a hereditary predisposition to cancer. The hereditary predisposition may assume many forms, from immunologic abnormalities to chromosomal instability to defects in cellular regulation to the harboring of temperate viruses in the host genome through successive generations. Given these sorts of hereditary predisposition, a superimposed infection, chemicals or radiation may trigger the neoplastic growth. The above statements are purely speculative, of course, and are intended only to illustrate possible mechanisms. Documenting these or other mechanisms in higher animals, specifically in man, remains a task for the future.

Case History. This six-year-old boy presented to his primary physician with a history of fever, bruising, and listlessness for a period of about a week. The physician obtained a peripheral blood count that revealed a low white blood cell count and immature forms. The patient was referred to the university medical center where the mother confided to her consultant physician that she had suspected the diagnosis of leukemia before taking the child to the doctor, because this was the way her daughter by a previous marriage had behaved before she had been diagnosed as having leukemia.

A bone marrow study confirmed the diagnosis of acute stem cell leukemia of childhood and standard therapy was begun. Several months later the paternal grandmother was diagnosed as having acute myelogenous leukemia. The grandmother's clinical course was rapidly downhill and she

died within six weeks. The half-sister of the proband had died before he was born with a rather fulminant course lasting six months (see Fig. 23-1).

This mother of four children by two fathers was understandably deeply distressed by having a second child with leukemia, and wanted to know what the chances were of her remaining children having this disease. She had not been contemplating future pregnancies. She was counseled that the risk was still very small, but that there were no data regarding the risk to a third sib after two affected sibs or half-sibs. The risk after one affected sib is increased fourfold (to 1/720) over the population risk of 1/2880 for leukemia in childhood.[5]

Her son survived with leukemia for almost two years. Shortly after his death she returned to the center with another son who had a low-grade fever and was acting listless. An evaluation for leukemia was undertaken. This time the family was happily assured that this child did not have leukemia.

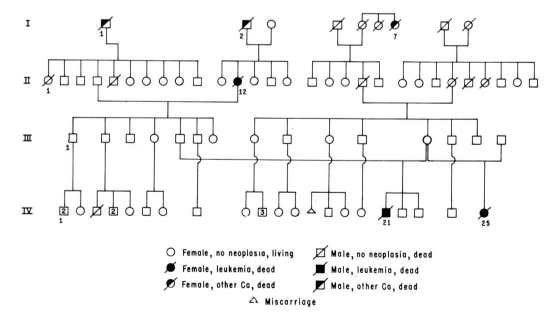

Figure 23-1. Pedigree of the family with leukemia described in the case history.

CHROMOSOMAL ABERRATIONS AND CANCER

Table 23-1 lists several conditions in which malignancies and chromosomal abnormalities are associated. In Down syndrome, the risk of leukemia is increased 30 times to 1/95 over the population risk of childhood leukemia of 1/2880. The Philadelphia chromosome has been mentioned in Chapter 3. This is a long-arm deletion of chromosome 22 (22q—), as established by QM fluorescence, which appears during exacerbation of chronic myelogenous leukemia in some patients and generally disappears during remission.

Three syndromes produced by single mutant genes are accompanied by chromosomal breaks and increased frequency of malignancy: Bloom syndrome, Fanconi pancytopenia and ataxia-telangiectasia, all autosomal recessive disorders. The risk of malignancy in Bloom syndrome appears to be as high as one in eight.

So-called preleukemic patients (myeloproliferative syndrome, intractable anemia, leukopenia, pancytopenia) usually exhibit some sort of aneuploidy prior to manifesting the diagnostic findings of leukemia.

SINGLE MUTANT GENES AND CANCER

A number of mendelizing disorders have been identified in which neoplasms are the sole phenotypic manifestations or are important features of syndromes.[1] These disorders are listed in Table 23-2. Those entities in which malignancies are the only manifestation are found exclusively under

TABLE 23-1. Conditions in Which Chromosomal Aberrations and Malignancy are Associated

Condition	Chromosomal Abnormality	Malignancy
Ataxia-telangiectasia	Multiple breaks	Lymphoma
Bloom syndrome	Multiple breaks	Leukemia
Down syndrome	21 trisomy	Leukemia
Fanconi pancytopenia	Multiple breaks	Leukemia
Philadelphia chromosome	22q—	Leukemia

TABLE 23-2. Single Mutant Genes and Cancer

Autosomal Dominant	Autosomal Recessive
Adenocarcinomatosis	Albinism
Chemodectoma	Ataxia-telangiectasia
Exostoses, multiple	Bloom syndrome
Neurofibromatosis	Chédiak-Higashi syndrome
Nevoid basal cell carcinoma syndrome	Fanconi pancytopenia
Pheochromocytoma	Xeroderma pigmentosa
Polyendocrine adenomatosis	
Polyposis I	
Polyposis III (Gardner syndrome)	X-Linked
Retinoblastoma	Burton agammaglobulinemia
Tuberous sclerosis	Wiskott-Aldrich syndrome
Tylosis	
Von Hippel-Lindau syndrome	

the autosomal dominant heading. Certainly, a dominant mode of inheritance is the entirely justifiable interpretation of given family pedigrees with these neoplasms. However, the possibility of a simulation of mendelism within so-called cancer families must also be considered, especially for those neoplasms in which the majority of cases are sporadic. Vertical transmission of virus could also be considered in this context.

Neoplasms occur as important features of a number of single mutant gene syndromes, autosomal dominant and recessive as well as X-linked. In these disorders one may visualize that the neoplasm is a consequence of the pleiotropic effect of a single mutant gene affecting many systems. A fundamental disturbance in cell regulation appears to be a reasonable etiologic consideration in many of these syndromes with associated neoplasms.

FAMILIAL, NONMENDELIAN, NONCHROMOSOMAL MALIGNANCIES

For decades, medical students have been taught to ask about cancer when taking the family history, and for decades they have obtained histories revealing that many neoplasms tend to recur in families in a nonmendelian mode: cancers of the stomach, lung, thyroid, breast, uterus; neuroblastoma; medulloblastoma; Hodgkin's disease; lymphoma and leukemia. Two of these malignancies that have been found to recur in families will be discussed.

Leukemia. Videbaek in 1947[7] published a study of 209 families ascertained through a proband having leukemia and concluded that there was a hereditary basis in this disease. His study was criticized because his control group contained fewer cases of leukemia than did the general population. The major problem with his study from the point of view of contemporary genetic analysis would be with his efforts to interpret his data in mendelian terms. Subsequent studies by a number of investigative teams have led to the general conclusion that there are significant familial aggregates in

leukemia, although at least one fairly recent study completely discounts a genetic role in acute childhood leukemia.[6]

As mentioned earlier, the risk of leukemia is increased in at least one chromosomal anomaly, Down syndrome. Suggestions that an increased frequency of leukemia may exist in other chromosomal syndromes (Klinefelter and 13 trisomy) have been very tentative. The risk of leukemia in Bloom syndrome may be as high as one in eight, but the majority of cases are nonchromosomal and nonmendelian. The risk of recurrence of leukemia in an identical twin is one in five and in a sib is one in 720.

The etiologic role of nongenetic risk factors, such as ionizing radiation, benzene, and viruses (which, although not established in the human subject, clearly operate in animal models), cannot be ignored. Leukemia could prove to be an excellent model for studying the interaction of genetic and environmental factors in neoplasia.

Breast Cancer. This disease was subjected to a comprehensive genetic analysis by Jacobsen in 1946.[3] A large number of studies have followed. It would appear that at least two forms of breast cancer must be distinguished[2]: (1) a premenopausal frequently bilateral form with a tendency to occur in persons with blood group O; (2) a postmenopausal unilateral form often associated with diabetes, hypertension and obesity, but not significantly more frequent in type O individuals. While there is no evidence of mendelian inheritance in breast cancer, an increased recurrence risk to first-, second- and third-degree relatives of patients with bilateral breast cancer has been demonstrated. The risk of developing breast cancer is 3.6 times higher for the daughter of a mother with bilateral breast cancer than for a daughter of a mother with unilateral disease.

REFERENCES

1. Anderson, D. E.: Genetic varieties of neoplasia. *In* Genetic Concepts and Neoplasia. Baltimore, Williams & Wilkins, 1970. p. 85.

2. ———: Some characteristics of familial breast cancer. Cancer, 28:138, 1971.
3. Jacobsen, O.: Heredity in Breast Cancer. Copenhagen, Nyt Nordisk Forlag, 1946.
4. Miller, R. W.: Relation between cancer and congenital defects in man. New Eng. J. Med., 275:87, 1966.
5. ———: Persons with exceptionally high risk of leukemia. Cancer Res., 27:2420, 1967.
6. Steinberg, A. G.: The genetics of acute leukemia in children. Cancer, 13:985, 1960.
7. Videbaek, A.: Heredity in Human Leukemia. Copenhagen, Nyt Nordisk Forlag, 1947.

Chapter 24

CARDIOVASCULAR DISEASE

The familial aspects of cardiovascular disease are well recognized. From the beginning of their clinical clerkships, medical students learn to ask the routine questions in obtaining the history: is there heart disease, high blood pressure, stroke, diabetes in the family? Frequently the questions are asked in such a routine manner that a positive answer is not awaited. This is especially true of history-taking in families with congenital heart diseases. Very often the respondent does not know, for instance, that a cousin died in infancy with transposition of the great vessels. The respondent only knows that the cousin (sibling, aunt) died in infancy. All too often, however, the respondent does know that a relative has a heart lesion—if given the time to answer. To demonstrate this point to students and house officers, we will frequently ask the parent of a child with a congenital heart lesion who has a relative whom we have also treated for a heart defect: "Is there anyone else in the family with congenital heart disease?" More often than not, if the question is asked hurriedly, the answer is a hurried no. Then we will ask: "Well, what about his cousin, Joe, Didn't he have a heart operation here about six years ago when he was a baby?"

Patients try to cooperate and to please their busy physicians. Sometimes this takes the form of giving a quick answer (which may be wrong) to "save the physician's valuable time." An occasional patient will get into the spirit of providing a pleasingly positive family history by creating established diagnoses in relatives when none, in truth, exists. Both types of "memory bias" must be avoided in history-taking. The point is that family histories of cardiovascular diseases as recorded in patients' charts are of little or no value. Even if a statement of a positive family history for a congenital heart disease appears in a chart, it is of minimal value unless the degree of relationship to the proband (sib versus third cousin) is stated and the precise anatomic diagnosis established. Family histories for research purposes must be taken by experienced investigators.

CONGENITAL HEART DISEASES (CHD)

As has been emphasized in previous chapters, there are essentially three possible genetic bases for a given disease: single mutant gene, chromosomal and multifactorial. The history of etiologic investigation into congenital heart diseases has followed the devious course pursued by studies of other diseases of complex genetic causation.

Positive family histories in the early decades of this century were interpreted in mendelian terms. Prior to 1959, if a disease was thought to have a genetic basis, it was a mendelian basis that was considered. Hippocrates and the Doctrine of Diathesis had somehow become obscured. In 1959, the first chromosomal aberration syndromes were recognized and an effort was made to explain congenital heart diseases on the basis of chromosomal anomalies. Most recently the cycle has returned to Hippocrates and data have been accumulated that suggest that most congenital heart lesions are not caused by single mutant genes nor by chromosomal aberrations, but appear to be the product of a hereditary predisposition (diathesis) often made manifest by an environmental trigger.

To give an overall picture of what proportion of congenital heart diseases fall into which genetic categories, Table 24-1 presents our experience, which is consistent with the experience of other investigators. From our cardiac clinic we have reported that less than 1% of congenital cardiovascular lesions in children are caused by a single mutant gene. Since we are now inclined to categorize Ullrich-Noonan syndrome as a mendelian disorder, this figure is doubled. We would say that 2% of congenital heart lesions are of single mutant gene etiology.

TABLE 24-1. Genetic Basis of Congenital Heart Diseases as Presently Visualized

Genetic Basis	Examples	Percentage
Single mutant gene	Ullrich-Noonan syndrome, IHSS	2
Chromosomal	Down, Turner syndromes	4
Multifactorial	"Nonsyndrome" VSD, ASD	94

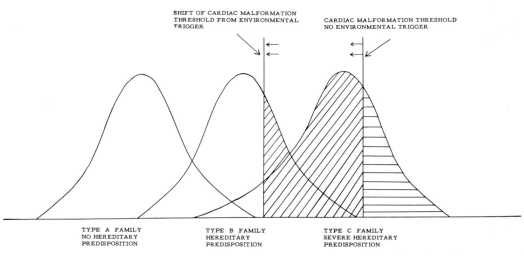

Figure 24-1. Predisposition to congenital heart diseases as represented by three hypothetic types of families. The type A family is not predisposed; the type B family represents the degree of predisposition found in the majority of families with congenital heart defects; and the type C family is the rare family with severe predisposition. In the type C family some congenital heart lesions can occur even without an environmental trigger. In the type B family congenital heart lesions do not occur unless an environmental trigger pushes the developmental threshold to the left. The type A family is not predisposed and even an environmental trigger cannot move the threshold line far enough to the left (or move the curve far enough to the right) to produce a congenital cardiac malformation.

About 4% are associated with chromosomal aberrations and the remaining 94% are presumed to be the result of a genetic-environmental interaction as conceptualized by multifactorial inheritance.

Multifactorial Inheritance

This is believed to be the major genetic category in the etiology of congenital heart diseases.[7] It brings together the previously recognized genetic (familial) and the environmentally influenced (e.g., rubella, thalidomide) cases. In the not-too-distant past the genetic and environmental causes of congenital cardiovascular disease were looked upon as conflicting etiologic interpretations. It is now becoming increasingly obvious that a genetic predisposition to congenital cardiovascular maldevelopment exists in certain families of man and in other animal species, such as mouse and dog.

This predisposition may be visualized in Figure 24-1, in which are inscribed three distribution curves.[8] Each one represents a hypothetic genotype with predisposition to a congenital heart lesion—let us say, ventricular septal defect (VSD). The type A family has no hereditary predisposition (i.e., it is genetically resistant); the type B family, a moderate predisposition; and the type C family, a marked predisposition. To the far right of the figures is a vertical line representing the threshold of cardiac malmalformation *if there is no adverse environmental influence*. The threshold may be moved to the left (or the distribution to the right) by an environmental trigger such as dextroamphetamine or hypoxemia. The important thing is the relationship of the threshold to the distribution.

The type A family is not at risk even when there is maternal exposure to an environmental trigger at the vulnerable period of cardiac development, because their distribution is relatively far from the threshold and most environmental triggers do not push the threshold far enough to the left (or distribution to the right) to cause a congenital heart defect.

To the type B family, it is another story. If there is no adverse environmental influence (threshold to the far right), a congenital heart disease does not occur. However, add an environmental trigger and the developing heart is at risk—the threshold moves to the left and produces cardiac maldevelopment in a small proportion of offspring. Type B families represent the vast majority of cases of congenital heart disease.

The type C family illustrates another more marked hereditary predisposition. In this hypothetic example not only does there appear to be greater risk (with a high frequency of affected offspring) from exposure to environmental triggers, but spontaneous cardiac maldevelopment may occur without a major adverse influence from the environment. This may be exemplified by an isogenic animal homology such as the C57/BL6 mouse, which spontaneously has a frequency of VSD of about 1%. This frequency is increased to 11% by dextroamphetamine administration.[10] What should be recognized is that there are a significant number of high-risk families in which a majority of first-degree relatives have congenital heart lesions. The recognition of the prognostic implications of the marked predisposition represented by the type C family is essential if the cardiologist is to offer accurate genetic counseling. The recurrence risks are not the low figures presented in Tables 24-2 and 24-3, which are based on the presence of a lesion in only one first-degree relative.

The use of family and twin studies and animal homologies to investigate genetic hypotheses has been presented in Chapter 17, and the data that favor multifactorial inheritance in the majority of cases of congenital heart disease have been detailed in the literature.[7] Therefore, this section will be devoted to empiric and theoretic recurrence risk figures for use in genetic counseling and to the presentation of selected clinical examples.

The calculation of recurrence risk figures (or rather recurrence risk approximations) has been arrived at rather simply. Assuming that congenital heart lesions are indeed produced through a multifactorial mode of inheritance, the recurrence in a first-degree relative of an individual having a congenital heart lesion would be approximated by the square root of the population frequency ($\sqrt{p}$). The population frequency of a specific defect is determined by taking the incidence of congenital heart diseases in the pediatric age group in a large population (e.g., the North American population) and multiplying this by the proportion of the specific defect to all defects in an accurate and representative pediatric heart registry. Combining two large studies, for instance, yields an approximate frequency of congenital heart disease in the North American pediatric population of 1%.[6,15] From the figures of the Cardiac Registry of the Toronto Hospital for Sick Children,[5] ventricular septal defect represents 25% of congenital heart diseases in children. Taking 25% of 1%, the population frequency of VSD should be 0.25% (2.5 per 1000).

The next step is to take the square root of 0.25% (0.0025) to determine the theoretic recurrence risk in first-degree relatives of patients with VSD: $\sqrt{0.0025}$ equals 0.05. Therefore, the recurrence risk in VSD is 0.05 or 5% *if there is only one affected first-degree relative.* However, this approach is based on the assumption of multifactorial inheritance, and the estimate is purely theoretic. It is gratifying to see that empiric observations provide a very similar estimate.

One of the implications of the multifactorial threshold model is that the recurrence risk increases sharply with the number of affected first-degree relatives. If there are two affected first-degree relatives, the risk is at least tripled. For three or more affected first-degree relatives, the risk appears to become extremely high, although the number of such families upon which this impression is based is small.

Tables 24-2 and 24-3 list the theoretic recurrence risks for 13 congenital cardiovascular malformations together with empiric recurrence risks derived from a study of 1478 families having a proband with a congenital heart disease.[8,9] It should be noted that predicted and observed recurrence risks are in close agreement. It is preferable in genetic counseling to use empiric recurrence risks when they are available and to reserve theoretic risks for those cases

TABLE 24-2. Observed and Expected Recurrence Risks in Siblings of 1478 Probands with Congenital Heart Lesions

| | | Affected Siblings | | |
Anomaly	*Probands*	*No.*	*%*	*Exp. ($\sqrt{p}$)*
Ventricular septal defect	212	24/543	4.4	5.0
Patent ductus arteriosus	204	17/505	3.4	3.5
Tetralogy of Fallot	157	9/338	2.7	3.2
Atrial septal defect	152	11/342	3.2	3.2
Pulmonic stenosis	146	10/345	2.9	2.9
Aortic stenosis	135	7/317	2.2	2.1
Coarctation of aorta	128	5/272	1.8	2.4
Transposition of great vessels	103	4/209	1.9	2.2
Atrioventricular canal	73	4/151	2.6	2.0
Tricuspid atresia	51	1/96	1.0	1.4
Ebstein's anomaly	42	1/96	1.1	0.7
Truncus arteriosus	41	1/86	1.2	0.7
Pulmonic atresia	34	1/77	1.3	1.0
Total	1478	95/3376		

(From Nora, J. J.: Etiologic factors in congenital heart diseases. Pediat. Clin. N. Amer., 18:1059, 1971)

TABLE 24-3. Observed and Expected Recurrence Risks in Offspring of 210 Probands with Congenital Heart Lesions

| | | Affected Offspring | | |
Anomaly	Probands	No.	%	Exp. $(\sqrt{p})$
Ventricular septal defect	57	6/162	3.7	5.0
Patent ductus arteriosus	42	4/117	3.4	3.5
Atrial septal defect	73	5/190	2.6	3.2
Pulmonic stenosis	38	3/102	2.9	2.9
Total	210	18/571		

(From Nora, J. J., *et al.*: Empiric recurrence risks in common and uncommon congenital heart lesions. Teratology, 3:325, 1970.)

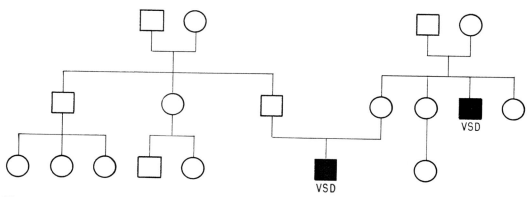

Figure 24-2. Type B family with common lesion (VSD) and low recurrence risk.

in which empiric data are lacking. Thus, the empiric recurrence risk for tetralogy of Fallot in a first-degree relative is known and is 2.7%. The empiric recurrence risk for anomalous left coronary artery (ALCA) is not known, but the frequency of ALCA in a congenital heart registry (0.25%) multiplied by the frequency of congenital heart anomalies in the population (1%) yields an approximation of the population frequency of 0.000025. The square root of 0.000025 is 0.005 (0.5%) which is, until proved otherwise, a reasonable prediction of the recurrence risk.

In general, common lesions recur in first-degree relatives more commonly (2 to 4.4%) than uncommon lesions ($\approx$ 1%), and this is the figure that is derived from $\sqrt{p}$. Therefore, the cardiologist needs to know that the range of recurrence of heart anomalies is from the order of 1% for uncommon lesions to 4.4% for the most common mal-

formation (VSD), and that the defect fits the model of a multifactorial distribution with developmental threshold.

Clinical Examples. *Common Lesion in a Type B Family With One Affected First-degree Relative.* A young couple has just discovered, to their great distress, that their first-born child has a ventricular septal defect. They want to know why and what the chances are that this will happen again. The cardiologist obtains the genetic history recorded in Figure 24-2. The only other individual in the family with a congenital heart lesion is an uncle who had his ventricular septal defect repaired ten years earlier.

The mother acknowledged that, like so many mothers of both normal and malformed infants, she had a number of potentially teratogenic exposures during the first trimester of her pregnancy, including a minor respiratory infection (which was treated with an antihistamine, a decongestant and aspirin). She had had a chest x-ray for an employment physical at a time when she was not quite sure whether or not she was pregnant. Finally, she confessed that she was most concerned about the dextroamphetamine she had been taking for appetite suppression before she became pregnant and during the early weeks of her pregnancy. At her first prenatal visit to her obstetrician she had been advised to discontinue the dextroamphetamine, but she had already reached six weeks' gestation.

Pedigree analysis reveals that the only affected first-degree relative of any future offspring of this couple is the proband, so the parents are advised that the risk for their next child is small—of the order of 4.4%. The mother is further advised to take all reasonable steps to protect her future pregnancies from unnecessary teratogenic exposures. Although there may be little she can do to avoid polluted air, water and food (except by political pressure), she is urged to be extremely cautious about drug ingestion, especially during the first trimester of her pregnancy. It might be pointed out (perhaps not if her guilt feelings were to be unduly exacerbated) that although no specific environmental trigger can be confidently implicated in the etiology of her child's ventricular septal defect, there is evidence from both human and animal studies that dextroamphetamine may play a role in cardiovascular maldevelopment.[10,11]

Uncommon Lesion in a Type B Family With One Affected First-degree Relative. The third child and only son of this farm family died at three months of age with a cardiovascular anomaly (see Fig. 24-3), persistent truncus arteriosus, diagnosed by cardiac catheterization at two weeks of age and confirmed at necropsy. The parents were still hoping to have a son, but were concerned about the risk of having another child with a congenital heart defect.

Analysis of the pedigree failed to disclose a known cardiac anomaly in any other family member. The mother was able to recall several potentially teratogenic exposures in the first trimester including a respiratory infection (not established as being bacterial, but treated with penicillin tablets and a cough medicine containing four different pharmacologic agents). She consumed aspirin for headaches on a number of occasions. Several times during the first two months of her pregnancy she sprayed the barn with potent insecticides.

Figures for both predicted and empiric recurrence risks are available. The predicted $\sqrt{p}$ is 0.7% and the empiric figure, based on a rather small sample, is 1.2%. Certainly the recurrence risk is of the order of 1% and this is what the parents were told. The mother was also cautioned about drug exposure early in pregnancy unless indi-

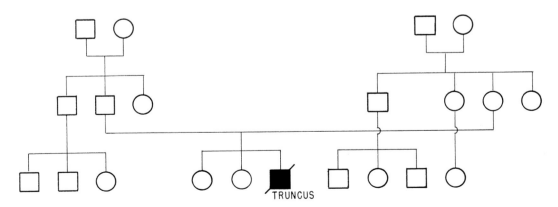

Figure 24-3. Type B family with uncommon lesion (truncus) and low recurrence risk.

cated on firm medical grounds. She was particularly warned about the inadvisability of exposure to plant and barn sprays (which may contain alkylating agents and other known teratogens and mutagens).

Common Lesion Recurring With High Frequency in First-degree Relatives (Type C Family). This family was well known to our clinic (Fig. 24-4). At least eight and probably nine closely related individuals had congenital heart lesions, mostly ventricular septal defects. The parents had lost their first child early in infancy before being referred for cardiovascular consultation. Their second child had benefited from a successful surgical closure of a ventricular septal defect at five years of age; and their third child died at two months of age following surgery for VSD, patent ductus arteriosus and coarctation of the aorta.

The parents had only one living child and sought advice because they wished to have another. On the basis of risk data obtained from a handful of such families the couple was advised that the risk could be very high, although no specific risk figure could be given. The possibility of adoption was suggested and the couple concurred. However, in three weeks a frantic call was received with information that the wife was pregnant and apparently had already been pregnant during the counseling session, although unaware of this at the time.

The parents elected not to terminate the pregnancy and the prediction of high risk was confirmed when their next baby also had a ventricular septal defect. Fortunately, this defect was small, has caused no disability and probably will not require surgery.

Uncommon Lesion Recurring With High Frequency in First-degree Relatives (Type C Family). This instructive sibship consists of seven children, four of whom had atrioventricular (AV) canal; three of these children died in infancy and early childhood with the disease and one was successfully repaired at five years of age (Fig. 24-5). A further tragedy in this family was that one of the three young children who had no evidence of heart disease died of digitalis poisoning, having consumed a bottle of his sister's digoxin.

The only two living children who did not have atrioventricular canal had an electrocardiographic abnormality found in this malformation: left axis deviation with counterclockwise frontal plane loop. It would appear that these two children had

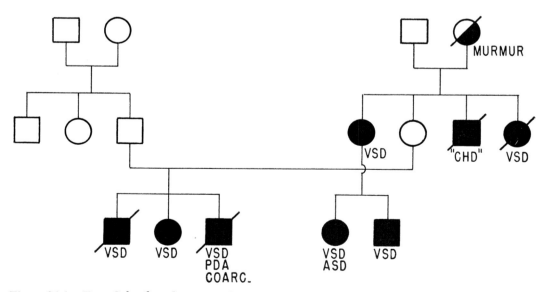

Figure 24-4. Type C family wth common lesion (VSD) and high recurrence risk.

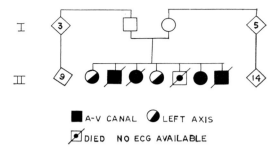

■ A-V CANAL ◑ LEFT AXIS

◪ DIED   NO ECG AVAILABLE

Figure 24-5. Type C family with uncommon lesion (AV canal) and high recurrence risk. (From Nora, J. J.: Etiologic factors in congenital heart disease. Pediat. Clin. N. Amer., 18:1059, 1971.)

the *forme fruste* of AV canal, i.e., the maldevelopment did not affect the septa and valves, but only the conducting system. No other family member could be discovered who had an atrioventricular canal or any other congenital heart lesion, although all members of the sibship who were studied had an abnormality of cardiac development or conduction.

Thus, it appears that even uncommon heart lesions such as AV canal (one-sixth as common as VSD, about 4% of patients

with congenital heart diseases) may occasionally recur in almost all members of a sibship if there is a particularly unfavorable predisposition. This re-emphasizes that the low recurrence risk figures apply if there is only *one* affected first-degree relative, but that the risk increases markedly with an increasing number of first-degree relatives who have either a common or uncommon cardiac malformation.

Genetic counseling of this family included the option that the father consider a vasectomy. The option was accepted.

Chromosomal Aberrations

As was stated earlier, only about 4% of congenital heart lesions are associated with chromosomal aberrations.[1,7] Early investigations sought to link chromosomal anomalies with isolated cardiac malformations (e.g., atrial septal defect), but it has become apparent that, when a congenital heart lesion exists in association with a chromosomal abnormality, it exists as part of a syndrome of multiple anomalies, such as Down syndrome or the XO Turner syndrome. Table 24-4 summarizes the frequency of occurrence and the characteristic

TABLE 24-4. Congenital Heart Diseases (CHD) in Selected Chromosomal Aberrations

Population Studied	Incidence of CHD	Most Common Lesions		
		1	2	3
General population	1%	VSD	PDA	ASD
4p—	40%	VSD	ASD	PDA
5p— (cri-du-chat)	25%	VSD	PDA	ASD
C mosaic	50%	VSD		
13 trisomy	90%	VSD	PDA	Dex
13q—	50%	VSD		
18 trisomy	99+%	VSD	PDA	PS
18q—	50%	VSD		
21 trisomy	50%	VSD	AV canal	ASD
XO Turner	35%	Coarc	AS	ASD

VSD	=	Ventricular septal defect	PS	=	Pulmonic stenosis
PDA	=	Patent ductus arteriosus	AV	=	Atrioventricular
ASD	=	Atrial septal defect	Coarc	=	Coarctation of aorta
Dex	=	Dextrocardia	AS	=	Aortic stenosis

types of cardiac defects for a number of chromosomal aberration syndromes. These syndromes are discussed in more detail in Chapters 3 and 4. Chromosomal syndromes such as XXY Klinefelter syndrome do not appear in the table because there is no firm evidence that congenital heart diseases occur more frequently in these disorders than in the general population.

Single Mutant Gene Syndromes

Diseases transmitted by single mutant genes account for about 2% of the total of cardiovascular anomalies. As with chromosomal disorders, the cardiac defects are present as part of a syndrome, such as the Ellis-van Creveld syndrome. Whether or not there exist any examples of discrete cardiac malformations caused by single mutant genes that are not associated with syndromes is debatable. It must require the products of a large number of genes to bring about truncoconal septation and it is reasonable to doubt that a single gene could be responsible for failure of a ventricular septum to close unless it is a single gene with a very specific small effect or more likely a gene of large effect, in which case a number of associated anomalies could be found. This returns us to the concept of the pleiotropic effect of a mutant gene of large effect.

One possible example of a single mutant gene in a familial heart lesion is that of

TABLE 24-5. Syndromes with Cardiovascular Involvement

Autosomal Dominant	Autosomal Recessive
Acrocephalosyndactyly (Apert)	Acrocephalopolysyndactyly II (Carpenter)
Cardiac arrhythmia, brachydactyly (Tabatznik)	Alkaptonuria
Cardiac arrhythmia, prolonged Q-T without	Bird-headed dwarfism (Seckel)
deafness (Romano-Ward)	Chondrodystrophia calcificans (Conradi)
Craniofacial dysostosis (Crouzon)	Cockayne
Deafness, M.I., freckles (Forney)	Cutis laxa
Ehlers-Danlos	Cystic fibrosis
Lymphedema (Milroy and Meige)	Dysautonomia (Riley-Day)
Marfan	Ellis-van Creveld
Neurofibromatosis	Fanconi pancytopenia
Osteogenesis imperfecta	Friedreich ataxia
Osler telangiectasia	Glycogenosis IIa, IIIa, IV
Treacher Collins	Homocystinuria
Tuberous sclerosis	Jervell and Lange-Neilsen
Ullrich-Noonan	Laurence-Moon-Biedl
Von Hippel-Lindau	Mucolipidosis III
	MPS IH, IV, V, VI
Unknown Etiology	Osteogenesis imperfecta
	Progeria
de Lange	Pseudoxanthoma elasticum
DiGeorge	Refsum
Goldenhar	Smith-Lemli-Opitz
Kartagener	TAR (thrombocytopenia absent radius)
Klippel-Feil	Weill-Marchesani
Poland	Werner
Robin	
Rubenstein-Taybi	*X-Linked*
Silver	
Sturge-Weber	Dermal hypoplasia, focal (Goltz)
Supravalvular aortic stenosis with	Incontinentia pigmenti
hypercalcemia	MPS II (Hunter)
	Muscular dystrophy (Duchenne and Dreifuss)
Environmental	
Rubella	
Thalidomide	

idiopathic hypertrophic subaortic stenosis (IHSS). This disease exceeds the predictions of the multifactorial inheritance hypothesis—the overall incidence in first-degree relatives being much higher than $\sqrt{p}$. However, IHSS is not an example of maldevelopment in the way that VSD is. It is an apparent progressive "overgrowth" of heart muscle that may not become manifest until adult life. Although this disease fails to meet the expectation for mendelian or multifactorial inheritance, it has been considered an autosomal dominant disorder on the basis of some rather striking pedigrees. In our experience, there are many instances of sporadic cases and familial cases *not* directly transmitted.

With the possible exception of IHSS, at the time of this writing we feel that there are no congenital heart lesions caused by single mutant genes that are not part of a syndrome. Table 24-5 provides a partial list of syndromes produced by single mutant genes, potent teratogens and of unknown etiology that have cardiovascular disease as a feature. The majority of these syndromes are discussed further elsewhere in this text.

CORONARY ARTERY DISEASE

The familial occurrence of coronary artery disease has long been recognized. Sir William Osler noted that both Matthew Arnold and his father suffered from angina pectoris. Levine, following observations made in the 1920's, recorded through successive editions of his textbook, *Clinical Heart Disease*, that the most important etiologic factor in coronary thrombosis was heredity.

Examples of familial aggregates abound in the literature as well as in the practice of almost any physician who treats patients with coronary artery disease. Twin studies, such as the National Danish Study, show a significantly higher concordance between monozygotic than dizygotic twins. A variety of animal homologies including rabbit, pigeon, dog and monkey have been found to be susceptible to atherosclerosis. There are few diseases, if any, in which the etiologic factors have been more vigorously investigated (and contested) than coronary artery disease. This high priority is entirely justified. Atherosclerotic diseases are unequaled as a cause of morbidity and mortality in Western society.

In preparing this chapter an effort was made to list some of the hereditary and environmental factors in the etiology of coronary artery disease (Table 24-6). It became obvious that these factors could not be categorized so simply. Although certain causes of coronary artery occlusion are secondary to factors that are predominantly hereditary (e.g., some patients with type IIa hyperlipoproteinemia, Hunter syndrome) or predominantly environmental (rubella syndrome), most causes do not comfortably fit under heredity or environment, but depend more on the interaction between factors. For example, considering personality, diabetes mellitus, hypertension and coro-

TABLE 24-6. Etiologic Factors in Coronary Artery Disease

Heredity	interaction	Environment
Metabolism		Diet
Cholesterol, etc.		Stress
Diabetes		Striving
Personality		Inadequate exercise
Hypertension		Overweight
Coronary artery anatomy		Cigarettes

nary artery anatomy under heredity is merely a judgment that, perhaps, the hereditary basis of these factors exceeds the environmental—although both are known to be important.

A very brief discussion of some of the so-called hereditary factors will be undertaken together with a consideration of how environment may interact with heredity. Since cardiovascular diseases are so widespread, need for their cure and prevention is most urgent. Although genetic manipulation may provide some eventual solution, the immediate attack on the problem has most judiciously been on the environmental factors as they interact with the hereditary predisposition.

Metabolism. The association of elevated serum cholesterol with atherosclerosis has been repeatedly documented, although there has not been broad agreement regarding its precise etiologic role. Other lipid abnormalities such as elevated triglycerides, beta-lipoproteins, pre-beta-lipoproteins, chylomicrons and total plasma lipids have been studied in an effort to define phenotypes of individuals and families at risk. Fredrickson has proposed a classification,[2] the most recent modification of which has been published as a World Health Organization Memorandum.[14] Table 24-7 lists the phenotypic characteristics of the current six hyperlipidemias and hyperlipoproteinemias.

All of these phenotypes have a tendency to recur in families, but the *relationship of the phenotype to the genotype is poorly understood*. In fact, we have seen as many as four of the six different phenotypes distributed among the first-degree relatives of the same family. We have also found families in which both biologic parents of the so-called "homozygous" type II child were without phenotypic manifestations of the "heterozygous" form of type II disease. We have recently seen the mother of a so-called "homozygous" type II child who had no detectable biochemical abnormality of a hyperlipidemia prior to sustaining a myocardial infarction at 30 years of age. The changes from one phenotype to another within the same individual, depending on diet or condition (e.g., pregnancy) or the disappearance or appearance of abnormal phenotypes with varying physiologic and pathologic states are well documented.

It is possible that a significant number of patients with type IIa disease have a single mutant gene abnormality. However, evidence is lacking for a firm mendelian basis for types IIb, III, IV and V as well as a sizable portion of IIa. If one could attack the problem of premature death from myocardial infarction and find the cause to be due mainly to a limited number of single gene mutations, methods for identifying patients at risk could be more easily devised. Unfortunately, the problem appears

TABLE 24-7. Classification of Hyperlipidemias and Hyperlipoproteinemias

Type	↑Chol.	↑ Trigly.	Electro.	Ultracent.	Chylo.
I	+			± VLDL	+
IIa	+		β	LDL	
IIb	+	+	β & pre-β	LDL & VLDL	
III	+	+	Broad β		
IV		+	pre-β	VLDL	
V	+	+	pre-β	VLDL	+

Chol.	=	Cholesterol	Chylo.	=	Chylomicron
Trigly.	=	Triglyceride	LDL	=	Low Density Lipoprotein
Electro.	=	Electrophoresis	VLDL	=	Very Low Density Lipoprotein
Ultracent.	=	Ultracentrifugation			

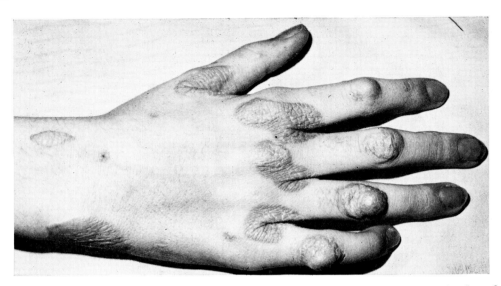

Figure 24-6. Typical xanthomatous skin lesions in child with severe homozygous type IIa hyperlipoproteinemia.

to be more complex than this and the mode of inheritance is almost certainly multifactorial in the vast majority of cases.

Although the Fredrickson system of phenotyping remains the most useful method at this time, it must be recognized that these phenotypes are probably far removed from actual genotypes; that there are significant pitfalls in defining true phenotypes; and that there is a great deal more heterogeneity and less specificity than the enumeration of the six phenotypes would imply.

Yet there is reason for optimism. Many patients at risk (whether their etiology is single gene or multifactorial) can be identified by current techniques, including such simple screening procedures as serum cholesterol and triglycerides. More elaborate phenotyping using lipoprotein electrophoresis and ultracentrifugation may be added to make use of the risk figures and dietary programs for specific phenotypes. Finally, environmental manipulation in the form of diet, exercise, weight reduction and other interventions can produce a lipid and lipoprotein profile that approaches normal in the majority of cases.

A dash of pessimism must be added. Long-term projects, such as the Framingham Study, have suggested that intervention in the older adult may be too late. The emphasis is now swinging to identification in infancy and childhood of the patient at risk.[4] The identification and treatment (when indicated) of the infant and child at risk introduce new problems to which a number of investigative teams are currently addressing themselves. Coronary artery disease has now become a pediatric problem.

Personality. The personality type of the individual predisposed to coronary artery disease has become increasingly obvious over the past several decades. A useful designation of the patient prone to coronary artery disease has been the **type A behavior pattern** of Friedman and Rosenman.[3]

Patients with type A behavior are usually male but the same sort of behavior pattern may be found in the coronary-prone female. By general appearance the type A individual presents with brisk self-confidence. He speaks and gestures forcefully. His work and activities are characterized by a high degree of drive, ambition, competitiveness and aggressiveness. He plays to win and loves to compete. Perhaps his most characteristic trait is his "sense of time-urgency." There never seem to be enough hours in the day to accomplish all that the man with a type A behavior pattern wishes.

It would seem that if such a man were to elect the life of a Trappist monk, the important interaction with an environment of stress and striving would be eliminated and the likelihood of coronary occlusion lessened. However, the same heredity that predisposes him by personality to be coronary-prone also predisposes him to select a competitive job (and to be a heavy cigarette smoker, to be too busy with striving to indulge in adequate physical exercise, etc.).

Other Factors. These include diabetes, which greatly accelerates the atherosclerotic process, and hypertension, which is accompanied by a three-fold increase in risk of future coronary disease in the 40 to 59 age group. The importance of the anatomy of the coronary arteries can easily be visualized when one considers the potential outcome of occlusion of a dominant left coronary artery or a single coronary artery. Stress and striving are accepted as the norm of modern living, but there is still some opportunity for the individual to elect another way of life. Certainly a large number of young people appear to be pointing out alternative approaches.

The recent emphasis on jogging and cycling may yet (for the younger patient) be able to reverse some of the deleterious effects of our pushbutton, spectator-oriented, sedentary society. The counter-advertising campaign of the American Heart Association and American Cancer Society may, at least, get people to question whether inhaling a cigarette really does bring springtime to their lungs and coronary arteries.

Numerous investigations have already yielded extensive (and sometimes contradictory) information about risk factors in coronary artery disease. At the time of this writing, the best recurrence risk figures are still rather limited in scope. The risk of death from early ischemic heart disease (early is defined as under 55 years of age for men and under 65 years for women) is 7% for individuals having a first-degree relative dying of early ischemic heart disease.[13] The risks for liability to coronary artery disease based on the clinical types of Fredrickson are now being investigated. For "heterozygous" patients with type IIa hyperlipoproteinemia, these risks are indeed impressive: the chances for onset of ischemic heart disease in men are 5.4% by age 30; 51.4% by age 50; and 85.4% by age 60. For "homozygous" patients with type IIa disease the prognosis is extremely grave, with many of these patients dying in their teens. The risks are somewhat less for types III, IV and V with respect to myocardial infarction, but the risk of cerebrovascular accidents is increased.[12]

Although many variables are still poorly understood, the best present hope is early and accurate identification of the patient at risk and successful manipulation of environmental factors participating in the genetic-environmental interaction leading to coronary artery disease.

RHEUMATIC FEVER

The familial aspects of rheumatic fever have been recognized for several decades, even to the extent that one prominent worker in the field attempted to interpret the family clusters of this disease in mendelian terms, concluding that this was an autosomal recessive disorder. Data from the National Danish Twin Study support a hereditary predisposition to rheumatic fever on the basis of higher concordance in monozygotic twins as compared to dizygotic twins, which is significant at a probability level of 0.01%. However, no data from twin or family studies provide evidence of mendelian inheritance of this disease and no active investigators in this area are willing to discount that the streptococcus is the environmental trigger in rheumatic fever.

Rheumatic fever appears to be an excellent example of a disease produced by a

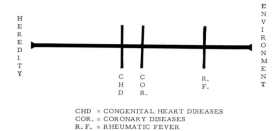

CHD = CONGENITAL HEART DISEASES
COR. = CORONARY DISEASES
R.F. = RHEUMATIC FEVER

Figure 24-7. Relative roles of heredity and environment in three categories of cardiovascular disease.

genetic-environmental interaction. Certain families have a hereditary predisposition, but rheumatic fever does not result unless there is an infection (almost always respiratory) with a group A beta-hemolytic streptococcus. (See Chapter 20 for immunologic considerations in rheumatic fever.)

Figure 24-7 illustrates the authors' present assessment of the relative contributions of heredity and environment to the etiology of three categories of cardiovascular disease discussed in this chapter. Congenital heart diseases are placed a little closer to the hereditary pole of the continuum, coronary artery diseases approximately in the middle, and rheumatic fever closer to the environmental pole.

ESSENTIAL HYPERTENSION

Evidence has been accumulated by a number of investigators to support the concept of a multifactorial mode of inheritance. Other investigators propose a monogenic etiology. Our review of the subject strongly favors multifactorial inheritance in the majority of cases, but does not exclude that a minority of patients may have hypertension attributed to single mutant genes.

An individual's systemic blood pressure, like his height and intelligence, appears to be determined by many genes. A "normal" distribution curve for systolic blood pressure in adults runs from 90 to 140 mm. Hg (and a diastolic curve from 50 to 90 mm. Hg). The tail at the lower end can extend further, but not as far as the tail at the

upper end of the curve, because a minimum blood pressure is required to sustain life. Thus it can be visualized that some individuals could have systolic blood pressures of 160, 180 or even 200 and be at the far end of a now skewed distribution curve.

This concept alone probably does not account for the relatively large number of people with hypertension. A polygenic predisposition to hypertension interacting with environmetal triggers (e.g., obesity, sodium, endogenous and exogenous vasoconstrictors), a genetic-environmental interaction, is as conceptually sound an etiologic proposal for hypertension as for congenital heart diseases, rheumatic fever and coronary artery diseases.

Of course, there are pathologic conditions that, when superimposed on a genetic predisposition to normal or even low blood pressure, will result in severe systemic hypertension. Renal diseases are in this category. However, this is no longer within the definition of essential hypertension.

REFERENCES

1. Emerit, I., de Grouchy, J., Vernant, P., and Corone, P.: Chromosomal abnormalities and congenital heart disease. Circulation, 36:886, 1967.
2. Fredrickson, D. S., and Levy, A. I.: Familial hyperlipoproteinemia. *In* Stanbury, J. B., Wyngaarden, J. B. and Fredrickson, D. S. (eds.): The Metabolic Basis of Inherited Disease. Ed. 3. New York, McGraw-Hill, 1972.
3. Friedman, M., and Rosenman, R. H.: Overt behavior pattern in coronary disease. JAMA, 173:1320, 1960.
4. Kannel, W. R., and Dawber, T. R.: Atherosclerosis as a pediatric problem. J. Pediat., 80:544, 1972.
5. Keith, J. D.: Incidence. *In* Keith, J. D., Rowe, R. D., and Vlad, P. (eds.): Heart Disease in Infancy and Childhood. New York, Macmillan, 1967.
6. Mitchell, S. C., Korones, S. B., and Berendes, H. W.: Incidence of congenital heart disease in 54,033 births. Circulation, 43:520, 1971.
7. Nora, J. J.: Multifactorial inheritance hypothesis for the etiology of congenital heart diseases: the genetic-environmental interaction. Circulation, 38:604, 1968.
8. ———: Etiologic factors in congenital heart diseases. Pediat. Clin. N. Amer., 18:1059, 1971.
9. Nora, J. J., McGill, C. W., and McNamara, D. G.: Empiric recurrence risks in common

and uncommon congenital heart lesions. Teratology, 3:325, 1970.

10. Nora, J. J., Sommerville, R. J., and Fraser, F. C.: Homologies for congenital heart diseases: murine models influenced by dextroamphetamine. Teratology, 1:413, 1968.

11. Nora, J. J., *et al.*: Dexamphetamine, a possible environmental trigger in cardiovascular malformations. Lancet, 1:1290, 1970.

12. Slack, J.: Risks of ischaemic heart disease in familial hyperlipoproteinemic states. Lancet, 2:1380, 1969.

13. Slack, J., and Nevin, N. C.: Hyperlipidemic xanthomatosis I: increased risk of death from ischaemic heart disease in first degree relatives of 53 patients with essential hyperlipidemia and xanthomatosis. J. Med. Genet., 5:4, 1968.

14. W.H.O. Memorandum: Classification of hyperlipidemias and hyperlipoproteinemias. Bull. W.H.O., 43:891, 1970. Circulation, 45:501, 1972.

15. Yerushalmy, J.: The child health and development studies, Berkeley and Oakland, California—description and selected findings. Excerpta Medica, Int. Cong. Ser. No. 191. Third International Conference on Congenital Malformations, p. 20 (abst.) 1969.

Chapter 25

GENETICS OF BEHAVIOR

Man's behavior is probably his most important phenotypic feature, but little is known of its genetic basis.[4] The literature on human behavioral genetics deals mostly with the psychoses and the behavioral changes resulting from mutational or chromosomal causes of mental retardation. Yet the psychologic effects of phenylketonuria or trisomy 21 will teach us no more about the genetics of normal behavior than tone-deafness will teach us about the genetics of musical ability, or throwing a spanner into a moving engine will teach us about its function. The same applies to major mutant genes in experimental animals such as the waltzing mouse or vestigial wing Drosophila.

One would expect that genes affecting "normal" behavior would be subtle in their effects and that the primary biochemical effect of the gene at the polypeptide level might be far removed from the behavioral effect. Thus the gene controlling the ability to taste phenylthiocarbamide presumably affects some enzyme, but it would be hard to deduce the existence of such a difference from a genetic study of preference for cabbage. Nevertheless, some functional defects resulting in behavioral differences do have a fairly simple genetic basis, such as the

specific dyslexias, and some have contributed significantly to the elucidation of normal function, e.g., the defects of color vision.

A number of **pathologic genes** have more or less specific effects on behavior. The phenylketonuric child (untreated) is hyperactive, irritable, has an uncontrollable temper, abnormal postural attitudes and agitated behavior. About 10% show psychotic behavior. Multiple discriminant analysis of a number of test scores permits discrimination of PKU children from those with other types of mental retardation, so the biochemical defect must have certain specific effects on behavior, from which we should be able to learn something. At least the spanner is always thrown into the same part of the engine, so the resulting damage may tell us something of the mechanism. Similarly, characteristic behavioral changes often precede the choreic movements in Huntington's chorea. Congenital cretinism, which may be recessively inherited, produces its familiar effects on personality. Perhaps the most striking example of a gene-induced behavioral defect is the bizarre tendency to self-mutilation in the Lesch-Nyhan syndrome. We are still far removed from a complete understanding of the relation between the gene-determined biochemical change and the behavioral response, but the rapid advances being made in neurobiochemistry may make this approach very rewarding.

Finally, information from animal experiments tells us that mutant genes known by their prominent effects on the physical phenotype, such as albinism, may have much more indirect and subtle effects on behavior. Thus a particular behavioral parameter, such as aggression, may be influenced by the indirect effects of a large number of genes with major effects on other parameters. In this sense the genetic basis of the behavioral parameter is polygenic.

Chromosomal aberrations also have effects on behavior.[1] A child with Down syndrome tends to be happier and more responsive to his environment than other children of comparable IQ, and he is often musical. Girls with Turner syndrome rate high on verbal IQ tests but low on performance and seem to have a deficit in perceptual organization. Males with an XYY chromosome complement seem to be predisposed to behavioral disturbances involving crimes against property rather than personal aggression, which may be attributed to excessive anxiety, although the picture is far from clear. Again, the series of casual links between the excess or deficiency of chromosomal material and the behavioral phenotype is entirely obscure.

There is such a wealth of literature on the genetics of **intelligence** that an adequate review would be longer than this book. The evidence is strongly in favor of a substantial genetic component. The degree of phenotypic correlation is at least as high as it is for physical traits such as height and weight. The picture is complicated by a high degree of assortative mating and the interaction of genotype and environment.

Much of the early work on the genetics of intelligence has considered it as an entity, measured more or less accurately by a variety of performance tests, more or less "culture free." More recently the trend has been toward identification and description of its various components, and this provides an opportunity for defining more specifically the genetic basis for these components. Vandenberg[6] has combined the results of several studies and concluded that heredity was most important for verbal ability and less so, in descending order of importance, for word fluency, perceptual speed, spatial perception memory, number ability and reasoning (as defined specifically for the purposes of the test). He suggests that the rather low degree of heritability for reasoning may be that, for several tests, the right answer may be reached by several routes that require different amounts of time. Identical twins often select different, equally correct routes, which tends to lower the concordance rate. We point this out mainly to illustrate the difficulty in interpreting this kind of data.

Specific **dyslexia,** or congenital word-blindness, is one of the few common behavioral disorders that shows a simple mode of inheritance, as first shown in the thorough study by Hallgren.[3] It is undoubtedly heterogeneous and there may exist a clinically indistinguishable nongenetic type. Affected children show the normal distribution of intelligence, but have specific reading and writing disabilities, such as confusion of letters p/q or b/d, and may have "nervous" symptoms, or turn out to be "problem children." There is an increased frequency of speech defects, such as stuttering, lisping, or retarded speech development, but probably not of left-handedness. The familial cases (which are the great majority) fit the expectation for autosomal dominant inheritance.

The **psychoneuroses** are so common that they might almost be considered normal; their genetic basis is correspondingly complex. There is considerable confusion even as to their definition. The few genetic studies available agree that the psychoneuroses are familial, with some degree of specificity for subtypes; i.e., if the proband has an anxiety state most of the affected relatives have an anxiety state, and there is a similar correspondence for hysteria and obsessional neurosis. This finding is corroborated by twin studies, but the importance of environmental factors is also demonstrated. Rosenthal[5] summarizes the situation in the following terms.

By and large we are limited in our conclusions about the heredity issue in neurosis because of the sparseness of studies, their relative lack of variety, their failure to take various diagnostic precautions, and the difficulty involved in assessing the role of environmental factors. However the overall evidence points to the likelihood that heredity plays a role in the development of psychoneurotic symptoms, but we can say very little about the genetics involved, except that various polygenic systems may be involved in a more or less low-keyed way. . . . Further studies with increased methodological sophistication may help us to understand more clearly the diathesis-stress interactions and their relation to subtype syndromes.

We have not attempted to give recurrence risk figures, since the data vary so widely from study to study that any attempt to average them would be bound to be misleading.

The situation for **homosexuality** is even less clear. Twin studies suggest that heredity plays an important role with respect to whether males become homosexuals, but family studies show a wide range of psychopathology in the families of homosexual probands, which raises the question of whether the homosexual behavior is secondary to such psychopathology or vice versa.

For **alcoholism** the situation is also complicated. Several family studies show a familial tendency; twin studies show monozygotic pairs have a higher concordance than dizygotic pairs, but dizygotic pairs also have a fairly high rate. One study, using adopted children of alcoholics, found a low rate of alcoholism in this group and concluded that the contribution of environmental factors is of overriding importance

with respect to whether addiction occurs. It may be that some aspects of drinking behavior are heritable and others not.

Family studies of **psychopathy** and **criminality** show that most children with antisocial behavior come from broken homes; thus it is impossible to tell from such studies how much of the antisocial behavior in these children is biologically transmitted and how much culturally acquired. Twin studies seem to have been devoted more to criminality than to the broader category of psychopathy. Monozygotic pairs show a higher concordance rate than dizygotic pairs, but it is clear that criminality must be a highly heterogeneous category. There are undoubtedly predisposing factors, such as EEG abnormalities, low IQ, chromosomal anomalies, and the so called "constitutional psychopathic state"—criminals tend to be predominantly mesomorphic. Each of these factors is under some degree of genetic control. This would account for at least part of the estimated heritability. However, the major group contributing to criminality are those classified as having a psychopathic or sociopathic personality, and the genetics of this condition is still almost completely obscure. In any case the role of the environment is clearly of major importance in criminality.

Finally, there is the question of **personality** and whether it has any genetic basis. The question is of some eugenic interest in this time of population crisis. For instance, if personality traits such as aggression and altruism were genetically determined one would expect the former to be selected for and the latter selected against, since the altruistic would be more likely to limit their family size than the aggressive.

According to Eysenck,[2] personality may be classified along two relatively independent dimensions: various grades of neuroticism or instability on the one hand, and extroversion-introversion on the other. Unstable extroverts are more likely to become delinquent; unstable introverts are more likely to become neurotic. Several twin studies have shown quite high heritability estimates for these dimensions, both by questionnaire and laboratory measurements. Family studies also show significant correlations between near relatives, and there seems little doubt that heredity is important in determining individual differences in personality. Just how important, and by what mechanisms, remains to be seen.

REFERENCES

1. Court Brown, W. M., Jacobs, P., and Price, W. H.: Sex chromosome aneuploidy and criminal behaviour. *In* Thoday, J. M., and Parkes, A. S. (eds.): Genetic and Environmental Influences on Behaviour. Edinburgh, Oliver and Boyd, 1968. pp. 180-193.
2. Eysenck, H. J.: Genetics and personality. *In* Thoday, J. M., and Parkes, A. S. (eds.): Genetics and Environmental Influences on Behaviour. Edinburgh, Oliver and Boyd, 1968. pp. 163-169.
3. Hallgren B.: Specific dyslexia (congenital word-blindness). A clinical and genetic study. Acta psychiat. neurol., Supp. 65:1-287, 1950.
4. McLearn, G. E.: Behavioural genetics. Ann. Rev. Genet. 4:437-468, 1970.
5. Rosenthal, D.: Genetic Theory and Abnormal Behaviour. New York, McGraw-Hill, 1970.
6. Vandenberg, S. G.: Primary mental abilities or general intelligence? Evidence from twin studies. *In* Thoday, J. M., and Parkes, A. S. (eds.): Genetic and Environmental Influences on Behaviour. Edinburgh, Oliver and Boyd, 1968. pp. 146-160.

Chapter 26

GENETIC COUNSELING

THE NEED FOR GENETIC COUNSELING

Genetic counseling usually begins with someone wanting to know whether a disease suspected of being genetic will recur in the near relatives of a patient with the disease. The role of the counselor is, firstly, to estimate P, the probability of recurrence. Some authorities believe that the task ends here, but we believe that the counselor, when asked, should be ready to assist the person concerned in deciding what to do and in taking the appropriate action.

Most counseling involves the occurrence of a particular disease in a child and the concern of the parents as to whether their future children might be similarly affected. For simplicity's sake, the following discussion will assume that this is the situation. However, other problems may be encountered. Parents may also want to know about the risk for affected children's children, or for the children of the unaffected brothers and sisters. A person contemplating marriage may be concerned about a specific disease or history of racial admixture in the fiancé's family. Cousins contemplating marriage may be worried about the possible genetic hazards of consanguinity. Occasionally the question may involve a child being considered for adoption and the presence of a disease or racial admixture in the family.

In certain populations in which a severe genetic disorder is unusually high, screening programs are now being initiated to detect heterozygotes and to encourage them not to marry other heterozygotes for the same gene. This involves "prospective" counseling rather than retrospective (when the affected child has already been born); it will require a quite different approach and raise quite different problems.

THE GENETIC COUNSELOR

In many cases the family doctor is the most appropriate person to do the counseling because he knows the family, its attitudes and socioeconomic background better than a consultant. However, he may have neither the genetic knowledge nor the time for perhaps several interviews, and in many cases the family does not have a family doctor. Finally, some cases may be so complex or require sufficiently specialized tests that the services of a professional genetic counselor are desirable.

At present a genetic counselor requires no formal qualifications. Some counselors have a higher degree, such as the Ph.D. in genetics, some have a medical degree, and some both. A good counselor needs a sound grasp of genetic principles, a wide knowledge of the scientific literature on diseases of possible genetic origin, and much sympathy, tact and good sense. Preferably he should be associated with a hospital, so that he can take advantage of its diagnostic resources and the expertise of its staff, and so that he is available to his colleagues and to patients' families. Those in need of genetic counseling are more likely to get it if the counselor is on the hospital staff than if they have to find one elsewhere. Often the family may not know that such a service is available unless they are referred to one by an interested doctor.

THE COUNSELING INTERVIEW

The first interview usually takes the better part of an hour or more; in addition to the collection of information, it allows the counselor to begin to get to know the parents and vice versa. For this reason it is best that the counselor take the family history rather than an assistant, time-consuming though it may be. It is also preferable to interview both parents; together they may present a more accurate family history than separately, and the counselor has a chance to get some impression of how they interact, which may be helpful later in the counseling process. This also guards against misinterpretation of information given by the counselor when it is communicated by the interviewed parent to the other parent. The facts given by the counselor should be written down and placed on record, in the patient's hospital chart, and in a letter to the family doctor, or in a letter to the parents, or both.

The first requirement, of course, is that the disease causing the concern is accurately diagnosed. This may already have been done, in which case the counselor needs only to be able to evaluate the reliability of the diagnosis and to know when to ask for confirmatory tests or opinions. In other cases the counselor may himself aid in making the diagnosis, either by performing special tests, such as examination of the chromosomes, or through his familiarity with diseases so rare that the practicing physician may not know of them. For instance, he must take into account the problem of genetic heterogeneity—the fact that diseases that present very similar features may have different causes and therefore different risks of recurrence. Further special tests and interpretation of the famliy history may permit a distinction to be made. Thus taking the family history may help to establish a diagnosis and is usually essential to the estimation of P, the probability of recurrence.

Taking the Family History. This involves construction of a pedigree and listing the patient's near relatives by sex, age and state of health, particularly with reference to the occurrence of relevant diseases in the family. A special form is used to ensure systematic recording of the data. It is often necessary to correspond with doctors and hospitals or to examine medical records directly to confirm diagnoses of possible relevant diseases occurring in family members. In most cases, carrying the family study beyond first cousins and grandparents is not useful, both because the information gets progressively less reliable with increasing distance of relationship, and because diseases occurring only in relatives more distantly removed than this are not likely to be relevant to the patient. Depending on the nature of the disease involved the counselor may want to amplify the family history by doing special examinations or tests on particular family members (e.g., to detect whether certain individuals are carrying a mutant gene or a chromosomal rearrangement).

The counselor may be able to estimate P reliably by the end of the first interview, and if the estimate is reassuringly low and the parents are happy about it, there may be no need for further interviews. However, if the risk is not reassuring or if the parents have any doubts about it or show any signs of uneasiness, a second interview is indicated. This may be necessary anyway if records have to be checked or special tests done. The interval provides an opportunity for the parents to absorb the information given, clarify their thoughts and define the questions they want to ask.

Establishing the Recurrence Risk. The process by which the counselor establishes the recurrence risk in question has been reviewed in Chapter 5 and elsewhere.[1,2,3] It involves placing the disease in one of four etiologic categories: diseases due to major mutant genes, chromosomal aberrations, major environmental agents and multifactorial causes. The recurrence risk can then be calculated from either mendelian laws or selection of the appropriate empiric estimate as outlined in previous chapters.

Interpreting the Recurrence Risk. The next step in the counseling process is to make certain that the parents know what the probability figure means in their situation. Some have trouble understanding the very concept of probability and some, even though they have an affected child, may not grasp the full implications of having another one.

Once clear about the meaning of the probability they have been given, the parents must convert the probability into a decision—whether to have another baby, seek sterilization, marry, adopt, or whatever their particular problem indicates. The counselor may be able to help the family reach a wise decision, but he should avoid making it for them. For instance, he can point out the various factors to be considered: the severity of the disease in relation to the risk of recurrence, the impact of the disease on the rest of the family, the social and moral pressures they may feel, the possibility of adoption or artificial insemination as an alternative to having their own children, the pros and cons of sterilization, and the possibility of monitoring the next pregnancy by amniocentesis.

The counselor should not try to impose his view of the appropriate decision. However, it is not enough simply to present the required probability and leave it at that. In the ensuing discussion the parents may ask the counselor what he would do in the same situation, in which circumstance he should say as best he can (without actually being in the same situation) what he thinks he might do. More than one of our counselees has expressed a wish in retrospect that we *had* been more directive, at least in emphasizing what an affected child meant in terms of daily living. "I understand the statistic in my head, but I don't *feel it.*"

Taking Action. The decision reached may demand definitive action. A decision not to have further babies of their own will requires further decisions by the parents about the use of contraceptives, sterilization, artificial insemination, adoption and so on. If contraception fails, the question of abortion may arise. Several recent developments have changed the situation radically with respect to this kind of decision.

The Pill. The advent of contraceptive pills has made it easier for those who wish to avoid having further children to do so. Diaphragms, condoms, and (even more so) "the rhythm" were sufficiently unreliable to make the prospect of another—potentially diseased—baby a constant menace. The pill has provided increased security, but on the other hand, for a young woman of 20 or more, the prospect of years "on the pill" and the fear of a single forgetfulness resulting in a high-risk pregnancy can be formidable.

Changing Attitudes to Abortion. There has been a radical change in social and legal attitudes toward abortion from a generally proscriptive to a generally permissive one. In some groups the mere fact that a pregnancy is unwanted is sufficient grounds for termination; in others there must be danger to the life or health of the mother, and in some there are no grounds for taking the life of an unborn human being. The counselor must respect the religious and moral attitudes of the parents, but in many cases these may be in conflict with the law or church. That is, the parents in good conscience may wish to have the pregnancy terminated, but may find it difficult to do so because of legal or religious restrictions. This situation has improved radically in many areas, but there are still many regions where the law does not allow parents who wish to prevent the birth of a child with a high risk of severe disease from taking the necessary steps.

Prenatal Diagnosis. There have been recent improvements in techniques for prenatal diagnosis. Certain gross malformations can be recognized before birth by special methods of x-ray or ultrasound examination, and methods are being developed whereby the embryo can be viewed directly by optical systems inserted into the uterus. Probably the most valuable approach is amniocentesis at 14 to 16 weeks of gestation. Examination of the amniotic fluid directly or of the fetal cells either directly or after culture can establish the diagnosis of some genetic disorders prenatally and convert an estimate of probability into virtual certainty that the baby will be affected or unaffected (Chapter 16).

Sex-linked Conditions. In the case of sex-linked conditions such as hemophilia, it is possible to examine the chromosomes of cultured cells and to determine whether they are XX or XY. If the mother carries the hemophilia gene, each son has a 50:50 chance of being a hemophiliac, whereas the daughters will be unaffected (although each has a 50:50 chance of being a carrier). Amniocentesis can establish whether the embryo is a female or a male, and the parents have the opportunity to seek termination of the pregnancy if it is male.

Chromosomal Aberrations. Culture of cells from the embryo and examination of their chromosomes allow diagnosis of chromosomal anomalies. Thus, in high-risk pregnancies, as when a parent has a chromosomal rearrangement or in mothers near the end of their reproductive period (when the risk of a chromosomal anomaly may be more than 1%), amniocentesis and prenatal diagnosis allow termination of a pregnancy that would inevitably result in a malformed and/or mentally retarded child, and allows high-risk parents to have only unaffected children.

Enzymatic Defects. Many genetic diseases are due to abnormal enzymes, and in an increasing number of cases the enzyme defect can be detected in fibroblasts cultured from the amniotic fluid. For example, parents who have had a child with infantile Tay-Sachs disease may be advised that there is a one-in-four risk of recurrence, but that amniocentesis and cell culture will allow diagnosis of the disease if the child falls into the affected class. Termination of the pregnancy would then prevent birth of a child destined to tragic death and allow the parents to try again until they had an unaffected baby. This procedure has already been a great boon to a number of families, and the number of diseases amenable to this approach is continually increasing as research progresses. However, although the procedure appears harmless in expert hands, there are many pitfalls in the diagnosis of rare diseases by enzymatic studies on cultures, particularly in relatively inexperienced laboratories. For this reason, steps are being taken to develop centers where samples from surrounding areas can be sent for the necessary tests. With modern methods of transport, material can be sent long distances, and a network of centers (such as the National Genetics Foundation Referral Centers) could provide the necessary services for a large country.

The Follow-up. One or more follow-up interviews are desirable for several reasons. Firstly, they may reinforce the parents' understanding of the information given and correct any misapprehensions resulting from reinterpretation of the information. Not infrequently follow-up interviews reveal that the figures given have been modified upwards or downwards, either through reinterpretation with the "aid" of friends and relations, or perhaps in response to the parents own wishes, subconscious or otherwise. For instance, when a one-in-four recurrence is translated into a three-to-one risk, one wonders whether this reflects the parents' desire not to have more children for any reason.

Finally, there are situations in which a mutant gene or chromosomal rearrangement segregating in the family places certain relatives at high risk. Such diseases as Huntington's chorea and multiple polyposis of the colon (dominant), hemophilia and Duchenne muscular dystrophy (sex-linked recessive) and chromosomal translocation may denote that certain family members other than the parents are at risk for developing the disease or having affected children. Seeing that these individuals receive counseling may be troublesome, involving questions of breach of confidence or invasion of privacy, but the counselor may also be criticized for failing to provide information that could possibly prevent a tragedy. With the help of the proband's parents and the appropriate family physicians, the task can usually be done.

Our family follow-ups have also reassured us that the opinion is false that "people are going to go ahead and have children no matter what you tell them." Some parents do seem willing to take what seems to us a rather inordinate risk, and some ignore the genetic hazards to the point of irresponsibility. However, the majority do heed the risks, and several surveys indicate that when the risk is low (less than 10%) most parents are prepared to take a chance even for a severe disease, but when the risk is high the majority take steps (however imperfect) to stop having children. Also, a crippling disease with long-term survival is regarded as more formidable than one that results in early death. It is important, however, to distinguish between parents who have been counseled routinely (e.g., as part

of a clinic procedure) and those who have actively sought counseling. Parents who have not sought counseling may not pay much attention to it. Those who have are usually grateful for the knowledge and heed it, making the counselor's task indeed rewarding.

HOW TO LOCATE A GENETIC COUNSELOR

As awareness of genetic counseling and what it can do becomes more widespread, the demand for it increases. Many medical schools and some large hospitals now have departments or divisions of medical genetics or have affiliations with a university genetics department through which referral to an experienced counselor can be arranged. Furthermore, an increasing amount of counseling may be done by specialty clinics with respect to their particular disease—diabetes clinics may provide counseling for diabetics, cystic fibrosis clinics for pancreatic cystic fibrosis, and so on.

Both the National Foundation-March of Dimes, 1275 Mamaroneck Avenue, White Plains, New York 10605, and the National Genetics Foundation, 250 West 57th Street, New York City, can direct those in need of counseling to an appropriate source. The National Genetics Foundation sponsors a series of Referral Centers that provide a variety of sophisticated diagnostic tests not routinely available. The time is coming, one hopes, when all those who are concerned about the genetic implications of a disease in themselves or their families will have access to expert counsel.

REFERENCES

1. Fraser, F. C.: Counseling in genetics: its intent and scope. Birth Defects: Original Article Series, VI (1): 7, 1970. New York, The National Foundation.
2. ———: Genetic counseling. Hospital Practice, 6:49, 1971.
3. Stevenson, A. C., and Davison, B. C. C.: Genetic Counselling. London, Heinemann, 1970.

Section III.

Syndromes and Malformations

Chapter 27

SYNDROMOLOGY

What is this face, less clear and clearer
The pulse in the arm, less strong and stronger . . . ?

T. S. Eliot, *Marina*

One of the most frustrating problems a genetic counselor meets is to decide whether a patient with multiple anomalies represents a syndrome or simply a coincidental association of several independent defects. The difference may be important, for both the genetic and the clinical prognosis. If a baby's hypospadias, webbed toes and cleft palate represent the Smith-Lemli-Opitz syndrome, the outlook is quite different than if these defects occurred together by chance. In the one case the risk of mental retardation is high and so is the risk of recurrence in sibs (one in four). In the other case these risks are comparatively low.

There is no problem if the etiology is defined, as in the case of a chromosomal trisomy or an enzyme defect. However, often this is not the case: no single diagnostic test is pathognomonic. The situation is further confused by differences of opinion as to what constitutes a "syndrome." Some take the "syndrome-by-definition" approach;

i.e., a syndrome is that association of defects described by whoever first described the syndrome, particularly if the syndrome is named after that person. This simplifies the matter for those who are interested mainly in categorizing, but presents difficulties to those interested in assigning causes or making prognoses, either clinical or genetic. In cases in which the etiology is known, such as the autosomal recessive gene causing the Laurence-Moon-Biedl syndrome or the 21 trisomy of Down syndrome, it is perfectly clear that the same etiology does not always produce the same effect. In the geneticist's jargon, the various features of the syndrome somewhat independently show reduced penetrance and variable expressivity. The sibs affected by the same gene that caused the Laurence-Moon-Biedl syndrome in the proband do not always have the same array of features.

This brings us to the "syndrome-by-etiology" approach, which holds that a syndrome should include all combinations of

anomalies known to be caused by the etiology of the syndrome. Thus, not all cases
of Marfan syndrome have arachnodactyly,
not all cases of Down syndrome have a
simian crease and not all cases of rubella
syndrome have a patent ductus arteriosus.
This is all very well when the etiology is
known, but in many syndromes the etiology
is not known. In such cases we are left in
the unsatisfactory position of having to
make an arbitrary judgment as to how
many and which features a patient must
have before he can reasonably be considered an example of the syndrome.

The syndrome-by-definition approach results in another difficulty—ascertainment
bias. If we decide arbitrarily that all cases
of a given syndrome must have all the features possessed by the original group of
cases, and if in fact the same etiology can
produce an array of defects not including
one or more of the original array, we are
ruling out as examples of the syndrome
some cases caused by the same etiology as
the cases we accept as examples of the
syndrome. This, to say the least, reduces
the value of the syndrome concept.

When a new syndrome is described, the
course of events often proceeds somewhat
as follows: Dr. Jones, in describing the first
group of cases, shows that they all have
features A, B, C and D, and that the individual features are rare enough that the
association is not likely to be coincidental.
Thus the association of features becomes
the "Jones syndrome." Other workers start
to notice and report cases of the syndrome,
and they show that in addition to A, B, C
and D, features E, F and G may also be
associated with the syndrome. Then someone observes a case with features, A, C, D,
E, F and G. Is this a case of the Jones syndrome? No, according to the syndrome-by-
definitionists," because it does not have B,
and Jones syndrome always has B. Why
does Jones syndrome always have B? Because if it does not have B it is not a case
of Jones syndrome. We hope the circular
reasoning is apparent! Thus there are those

who will not accept a patient as a case of
the Rubinstein-Taybi (or "broad-thumb-
and-great-toe syndrome") unless he has
broad thumbs, even though he might have
all the other characteristic features. As long
as this view prevails, the frequency of
broad thumbs in the Rubinstein-Taybi syndrome will always be 100%. We prefer the
view that probably no one feature is a *sine
qua non* of a syndrome. This seems to be
true in many syndromes of known etiology;
why should it not be true in syndromes that
unknown etiology?

Consider the history of Turner syndrome.
This syndrome was originally recognized
by the association of shortness, edema,
webbed neck and increased carrying angle
in female children. Sexual infantilism was
recognized later, and other features later
still. Sex chromatin and, later, karyotyping
revealed the cause of the syndrome. Only
then was it recognized that about half the
cases of Turner syndrome do not have
webbed neck, some are not strikingly short
and, in fact, an appreciable number of cyto-
logically diagnosed cases would not fit the
original criteria for Turner syndrome!

What can be done about this difficult
situation? The best solution would be to
discover the specific etiology of each syndrome. For instance, some may be the result of presently unrecognizable chromosome rearrangements, and others the result
of a specific prenatal insult at a particular
stage of gestation. Secondly, we can try to
understand the basis for the variability of
syndromes. One source may be the timing
of an embryologic insult, as demonstrated
for the rubella and the thalidomide syndromes. Another may be variation in the
genetic background. Are the relatively not
short cases of Turner syndrome not short
because they come from tall families? Do
persons who have Marfan syndrome without arachnodactyly fail to show arachnodactyly because they have an otherwise
short stocky build? Finally, we must be
aware of the ascertainment bias mentioned
previously, and recognize, for instance, that

cases of Turner syndrome diagnosed in a cardiology clinic will have the highest frequency of heart defects, whereas those diagnosed at birth will have the highest frequency of webbed neck and pedal edema, and those diagnosed in endocrinology clinics are most likely to be short. Being aware of these biases and keeping an open mind on the question of atypical syndromes will at least leave the way open toward a better understanding of syndromology.

REFERENCES

1. Pinsky, L., and Fraser, F. C.: Atypical malformation syndromes. J. Pediat., 80:141, 1972.
2. Warkany, J.: Syndromes. Amer. J. Dis. Child., 121:365, 1971.

Chapter 28

TABLES OF SELECTED SYNDROMES AND DISORDERS

The tables presented in this chapter were designed to provide a guide to syndromes and their etiologies. The names of the disorders are arranged alphabetically in the column to the far left, and the diagnostic features of each disease are arranged alphabetically across the page from left to right. The etiologies are coded for eight possibilities. Thus, one may scan a row of core features for a given syndrome and arrive at a reasonable clinical picture. One might also use the tables to deduce a tentative diagnosis from a given set of clinical features.

Some introductory remarks regarding our methods of tabulation: We have chosen to list only 157 disorders of the 216 mentioned in the text and of the thousands of entities that are of potential genetic interest. This choice was based upon the following criteria: they are common diseases; they are representative of diagnostic problems that come to the genetic counselor; or they are disorders that are informative at fundamental or clinical levels. The name of the disorder used in the table is not necessarily the name under which the syndrome was discussed in the text. Although we sought to avoid the excessive use of eponyms in the text, in the tables we have chosen those names that are used most commonly in practice (e.g., Goldenhar syndrome rather than oculo-auriculo-vertebral syndrome) or those that better fit the format of the table (e.g., 21 trisomy rather than Down syndrome). Alternative names may be found in the index or in the text (see the text page reference listed beside each name).

In categorizing the clinical features of the syndromes to be considered, the reader will appreciate the necessity to "lump" together some features; otherwise a listing of discrete features would be far too unwieldy to be useful. Obviously, many syndromes have a number of core features in common. For example, craniofacial receives a plus in the majority of chromosomal aberrations. How would this help one to arrive at a clinical picture of the syndrome? Although the specific craniofacial features may be different for each syndrome, craniofacial anomaly is a characteristic of the syndrome. The reader may refer to the text for the specifics of the anomaly itself.

In scoring for the presence or absence of a feature, we had to make decisions that might seem arbitrary to the reader. We decided not to weigh each feature from $++++$ though $+$ and $\pm$ to $-$; this would have made the columns impossible to read meaningfully. Thus the columns have been programmed either plus or blank, and a judgment was made regarding how important a feature must be in the syndrome to warrant a plus. For example, the authors are aware that mental retardation is not uncommon in Hunter syndrome (this would be a good place for $\pm$), but elected *not* to give retardation a plus to emphasize a point of differentiation from Hurler syndrome. These decisions have been made repeatedly with the full recognition that they are open to interpretation if not dispute.

Syndrome	Etiology	Cardiovascular	Cleft lip, palate	Craniofacial	Deafness	Digits	Ear	Endocrine-Metabolic	Eye	Gastrointestinal	Genitourinary	Hematology-Oncology	Hepatosplenomegaly	Immunology	Muscular	Neurologic (psych.)	Respiratory	Retardation	Shortness	Skeletal	Skin, Hair, Teeth, Nails
Fabry (186)	X-R							+	+							+					+
Fanconi pancytopenia (150)	R	+										+							+	+	
Fanconi I and II (150)	R							+			+								+	+	
Farber (166)	R							+								+		+	+	+	+
Fibrodysplasia ossificans (118)	D					+									+						
Forney (116)	D	+			+														+	+	+
Friedreich ataxia (153)	R	+							+							+				+	
Galactosemia (160)	R							+	+				+					+	+		+
Gangliosidosis GM(I) Type 1 (166)	R							+	+				+			+		+	+	+	
Gangliosidosis GM(I) Type 2 (166)	R							+	+							+		+	+	+	
Gangliosidosis GM(2) Type 2 (166)	R							+	+							+		+	+		
Gangliosidosis GM(2) Type 3 (166)	R							+	+							+		+	+		
Gaucher (166)	R							+					+			+				+	
Glycogenosis Ia, Von Gierke (162)	R							+		+	+		+						+		
Glycogenosis IIa, Pompe (162)	R	+						+					+		+	+		+	+		
Glycogenosis IIIa (162)	R	+						+					+		+						
Glycogenosis IV (162)	R	+						+					+			+					
Glycogenosis V, McArdle (162)	R	+						+			+				+						
Glycogenosis VIa, Hers (162)	R							+					+								
Glycogenosis VII, Tarui (162)	R							+			+				+						
Glycogenosis VIII, Thomson (162)	R							+							+						
Goldenhar (253)	U	+	+	+	+		+		+											+	+
Hartnup (146)	R							+								+					+

Abbreviations D=Autosomal dominant, R=Autosomal recessive, X-D=X-linked dominant, X-R=X-linked recessive, C=Chromosomal, E=Environmental effect predominates, U=Unknown, U(S)=Unknown but recurs in sibs

Syndrome	Etiology	Cardiovascular	Cleft lip, palate	Craniofacial	Deafness	Digits	Ear	Endocrine-Metabolic	Eye	Gastrointestinal	Genitourinary	Hematology-Oncology	Hepatosplenomegaly	Immunology	Muscular	Neurologic (psych.)	Respiratory	Retardation	Shortness	Skeletal	Skin, Hair, Teeth, Nails
Histidinemia (147)	R							+								+		+			
Holt-Oram (118)	D	+				+														+	
Homocystinuria (147)	R	+						+	+									+		+	+
Hyperuricemia (Lesch-Nyhan) (189)	X-R			+		+		+					+			+		+			+
Hypophosphatasia (163)	R							+					+					+		+	+
Incontinentia pigmenti (194)	X-D	+		+	+				+							+		+		+	+
Jervell, Lange-Nielsen (157)	R	+			+																
Jeune (160)	R					+					+							+		+	
Kartagener (251)	U(S)	+															+				
Klippel-Feil (251)	U(S)	+		+	+											+				+	+
Klippel-Trenaunay-Weber (253)	U			+																+	+
Laurence-Moon-Biedl (164)	R					+			+		+							+			
Leopard (116)	D	+			+				+										+		+
Leprechaunism (164)	R			+			+	+	+		+							+			
Lowe oculo-cerebro-renal (190)	X-R							+	+		+				+	+		+		+	
Maple syrup urine (148)	R							+			+					+		+			
Marfan (124)	D	+		+	+				+											+	
McCune-Albright (253)	U			+				+			+										
Metaphyseal dysostosis, Schmid (125)	D																		+	+	
Mucolipidosis I (166)	R			+					+	+			+					+	+		
Mucolipidosis II, I-cell (167)	R			+					+										+	+	+
Mucolipidosis III, Pseudo-Hurler (167)	R	+		+					+	+									+	+	+
MPS IH, Hurler (169)	R	+		+				+	+				+					+	+	+	+

Abbreviations D = Autosomal dominant, R = Autosomal recessive, X-D = X-linked dominant, X-R = X-linked recessive, C = Chromosomal, E = Environmental effect predominates, U = Unknown, U(S) = Unknown but recurs in sibs

Syndrome	Etiology	Cardiovascular	Cleft lip, palate	Craniofacial	Deafness	Digits	Ear	Endocrine-Metabolic	Eye	Gastrointestinal	Genitourinary	Hematology-Oncology	Hepatosplenomegaly	Immunology	Muscular	Neurologic (psych.)	Respiratory	Retardation	Shortness	Skeletal	Skin, Hair, Teeth, Nails
MPS IS, Scheie (171)	R	+		+				+								(+)				+	
MPS II, Hunter (190)	X-R	+		+	+			+					+						+	+	
MPS III, Sanfilippo (171)	R	+						+					+			+		+		+	
MPS IV, Morquio (171)	R	+		+				+	+										+	+	
MPS VI, Maroteaux-Lamy (172)	R			+				+	+										+	+	
Muscular dystrophy (191, 173)	X-R, R,D	+													+	+					
Myotonic dystrophy, Steinert (126)	D	+		+				+	+		+				+	+					+
Nail-patella (127)	D							+	+											+	+
Neurofibromatosis (127)	D	+						+	+			+	+			+				+	+
Neuromas, multiple mucosal (128)	D			+				+					+								
Niemann-Pick (166)	R							+					+			+		+			
Noack (111)	D	+		+																	
Oculo-dento-digital (ODD) (130)	D		+	+	+	+			+												+
Oral-facial-digital (OFD) I (195)	X-D		+	+												+		+			+
Oral-facial-digital (OFD) II (195)	R		+	+	+	+										+					
Osler hereditary telangiectasia (133)	D									+							+				+
Osteogenesis imperfecta (129)	D	+		+	+			+	+										+	+	
Osteogenesis imperfecta (130)	R	+		+															+	+	
Osteopetrosis (174)	R			+	+				+			+	+							+	+
Osteopetrosis (174)	D			+																+	+
Pendred (156)	R				+			+													
Phenylketonuria (149)	R							+									+		+		+
Poland (254)	U	+				+									+					+	

Abbreviations D=Autosomal dominant, R=Autosomal recessive, X-D=X-linked dominant, X-R=X-linked recessive, C=Chromosomal, E=Environmental effect predominates, U=Unknown, U(S)=Unknown but recurs in sibs

Syndrome	Etiology	Cardiovascular	Cleft lip, palate	Craniofacial	Deafness	Digits	Ear	Endocrine-Metabolic	Eye	Gastrointestinal	Genitourinary	Hematology-Oncology	Hepatosplenomegaly	Immunology	Muscular	Neurologic (psych.)	Respiratory	Retardation	Shortness	Skeletal	Skin, Hair, Teeth, Nails
Polycystic kidneys (174)	R			+			+			+	+					+					
Polycystic kidneys (174)	D	+								+	+										
Polyposis I, familial (131)	D									+		+									
Polyposis II, Peutz-Jeghers (131)	D									+											+
Polyposis III, Gardner (131)	D			+						+		+									+
Porphyria, erythropoietic (175)	R							+				+	+	+							+
Porphyria, hepatic (132)	D							+				+				+					+
Prader-Willi (254)	U							+	+	+						+		+	+	+	+
Progeria (176)	R	+		+					+										+	+	+
Prune belly (255)	U									+	+				+						
Pseudoxanthoma elasticum (177)	R	+							+	+						+					+
Riley-Day (157)	R	+							+	+						+		+			+
Rickets, hypophosphatemic (193)	X-D							+											+	+	+
Robin (255)	U(S)			+												+					
Rothmund (175)	R							+	+											+	+
Rubella, congenital (281)	E	+			+		+			+		+	+			+		+	+	+	
Rubenstein-Taybi (255)	U(S)	+		+	+				+	+								+	+		
Seckel (157)	R	+		+						+								+	+	+	
Sickle cell disease (151)	R	+										+								+	+
Silver (256)	U	+		+	+	+				+									+	+	+
Sjögren-Larsson (157)	R								+							+		+	+	+	+
Smith-Lemli-Opitz (178)	R	+		+	+					+								+	+	+	
Spherocytosis (132)	D											+	+								+

Abbreviations D = Autosomal dominant, R = Autosomal recessive, X-D = X-linked dominant, X-R = X-linked recessive, C = Chromosomal, E = Environmental effect predominates, U = Unknown, U(S) = Unknown but recurs in sibs

Syndrome	Etiology	Cardiovascular	Cleft lip, palate	Craniofacial	Deafness	Digits	Ear	Endocrine-Metabolic	Eye	Gastrointestinal	Genitourinary	Hematology-Oncology	Hepatosplenomegaly	Immunology	Muscular	Neurologic (psych.)	Respiratory	Retardation	Shortness	Skeletal	Skin, Hair, Teeth, Nails
Spondyloepiphyseal dysplasia (133)	D																		+	+	
Spondyloepiphyseal dysplasia, late	X-R																		+	+	
Sturge-Weber (256)	U															+		+			+
Supravalvular aortic stenosis-hypercalcemia (248)	U(S)	+		+				+	+	+								+			+
Tay-Sachs (166)	R							+	+							+					
Testicular feminization (192)	X-R							+			+										+
Thalassemia major (152)	R	+		+								+	+							+	+
Thalidomide syndrome (283)	E	+		+	+	+	+													+	
Thyroid, genetic defects (154)	R	+		+				+			+				+			+	+	+	+
Treacher Collins (122)	D	+	+	+	+		+		+	+										+	
Tuberous sclerosis (133)	D	+		+					+		+	+				+				+	+
Tyrosinemia, hereditary (150)	R							+		+	+								+	+	
Ullrich-Noonan (134)	D	+		+	+	+	+	+	+		+								+	+	+
Von Hippel-Lindau (137)	D	+							+		+					+					
Waardenburg (138)	D			+	+				+												+
Weill-Marchesani (178)	R	+		+		+			+										+	+	
Werdnig-Hoffmann (173)	R														+	+	+				
Werner (177)	R	+						+	+	+	+					+	+		+	+	+
Wilson (163)	R							+	+	+						+					
Wiskott-Aldrich (193)	X-R											+		+							+

Abbreviations D = Autosomal dominant, R = Autosomal recessive, X-D = X-linked dominant, X-R = X-linked recessive, C = Chromosomal, E = Environmental effect predominates, U = Unknown, U(S) = Unknown but recurs in sibs

Appendix A

ANALYSIS OF CHROMOSOMES

FLUORESCENT BANDING TECHNIQUES

A standardized system of identification of the human somatic karyotype based on the fluorescent pattern is described. Because most laboratories do not have available the equipment for densitometric measurements, the decription has been confined to visually recognizable patterns, but confirmed by comparison with the densitometric results of Caspersson *et al.*[1]

General Aspects of Terminology. The previously used definitions by length, centromeric index, autoradiography, or secondary constrictions that exist for chromosomes number 1, 2, 3, 4, 5, 9, 13, 14, 15, 16, 17, 18, and Y have been accepted.[2] (X chromosomes in numbers greater than one can be identified by their late replicating characteristics.) The numbers of the remaining autosomes are based on their fluorescent banding pattern as given by Caspersson *et al.*[1] The chromosome associated with Down syndrome, although smaller than number 22, has been retained as number 21.

Descriptive Terms. In the description that follows, "A" are the diagnostic features

Adapted from: Paris Conference (1971): Standardization in Human Cytogenetics. Birth Defects: Original Article Series, VIII: 7, 1972. The National Foundation, New York.

that can be seen in a fluorescent metaphase of fair technical quality, "B" are the details that are usually only visible in cells of good quality. When these details are not included in the text they are identical to "A." "C" denotes features that may vary in fluorescent intensity and/or length between individuals and between homologues.

Intensity of Fluorescence. Some mitoses show considerable nonuniformity in that two homologous chromosomes differ greatly in overall fluorescence and relative length. Identification must therefore be based on the fluorescent banding pattern of a chromosome rather than on its overall intensity. However, the latter may serve as a secondary criterion if due allowance is made for nonuniformity. In the descriptions the following terms have been used to indicate the approximate intensity of fluorescence:

Negative—no or almost no fluorescence
Pale —as on distal 1p
Medium —as the two broad bands on 9q
Intense —as the distal half of 13q
Brilliant —as on distal Yq

Proposed System of Identification for Individual Chromosomes. In the following section, only major fluorescent bands will be referred to, even though in some cells these may appear to consist of several

C q: The brilliant fluorescent segment on the end of q may vary in length and may be subdivided into two or more bands. The normal variation in length of the chromosome is associated with variation in length of the brilliant segment.

GIEMSA BANDING TECHNIQUES

In this section the results obtained by G, R, and C techniques are reported. In all instances, Q-banding is used as the reference method in order to establish the identity of the chromosomes and their characterization.

Banding Patterns Obtained by G-, R- and C-staining Methods

Chromosome No.	G	R	C
1	As for Q *except* C-band stains deeply	Reverse of G	Large, extends from centromere into q
2	As for Q	" "	Small
3-8	As for Q	Reverse of G	Medium
9	" "	Reverse of G except for C-band	Large, extends from centromere into q
10	" "	Reverse of G	Medium
11	" "	" "	Medium, but larger than 10 or 12
12	" "	" "	Medium
13	" "	" "	Medium, but sometimes bipartite
14-15	" "	" "	Medium
16	As for Q *except* C-band stains deeply	Reverse of G	Large, extends from centromere into q
17	As for Q	" "	Medium
18	" "	" "	Medium, but larger than 17
19-22	As for Q	Reverse of G	Medium
X	" "	" "	Medium
Y	Variable	Variable	Very small C-band at the centromere, plus large C-band on distal end of q

Comments on Proposed System of Identification. (1) Comparison of staining results.

There was uniform agreement that the G- and R-staining techniques gave comparable results to those obtained by Q-staining apart from the following exceptions (h = secondary constriction):

The G- and R-methods do not in general clearly demonstrate the variant bands which are visible with the Q-method near the centromeres of chromosome numbers 3, 4, 13, 14, 15, 21 and 22.

The morphologic variability of satellite size and density is reflected in the Q-, G- and C-staining techniques by size and staining intensity.

Chromosome Region	Q	G	R	C
1qh	negative	+	−	+
9qh	negative	−	−	+
16qh	negative	+	−	+
distal Yq	brilliant	variable	variable	+

(2) R bands.

The lightly stained bands in the G-staining technique are darkly stained by the R-band technique. The one exception is the secondary constriction region of chromosome 9, which is lightly stained by both techniques. The ends of chromosomes stain darkly with the R-band technique.

(3) Variable features.

The C-bands in chromosomes 1, 9, 16 and Y (distal band in q) are all associated with obvious morphologic variation.

(4) Late or early replicating X chromosomes cannot be distinguished by the Q-, G-, R- and C-staining methods.

REFERENCES

1. Caspersson, T., Lomakka, G., and Zech, L.: 24 fluorescence patterns of human metaphase chromosomes—distinguishing characters and variability. Hereditas, 67:89-102, 1971.
2. Chicago Nomenclature: Birth Defects: Original Article Series II: 2, 1966. The National Foundation, New York.

Appendix C

GENERAL SOURCES OF INFORMATION ON MEDICAL GENETICS

Review Article Series

1. Harris, H., and Hirschhorn, K. (eds.): Advances in Human Genetics. New York, Plenum Press.
2. Steinberg, A. G., and Bearn, A. G. (eds.): Progress in Medical Genetics. New York, Grune & Stratton.

Mendelian Traits

3. McKusick, V. A.: Mendelian Inheritance in Man. A catalogue of autosomal dominant autosomal recessive and X-linked phenotypes. 3rd ed. Baltimore, John Hopkins Press, 1971. (The most complete catalogue of mendelian traits, with references.)
4. Stanbury, J. B., Wyngaarden, J. B., and Fredrickson, D. S. (eds.): The Metabolic Basis of Inherited Disease. 3rd ed. New York, McGraw-Hill, 1972. (A detailed description of the major inborn errors of metabolism and their underlying biochemistry.)

Syndromes and Birth Defects

5. Fraser, F. C., and McKusick, V. (eds.): Congenital Malformations. Amsterdam, Excerpta Medica, 1970. (Proceedings of a symposium on the biologic, clinical and epidemiologic aspects of birth defects.)
6. Geeraets, W. J.: Ocular Syndromes. 2nd ed. Philadelphia, Lea & Febiger, 1969. (A well-catalogued but not illustrated collection of syndromes involving, but by no means limited to, the eye.)
7. Gellis, S. S., and Feingold, M.: Atlas of Mental Retardation Syndromes. Visual diagnosis of facies and physical findings. Washington,

D.C., U.S. Government Printing Office, 1968. (Another illustrated atlas devoted to syndromes involving mental retardation.)
8. Gorlin, R. J., and Pindborg, J. J.: Syndromes of the Head and Neck. 2nd ed. New York, McGraw-Hill, 1971. (An atlas overlapping Smith's somewhat, but with more emphasis on adults.)
9. Jablonski, S.: Illustrated Dictionary of Eponymic Syndromes and Diseases and Their Synonyms. Philadelphia, W. B. Saunders, 1969. (A handy guide through the confusion created by the wealth of eponyms attached to syndromes.)
10. V. McKusick (ed.): International Conferences on the Delineation of Syndromes. The National Foundation-March of Dimes. (A series of conference proceedings profusely illustrated; each volume is more or less devoted to one or more organ systems, plus one on chromosome syndromes.)
11. Smith, D. W.: Recognizable Patterns of Human Malformations. Philadelphia, W. B. Saunders, 1970. (An excellent review of the problems of "dysmorphogenesis" and catalogue, well-illustrated and annotated, of syndromes, particularly those of the pediatric group.)
12. Warkany, J.: Congenital Malformations. Chicago, Year Book Medical Publishers, 1971. (An exhaustive source book of information and wisdom.)

Chromosomes

13. Paris Conference (1971): Standardization in Human Cytogenetics. Birth Defects: Original Article Series, VIII: 7, 1972. The National Foundation, New York.